AF682586

RENAL AND UROLOGIC DISORDERS

PRIMARY AND SECONDARY GLOMERULONEPHRITIS

SIGNS, SYMPTOMS AND TREATMENT

RENAL AND UROLOGIC DISORDERS

Additional books in this series can be found on Nova's website under the Series tab.

Additional e-books in this series can be found on Nova's website under the e-book tab.

RENAL AND UROLOGIC DISORDERS

PRIMARY AND SECONDARY GLOMERULONEPHRITIS

SIGNS, SYMPTOMS AND TREATMENT

FOTEINI LAMPRIANOU

NOVA BIOMEDICAL

New York

Copyright © 2015 by Nova Science Publishers, Inc.

All rights reserved. No part of this book may be reproduced, stored in a retrieval system or transmitted in any form or by any means: electronic, electrostatic, magnetic, tape, mechanical photocopying, recording or otherwise without the written permission of the Publisher.

For permission to use material from this book please contact us:
nova.main@novapublishers.com

NOTICE TO THE READER

The Publisher has taken reasonable care in the preparation of this book, but makes no expressed or implied warranty of any kind and assumes no responsibility for any errors or omissions. No liability is assumed for incidental or consequential damages in connection with or arising out of information contained in this book. The Publisher shall not be liable for any special, consequential, or exemplary damages resulting, in whole or in part, from the readers' use of, or reliance upon, this material. Any parts of this book based on government reports are so indicated and copyright is claimed for those parts to the extent applicable to compilations of such works.

Independent verification should be sought for any data, advice or recommendations contained in this book. In addition, no responsibility is assumed by the publisher for any injury and/or damage to persons or property arising from any methods, products, instructions, ideas or otherwise contained in this publication.

This publication is designed to provide accurate and authoritative information with regard to the subject matter covered herein. It is sold with the clear understanding that the Publisher is not engaged in rendering legal or any other professional services. If legal or any other expert assistance is required, the services of a competent person should be sought. FROM A DECLARATION OF PARTICIPANTS JOINTLY ADOPTED BY A COMMITTEE OF THE AMERICAN BAR ASSOCIATION AND A COMMITTEE OF PUBLISHERS.

Additional color graphics may be available in the e-book version of this book.

Library of Congress Cataloging-in-Publication Data

ISBN: 978-1-63463-541-7

Library of Congress Control Number: 2014955557

Published by Nova Science Publishers, Inc. † New York

To my beloved husband Nikos, for all the patience and support

Contents

Preface

Glomerulonephritis is a term referring to direct injury of the glomeruli with resulting disturbances of normal glomerular function, progressively leading to renal failure. The nature of glomeruli damage determines the intensity and gravity of clinical manifestations of the disease. It may manifest with isolated hematuria proteinuria, edema, hypertension, oliguria, or anuria, or present two or more of these symptoms giving rise to nephritic or nephrotic syndrome.

Glomerulonephritis are classified as primary, where glomerular damage is the prime disturbance, with extra renal manifestations as consequence of the renal impairment, and secondary, following systemic disorders, infections, or exposure to certain drugs. However there are various classifications of glomerulonephritis according to clinical, etiological, and histological patterns.

In this book, glomerulonephritis are grouped according the presence or absence of proliferative histological alternations into primary and secondary proliferative and non-proliferative types.

Although noteworthy progress has been made in the past years in the symptomatic and specific treatment of each glomerulonephritis, therapy of both primary and secondary glomerulonephritis can be challenging. Management of these patients requires early diagnosis, expert knowledge of the immunosuppressive agents and other drugs currently available for the treatment of each glomerulonephritis, consideration of possible adverse reactions to these drugs, alternative therapeutic strategies in cases of hyporesponsiveness or non responsiveness of the patient to the treatment, and possible relapses of the disease.

This book reviews knowledge of the main primary and secondary glomerulonephritis, with emphasis on current therapeutic strategies and practical recommendations. Each chapter deals with etiopathogenesis, epidemiology, pathology, clinical manifestations, natural history, and therapeutic options of the most common primary and secondary glomerular diseases, with exception to the last chapter that covers inherited diseases with renal involvement. An atlas of the pathology of the glomerular diseases discussed completes this work. The goal of this work it is to provide a practical and useful tool for the day-to-day management of patients with primary or secondary glomerular disease.

Special thanks to Prof. Nakopoulou Lydia for the beautiful pathologic illustrations that complement this book.

Section A.
Introduction to Glomerulonephritis

Chapter I

Introduction to Glomerulonephritis

Abstract

The term glomerulonephritis applies to a group of glomerular diseases characterized by structural and functional disturbances of the glomeruli that can be urine abnormalities or clinical syndromes, including nephrotic and nephritic syndrome. Etiopathogenesis can vary, but it has become increasingly apparent that immune humoral and cellular mechanisms are the basis of the disease. Diagnosis of different types of glomerulonephritis can be established by renal biopsy, although clinical manifestations often direct to a specific glomerular disease, sparing biopsy performance. Treatment may be challenging, therefore symptomatic and disease-specific approach is required.

In this chapter, we will discuss classification, etiopathogenesis, clinical manifestations, and diagnosis of glomerularolonephritis. Also, a brief reference to therapeutic approaches will be made.

Definition, Classification and Pathogenesis

Glomerular disease is a term referring to a group of disorders of different etiopathogenesis, characterized by direct injury of the glomeruli, resulting in structural and functional disturbances. The nature of glomerular damage, determines intensity and gravity of clinical manifestations as well as the possibility of remission of the disease or it's progression to renal failure. Although the term glomerulonephritis applies to glomerular diseases attributable to inflammatory and immune processes, nowadays it is used as a nonspecific title for most of the glomerular diseases.

Glomerulonephritis are divided in two main classes. *Primary*, where the glomerular damage is the prime disturbance, where external manifestations are a consequence of the renal impairment, and *secondary*, where glomerular damage results from systemic disorders, infections or exposure to certain drugs. Classification of glomerulonephritis though is more complicated than that. Given the complexity of clinical manifestations, the fact that different glomerular histopathology can present similar signs and symptoms, and that in patients having the same histopathology, glomerular disease manifests differently, it must be noted that evaluation of clinical symptoms alone is not of diagnostic value or indicative of a particular type of glomerulonephritis, and that classification of glomerulonephritis and diagnosis has to be based on both clinical and histopathological grounds. Clinical presentation of glomerulonephritis can vary from asymptomatic urinary abnormalities to nephritic syndrome to severe nephrotic syndrome with marked protein excretion and edema. Clinical manifestations and syndromes will be described separately in this chapter. (Table 1)

Table 1.1. Clinical manifestations of Glomerulonephritis

Asymptomatic Microscopic Hematuria	
Primary	**Secondary**
IgA Nephropathy Mesangial Proliferative Glomerulonephritis Focal Segmental Glomerulosclerosis (FSGS)	Alport Syndrome Thin Basement Membrane Nephropathy
Macroscopic Hematuria	
Primary	**Secondary**
IgA Nephropathy	Alport Syndrome Thin Basement Membrane Nephropathy
Nephritic Syndrome	
Primary	**Secondary**
Membranoproliferative Glomerulonephritis Mesangial Proliferative Glomerulonephritis Focal Segmental Glomerulosclerosis	Amyloidosis Diabetic Nephropathy
Nephrotic Syndrome	
Primary	**Secondary**
Minimal Changes Glomerulonephritis Focal Segmental Glomerulosclerosis Membranous Glomerulonephritis Membranoproliferative Glomerulonephritis	Light Chain Deposition Disease Diabetic Nephropathy Lupus Nephritis Amyloidosis

The histopathologic classification relies on the morphology of the gromeruli when examined by light microscopy, immunofluorescence, and electron microscopy. Based on the extension of glomerular damage, glomerulonephritis can be classified as *focal*, concerning only some of the glomeruli, *diffuse*, affecting all glomeruli, or *segmental*, where only parts of an affected glomerulus present alternations. Other histopathologic classifications proposed, regard the nature of glomerular injury including proliferation of epithelial, endothelial or mesangial cells, injury of the glomerular basement membrane, and sclerosis of glomerular capillaries. In this context, glomerulonephritis are grouped according to the presence or absence of proliferative histological alternations. (Table 2)

Table 1.2. Classification of Glomerulonephritis according to proliferative histopathologic alternations

Primary Non Proliferative	**Primary Proliferative**
Minimal Changes Glomerulonephritis Focal Segmental Glomerulosclerosis Membranous Glomerulonephritis	IgA Nephropathy (Berger's Disease) Post-Infectious Glomerulonephritis Membranoproliferative glomerulonephritis Rapidly Progressive Glomerulonephritis
Secondary Non Proliferative	**Secondary Proliferative**
Diabetic Nephropathy Amyloidosis Fabry Disease Alport Syndrome	Lupus Nephritis Hepatitis B associated Glomerulonephritis Hepatitis C associated Glomerulonephritis

Incidence and Prevalence

Incidence of glomerulonephritis is hard to evaluate given that most of end stage renal disease (ESRD) patients, at the time of initiation of renal replacement treatment, are not diagnosed. However, according to the 2013 annual report of the US Renal Data System, after studying 573,815 ESRD patients for the years 2007-2011, researchers concluded that 6.7% (37,004) of these patients were diagnosed with primary glomerulonephritis, 45.7% (252.870) with diabetic nephropathy (secondary glomerulonephritis), and 2.1% (11,629) of patients with other secondary glomerulonephritis [1]

Racial differences have also been noticed. 375,952 of the 573,815 patients were white (65.5%) and 160,869 were African American (28%). Primary glomerulonephritis and diabetic nephropathy seem to prevail among white people. From the 37,004 presenting primary glomerulonephritis, 67.5% were white and 23.4% were African American. Patients with diabetic nephropathy (252.870) were mostly white (65.4%) while African Americans represented only 27.4% of this population. Secondary glomerulonephritis (11,629 in total) seem to generally follow this pattern (64.4% to 29.6%), with the only exception being the prevalence of lupus nephritis (5,497 patients in total) among African Americans, 48.5% to 42.8% of white patients. [1]

Pathophysiology

During the past decades, it has become increasingly apparent that most of the glomerular diseases have an autoimmune nature and may develop as a dysfunction of the immune system, expressed as an exaggerated response of the immune system to an endogenous antigen or as a limited response to an esogenous antigen. Immune response in glomerulonephritis, includes both humoral and cellular mechanisms.

Humoral mechanisms are responsible for the formation of immune complexes of antigens and antibodies in the glomeruli, while cellular mechanisms are in charge of the production, multiplication, and migration of activated cells of inflammation (neutrophils, macrophages and monocytes) from the circulation at the site of formation of the immune complexes.

Formation of immune complexes depends on the molecular weight and charge of the antigens, the chemical structure and charge of the antibodies and the ratio of circulating antigens/antibodies. Antigens present epitopes on their surface that act as sites of connection to the antibodies. These epitopes can be recognized and connected to more than one antibody at the same time with resulting formation of a net, characteristic of the glomerulonephritis with depositions.

The circulating antibodies can connect to a normal glomerular component (endogenous antigen) and form immune complexes *in situ,* with a non glomerular antigen that has circulated and was trapped on the renal structures (esogenous antigen), or immune complexes can be formed in the circulation and passively reach the renal structures.

In normal conditions, immune complexes are removed from the circulation by the phagocytes with endocytosis and transferred into organs like the spleen or liver, with progressive reduction of antibody production. In cases of abnormal immune response, immune complexes are formed in excessive quantity and with certain characteristics (molecular weight, charge, chemical configuration) that make their removal from the circulation insufficient or impossible. Then, the circulating immune complexes reach various organs, including the kidney, and deposit on the capillaries, promoting inflammation and tissue damage.

However, deposition of the immune complexes can be altered by numerous factors other than antigen and antibody characteristics, including arterial blood pressure, nutritional status, renal blood flow, and intraglomerular pressure. Hormonal disorders such as diabetes and release of catecholamines may also contribute.

Once the immune complexes are deposited on the tissues, they activate the complement cascade with resulting production of chemotactic factors that induce infiltration of leucocytes monocytes and mastocytes. Leucocytes and monocytes produce proteolytic enzymes, oxygen radicals, and cytokines that provoke proliferation of mesangial and epithelial cells, expansion of the mesangial matrix and modification of the glomerular basement. Mastocytes release vasoactive substances that modify capillary permeability, renal blood flow, and the GFR.

Activation of the complement cascade can take place in 3 different pathways, the classic pathway, the alternative pathway, and the manose-lectin pathway.

All three ways converge to a common final pathway that has both destructive and protective properties. Formation of the complex C5b-9 in the final common pathway, and its accumulation results in the membrane attack complex (MAC), capable of creating pores on the cell membrane because of its lytic properties. MAC also activates cells to secrete cytokines, oxidants, and extracellular matrix. For these properties, MAC is considered a particularly important mediator of glomerular injury.

As previously mentioned, the complement system also has protective properties. In fact, activation of the classic pathway inhibits formation of large size immune complexes. The resulting smaller circulating complexes are more soluble, thus easier to remove from glomerular deposition sites, easier to be phagocyted and moved to the spleen, transferred by the erythrocytes. This mechanism of defense is called "primate erythrocyte immune complex clearing mechanism". [2, 3]

In any case, activation of the final common pathway of the complement system is not absolutely necessary for induction and progression of renal injury, given that complement factors C3, C4 and C5 induce accumulation of neutrophils and monocytes at the endothelium, production of proteases, ecosanoids and oxidative substances that aggravate renal injury. [2]

Progression of glomerular injury to glomerular sclerosis involves activation of various types of cells, including endothelial, epithelial and mesangial cells, monocytes leucocytes and platelets, which leads to production and release of cytokines, vasoactive and growth factors, promoting hyperplasia of mesangial cells and increased production of mesangial matrix. [4] Mesangial cells also transform to myofibroblast-like cells that proliferate and produce extracellular matrix. Uncontrolled mesangial proliferation and excessive production of mesangial matrix lead to tissue fibrosis, scarring, and glomerulosclerosis. [4]

Injury of podocytes, and their inability to replicate, leads to exposure of the glomerular basement membrane (GBM) and permits its interaction with parietal epithelial cells. Capsular adhesions between GBM and parietal epithelium result in glomerulosclerosis and inadequate filtration with accumulation of amorphous material, disruption of the glomerular-tubular continuity with consequential tubular atrophy and interstitial fibrosis. Tubular cells are also activated and transformed into a myofribroblast phenotype with excessive production and deposition of extracellular matrix that contributes to fibrosis. [5]

Damage of peritubular capillaries and postglomerular arterioles produce ischemia and hypoxia, stimulating tubular cells and fibroblasts to produce extracellular matrix, with consequent exacerbation of fibrosis. [6, 7] Recently, tubulointerstitial lesions were strongly correlated with lymphatic neoangiogenesis. Increase on number of lymphatic vessels depending on the degree of tissue damage and was more accentuated in areas of fibrosis than in areas of inflammation, suggesting contribution of lymphangiogenesis to the progression of tubulointerstitial fibrosis. [8]

The pathogenic pathways, mentioned above, correspond to the main and general mechanisms of glomerular damage. Pathogenesis of different types of glomerulonephritis will be described in the respective chapters. However, pathogenesis of glomerular diseases is not totally clarified yet and pathways of progression of the disease to renal failure are still under investigation.

Clinical Manifestations of Glomerulonephritis

Glomerulonephritis may manifest as clinical syndromes, including:

- Nephrotic syndrome characterized by marked proteinuria, higher than 3,5g/24h
- Nephritic syndrome, with oliguria and proteinuria, less than 3g/24h.
- Often, glomerulonephritis may present as urine abnormalities, including:
- Asymptomatic microscopic hematuria
- Asymptomatic non-nephrotic proteinuria
- Asymptomatic proteinuria with hematuria
- Macroscopic hematuria

1. Nephrotic Syndrome

Nephrotic syndrome is a heterogeneous group of pathognomonic disorders by:

- Proteinuria >3,5 g/24h in adults or > 40 mg/h per m^2 in children
- Hypoalbuminemia <3,5g/dl
- Edema
- Hypercholesterolemia and lipiduria
- Hypercoagulability

The main damaging mechanism causing nephrotic syndrome, independently from the type of glomerular disease, is the dysfunction of the normally highly selective glomerular filtration barrier (GFB), which allows massive urinary losses of molecules, including albumin.

GFB consists of the fenestrated glomerular endothelium, the glomerular basement membrane (GBM), and the podocytes with their foot processes. Podocytes are voluminous highly differentiated epithelium cells with cell bodies floating within the urinary space. The foot processes of neighboring podocytes are interdigitated, leaving between them filtration slits, bridged by the slit diaphragm, a zipper like structure formed by proteins that are connected to the cytoskeleton of the foot processes. [9]

Podocytes are considered the most important segment of GFB and mainly responsible for the establishment of nephrotic syndrome, because of their susceptibility to different damaging substances and processes, such as NSAIDS, toxins, antibodies, cytokines, reactive oxygen species (ROS), activation of the complement, hemodynamic instability and others.

Once exposed in the above-mentioned stimuli, podocytes are incapable of preserving their normal morphology. Structural changes of podocytes or their foot processes, effect the interaction with the GBM and fenestrated endothelium with resulting alternation of their normal architecture and function of GFB. These changes include hyperplasia and hypertrophy of podocytes, fusion and effacement of the foot processes, formation of pseudocystis and detachment of the podocytes off the GBM. [10, 11]

Structural elements of the slit diaphragm and the cytoskeleton of the podocytes, such as nephrin, podocin, actin cytoskeleton (α-actin-4), myosin, and the CD2 associated protein (CD2AP) are responsible for polarity, cytokinesis, integrity, and survival of the podocytes. Emerging data on the role of genetics in nephrotic syndrome suggests that genetic mutations of proteins of the slit diaphragm may play a significant role in the onset and progression of nephrotic syndrome, mostly in children.

NPHS1 encodes nephrin, the main component of slit diaphragm. Mutation of NPHS1 may determine the onset of congenital nephrotic syndrome (CNS) of the Finnish type or early onset of steroid-resistant nephrotic syndrome (SRNS). [12, 13] NPHS2 encodes podocin, and its mutation determines CNS, juvenile and adult autosomal recessive SNRS. [14-16] Mutation of the CD2AP gene, that encodes the CD2 adaptor protein, a protein that anchors the slit diaphragm to the actin cytoskeleton of the podocyte, may cause early onset of SRNS and FSGS. [17] Mutation of MYH9, a gene encoding myosin, a protein in charge of the podocyte movement, has been associated with FSGS. [18] Recently ADCK4, an aarF domain containing kinase, a protein that participates in coenzyme Q10 (CoQ10) biosynthesis has been identified in the podocyte mitochondria and foot processes in rats and in humans. Mutation of the ADCK4 gene resulted in reduced CoQ10 levels and reduced mitochondrial respiratory enzyme activity in rats with SRNS. In human patients with SRNS and mutation of ADCK4, treated with CoQ10, a partial remission of the nephrotic syndrome was noticed. [19] Finally, a recent cohort study of childhood nephrotic syndrome, the INSIGHT study, suggests that both genetic and environmental factors are involved in the development and course of the nephrotic syndrome. [20] This ongoing Canadian study recruited 211 patients and targets to at least 350, with the aim being the determination of the genetic risk factors related to nephrotic syndrome and understanding of environmental, clinical and social impacts of the disease on the patient and family. Even though results are not yet finalized, researchers believe that this study will lead to a better screening of the disease and better treatment strategies.

Causes of NS include different glomerular disease, primary, and secondary, which prevalence varies with the age. In childhood minimal change disease (MCD) seems to prevail while in adults, FSGS is the most common cause. [21, 22]

Primary causes of nephrotic syndrome are:

- Minimal change disease (MCD)
- Focal segmental glomerulosclerosis
- Membranous nephropathy

Secondary causes include:

- Diabetes
- Systemic Lupus Erythematosus
- Amyloidosis
- Infections (Hepatitis B and C, HIV)
- Preeclampsia
- Hereditary nephropathies

i. Nephrotic Range Proteinuria

Nephrotic range proteinuria is defined as urinary excretion of protein greater than 3,5g/24h in adults or greater than > 40 mg/h per m^2 in children. Dysfunction of the GFB determines loss of the negative charge selective barrier, allowing negatively charged small molecular weight proteins to be excreted. Structural changes affect the diameter of both pores and slit diaphragm cancelling the size selective barrier with resulting urinary loss of high molecular weight proteins such as albumin.

Lately, the proximal tubule is being considered as playing a role on proteinuria. [23] Reabsorption of filtered albumin takes place on the brush border of the proximal tubule, with a receptor-mediated process that may involve megalin/cubilin receptors. [24, 25] Reduced expression of the receptors on the brush borders results in perturbation of reabsorption processes and contribute to nephrotic range proteinuria. [26]

Proteinuria can be *selective*, with excretion of albumin without significant loss of other proteins, usually in glomerular diseases with minor structural damages of the glomeruli, such as MCD or *non selective,* with massive loss of albumin and other proteins, usually in glomerular diseases with extensive damage of the GBM, including glomerular diseases characterized by deposition of immune complexes and hereditary nephropathies. The magnitude of proteinuria is associated with the severity and progression of kidney disease. [27]

ii. Hypoalbuminemia

Albumin levels lower than 3g/dL is the consequence of urinary loss of albumin and increased renal catabolism. In nephrotic states, the liver tries to compensate loss by increasing synthesis of albumin. In most cases, loss exceeds production, rending the compensatory mechanism insufficient.

Another important mechanism contributing to hypoalbuminemia is the reabsorption of great quantities of filtered albumin in the proximal tubules. Megalin/cubilin receptors are expressed on the brush border of the epithelial cells of the proximal tubule. Albumin is bound to cubilin and the complex formed, with the help of megalin, is internalized, and transferred to lysosomes for degradation. [28] The amount of albumin degraded can't return to the blood stream aggravating the hypoalbuminemia.

iii. Edema

Edema is common in nephrotic syndrome, especially in excessive proteinuria and hypoalbuminemia, with levels lower than 2,5g/dL. It is usually the symptom of glomerular disease that preoccupies undiagnosed patients and induces them to seek medical advice.

There are two main pathophysiologic mechanisms involved in nephrotic edema formation: The *underfilling mechanism*, where edema is the consequence of low serum albumin, and the *overfilling mechanism* characterized by sodium retention.

In the underfilling mechanism, low serum albumin levels establish a decreased plasma oncotic pressure, which allows movement of fluids from capillaries to the interstitium according to Starling forces. Consequent reduction of circulating plasma volume stimulates activation of the renin-angiotensin system with increase of aldosterone that causes sodium retention in the distal tubule. Release of antidiuretic hormone (ADH) is also increased, with consecutive water retention by the kidney. Water and sodium retention is an attempt to compensate hypovolemia but their accumulation to the interstitium, because of inadequate lymphatic flow, aggravates edema.

In the overfilling mechanism, renal sodium retention occurs because of a primary defect on distal nephron and duct to excrete sodium. This mechanism is more related to proteinuria than to intravascular volume or protein serum levels. In fact, sodium retention can be observed before hypoproteinemia is established. [29] It is believed that proteolytic enzymes reaching the distal nephron and the tubular lumen increase the expression of epithelial sodium channels (ENaC) at the collecting duct with resulting retention of sodium. [30] Retention of sodium determines normal, or in some cases, increased blood volume (overfill), which provokes fluid transudation from the vascular department to the interstitium, and edema.

The increased blood volume suppresses the antidiuretic hormone release and the rennin-angiotensin system activation, leading to hypertension.

iv. Hyperlipidemia and Lipiduria

Hyperlipidemia is a common feature of nephrotic syndrome attributed to enhanced synthesis and decreased catabolism of lipoproteins. Hypoalbuminemia, due to excessive urinary loss, activates hepatic synthesis of proteins, including lipoproteins, while reduced plasma levels of lipoprotein lipase fail lipid catabolism. [31]

Low-density lipoproteins (LDL), very low-density lipoproteins (VLDL), and intermediate density lipoproteins (IDL), are usually increased in nephrotic syndrome but high-density lipoproteins (HDL) remain invariant. Lipoprotein (α) and apolipoproteins B and CIII are also increased.

This perturbation of lipid metabolism in nephrotic syndrome increases the potential risk for atherosclerotic cardiovascular events, especially when associated with other risk factors such as obesity, diabetes, hypertension, and smoking.

Experimental data suggest that hyperlipidemia contributes to renal disease progression [32] and that use of statins could have a protective effect, retarding glomerular disease, but there are no clinical studies to unequivocally prove it. [33]

Lipiduria results from elevated filtration and excretion of lipoproteins in nephrotic range proteinuria. It can be seen in urine sediment in cellular debris or as fatty bodies and waxy casts. It must be noted that lipiduria is not linked to the grade of hyperlipidemia but to the degree of proteinuria.

v. Hypercoagulability

Alternation of the coagulation cascade and enhanced platelet aggregation are common features in nephrotic syndrome, in both adult and children. Although hypercoagulability has been considered a complication of nephrotic syndrome, its high prevalence among nephrotic patients make authors regard it as an integral part of the nephrotic syndrome pentad.

The hypercoagulable and thrombophilic state in nephrotic syndrome are correlated to the degree of hypoalbuminemia. [34] Serum albumin concentration inferior to 2,5g/dl seem to be associated with increased risk for thromboembolic events.

The pathophysiology of this thromboembolic state seem to be multifactorial but the main mechanism consists in urinary loss of proteins of the coagulation cascade, such as protein C, protein S and antithrombin III. [35] Also, reduced blood levels of coagulation factors IX (or Christmas factor), XI, and XII (or Hageman factor) have been described.

Thrombotic events taking place in nephrotic syndrome include renal vein thrombosis (RVT). In the past years, RVT was considered a cause of nephrotic syndrome, but nowadays is considered a complication of nephrotic syndrome, and this has changed because patients without RVT could present nephrotic syndrome and vice versa.

Coagulability disorders are most prominent in membranous nephropathy, in membranoproliferative glomerulonephritis and in minimal change disease (MCD). [35] Incidence of RVT is also increased in membranous nephropathy, indicating that not all nephropathies present the same tendency to thromboembolic events. [35]

2. Nephritic Syndrome

Acute nephritic syndrome or acute glomerulonephritis is a combination of signs and symptoms, related to immunologic mechanisms that trigger acute glomerular inflammation and proliferation with resulting damage of the GBM, mesangium or endothelium and consecutive reduction of GFR.

Typical presentation of nephritic syndrome is the sudden onset of hematuria with red blood cell casts and non-nephrotic range proteinuria lower than 3g/24h. This clinical picture is accompanied by oliguria (< 400ml of urine/24h) or anuria, renal salt and water retention with edema and weight gain within few days from the onset of the syndrome, and hypertension due to elevated circulating volume. Urinary protein losses vary, but they do not usually exceed 3g in 24 hours. Therefore serum protein levels are in general maintained within normal range. Edema is initial periorbital and later can become peripheral with swelling of hands and feet.

Other non-specific symptoms present in nephritic syndrome include blurred or abnormal vision, confusion, malaise, arthralgias, and abdominal pain.

The main causes underlying nephritic syndrome can be divided into *infectious* and *non-infectious*. Most common infectious cause of nephritic syndrome is streptococcus. Post streptococcal glomerulonephritis usually develops 1 to 3 weeks after infection by group A beta-hemolytic streptococcus following pharingitis or more often skin infections. Incidence is higher in children and its clinical presentation corresponds to the classic nephritic syndrome presentation.

Post infectious glomerulonephritis may also result from other bacteria, such as staphylococci, pneumococci, mycobacteria, Salmonella Typhi, Brucella Suis, and others. Viral causes also referred are cytomegalovirus, Coxsackie virus, Epstein–Barr virus (EBV), Hepatitis B virus (HBV, Hep B), and others. Other pathogens involved in post infectious glomerulonepnritis are Plasmodium malariae and falciparum, Toxoplasma gondii and Trypanosomes.

Non-infectious causes of nephritic syndrome include primary renal diseases, such as membranoproliferative glomerulonephritis and IgA nephropathy, systemic diseases like vasculitis, systemic lupus erythematosus (SLE), and Henoch–Schönlein purpura (HSP). Vaccines, irradiations, and administration of epidermal growth factor receptor (EGFR) inhibitors may also contribute. [36, 37]

Diagnosis and evaluation of nephritic syndrome are based on urinalysis and sediment examination. Presence of red blood cell casts, dysmorphic red blood cells (RBC), white blood cells, and cellular casts are indicative of acute glomerulonephritis. In particular, presence of RBC casts is considered pathognomonic. Urine protein concentration is, as mentioned, lower than 3g/24h and usually is around 2g/24h.

BUN and creatinine levels are elevated, indicating the degree of renal impairment and are often accompanied by increased blood concentration of potassium. Hematocrit can be decreased due to dilutional anemia.

Other laboratory tests allowing differential diagnosis are streptozyme test and complement serum levels. Antistreptolysin O (ASO) titer is increased in about 80% of the patients with post streptococcal glomerulonephritis (PSGN). Low complement levels, especially C3, are found in acute PSGN but they could also suggest systemic diseases such as systemic lupus erythematosus (SLE), endocarditis, shunt nephritis, and cryoglobulinemia. Antineutrophil cytoplasmatic antibodies (ANCA) and hepatitis B and C serology could also contribute to differential diagnosis.

Biopsy is not always necessary. If PSGN is suspected, biopsy could be avoided, while in atypical presentation of nephritic syndrome or rapidly progressive renal impairment, renal biopsy is required for definitive diagnosis.

Prognosis of nephritic syndrome can vary. When the disease behind nephritic syndrome is PSGN, prognosis is good, because in most of the cases and especially in children, it resolves completely. Only 1-3% of the cases evolve into chronic renal failure and only a few patients develop EDRD. In cases of non-poststreptococcal glomerulonephritis, early recognition of the underlying disease and initiation of adequate therapy are essential for limitation of renal impairment and prognosis of the disease. In some cases, patients show partial remission of the syndrome, presenting asymptomatic proteinuria and hematuria.

3. Urine Abnormalities

i. Asymptomatic Microscopic Hematuria

Microscopic hematuria is defined as the presence of more than 3 RBC per high-power field in a 's' centrifuged or spun urine sediment, [38] although other researchers define hematuria as the presence of more than 2 RBC, [39] or more than 1. [40] It is characteristic that urine color seems normal if observed by the naked eye and hematuria can be confirmed only after microscopic evaluation.

Microscopic hematuria can be *symptomatic* or *asymptomatic* according to presence or absence of accompanying pain, and *persistent* or *intermittent* based on the modality of its appearance.

Glomerular hematuria is thought to result from disruption of the glomerular filtration barrier (GFB), especially from abnormalities in the GBM of the glomerular capillary wall, which allow RBC to pass in the urinary space. Some of the RBC can be trapped in Tamm-Horsfall mucoprotein, with formation of RBC casts. Presence of dysmorphic RBC and RBC cast in urine analysis is indicative of glomerular disease.

Asymptomatic microscopic hematuria can be observed in many glomerular diseases. Most common causes are IgA nephropathy, PSGN and thin basement membrane nephropathy (TBMN). Rarely, persistent microscopic hematuria can be the only manifestation of necrotizing vasculitis, characterized by concomitant presence of elevated ANCA titer and necrotizing glomerular alternations. Etiology can be determined by renal biopsy but is usually avoided because in most of the cases asymptomatic microscopic hematuria manifests without proteinuria and with normal renal function.

Suspicion of necrotizing vasculitis is mandatory of renal biopsy. Early diagnosis permits early initiation of treatment, avoiding further necrotizing glomerular damages and progression to renal failure.

Besides necrotizing vasculitis and SLE, renal biopsy reveals, in most of the cases, mild non-specific alternations of the capillaries and mesangium and more rarely, tubulointerstitial damages. [41] Therefore, diagnostic value of renal biopsy in asymptomatic microscopic hematuria is considered controversial and its contribution to therapeutic strategies dubious.

ii. Asymptomatic Non-Nephrotic Range Proteinuria

Non-nephrotic range proteinuria is defined as urine protein excretion lower than 3,5 g/24h. It is usually caused by glomerular disease but it may also represent tubulointerstitial nephropathy and systemic diseases such as multiple myeloma or renal tumors.

Glomerular non nephrotic proteinuria can be *intermittent*, present in at least 50% of a random urine sample of a patient without any other symptoms or signs of renal disease, or *persistent*, present in all random urine samples.

Initially, renal function is normal and no other symptoms of renal impairment accompany asymptomatic proteinuria. Thus, biopsy is not indicated unless proteinuria exceeds 1gr/day and persists despite initiation of angiotensin-converting enzyme inhibitor (ACE-I) or angiotensin receptor blocker (ARB) therapy. Renal tissues may result as normal under renal biopsy, but mild glomerular injury, mesangial proliferation, and mild tubulointerstitial alternations may occur.

Persistent asymptomatic non-nephrotic proteinuria has a prognosis that varies from preservation of renal function, to hypertension and renal failure. Therefore, periodic evaluation of these patients with 24h urine collection and complete laboratory work up and daily control of blood pressure are required. Renal biopsy should be considered if decrease of GFR is noticed.

Other forms of asymptomatic non-nephrotic proteinuria include *functional* and *orthostatic* proteinuria. Functional proteinuria occurs in excessive exercise, fever, excessive stress, congestive heart failure, and others. It is attributed to hemodynamic disturbances of renal blood flow.

Orthostatic proteinuria is a non-nephrotic glomerular proteinuria, typically less than 2gr/24h, which is present only in the standing position and disappears in the recumbent position. When no proteinuria is observed in the morning, diagnosis of orthostatic proteinuria can be made. Prognosis is usually good, given that in more than 80% of the patients, orthostatic proteinuria is transient. Renal biopsy is not indicated, but if performed, thickening of the capillary wall and cellularity of mesangium can be noticed.

iii. Asymptomatic Proteinuria with Hematuria

Patients presenting asymptomatic proteinuria concurrently to hematuria have a higher risk of renal impairment, hypertension, and resulting renal failure. These patients should be evaluated every 6 to 12 months with urine analysis, 24h urine collection, and complete laboratory workup. Renal biopsy is indicated for definition of glomerular damage. Prognosis is usually bad, especially in elderly.

iv. Macroscopic Hematuria

Macroscopic hematuria is defined as a massive presence of RBC in the urine sediment or if the presence of blood in the urine can be observed by naked eye. Urine color is often brown or smoky grey, especially in acid environment, while red colored urine is observed in alkaline conditions.

Macroscopic hematuria can be of urinary tract origin, often escorted by pain or renal colic, or of glomerular origin, usually painless. Distinction of the origin of hematuria is essential for diagnostic and therapeutic purposes. Presence of RBC casts, dysmporphic RBC, acanthocytes, and smokey grey color suggest glomerular origin while red colored urine and presence of blood clots favor a urinary tract origin.

Also, the time of presentation of hematuria during urination may be helpful in determination of its origin. Presence of hematuria at the beginning of urination indicates urinary tract origin, most probably vescical, while hematuria during the entire urination time suggests glomerular origin.

Most common causes of macroscopic hematuria are IgA nephropathy, Alport's syndrome and thin basement membrane nephropathy (TBMN). Other frequent causes include acute glomerulonephritis, rapidly progressive glomerulonephritis, vasculitis, lupus nephritis, and acute interstitial nephritis.

In the past, macroscopic hematuria has been considered only a clinical marker of renal disease. Recent studies though, have shown that macroscopic hematuria may induce acute kidney injury. [42] Acute kidney injury occurs due to accumulation of RBC casts, tubular cells, and leucocytes in the tubules with successive intraluminal obstruction and acute tubular necrosis. Mesangial proliferation may also take place but is usually mild to moderate. [43, 44] The main pathophysiologic mechanism involved, is the direct tubular toxicity of hemoglobin, heme, and other molecules released from the RBC. Possibly, these molecules are connected to Tamm-Horsfall protein forming casts, accumulation of which promotes tubular obstruction.

Diagnosis requires urinanalysis, microscopic evaluation of the urinary sediment, and urologic evaluation with cystoscopy. If urinary tract abnormalities are excluded and macroscopic hematuria persists, renal biopsy is indicated.

General Considerations on the Treatment of Glomerulonephritis

Treatment of glomerular disease can be *disease-specific,* directed to the specific underlying disease, or *symptomatic*, including blood pressure adjustment, reduction of proteinuria, control of edema, treatment of hyperlipidemia, and management of the hypercoagulable state.

Both symptomatic and disease-specific treatment should be applied in order to obtain better outcome, taking into consideration the underlying pathophysiological alternations and potential complications.

Disease-specific treatment of each glomerulonephritis will be discussed in the respective chapters. This chapter focuses on general management principals.

i. Treatment of Hypertension

Management of hypertension in glomerular disease aims at reducing cardiovascular risk and events such as stroke, myocardial infarction, and congestive heart failure, at the delay of progression to renal insufficiency.

The target blood pressure in CKD and glomerulonephritis has been largely discussed but it hasn't been firmly established. Current recommendations of 2012 KDIGO (Kidney Disease: Improving Global Outcomes) guidelines suggest target blood pressure up to 130/80 mmHg if proteinuria is lower than 1 g/24h or 127/75mmHg if proteinuria exceeds 1g/24h. [45, 46]

Experimental and clinical studies consider angiotensin-converting enzyme inhibitors (ACE-I) and angiotensin receptor blockers (ARB) to be the first-choice therapy. [47, 48] These drugs tend to reduce proteinuria by interfering with the intrarenal hemodynamics, thus protecting the kidney from potential damaging effects of proteinuria and delaying progression to ESRD. [49, 50]

Combination of ARB and ACE-I is quite effective but it may reduce GFR, especially if used in patients with cardiac disease. [49] Thiazide and loop diuretics can also be used but they are often ineffective, especially when GFR is lower than 30 ml/min. However, their addiction to ARB/ACE-I therapy can be useful.

Refractory hypertension often requires a multi-drug approach, and in these patients, combination of ACE-I and/or ARB to diuretics, β-blockers or calcium channel blockers can be very helpful. Of note, β-blockers and calcium channel blockers are not associated with reduction of protein excretion. Moreover, calcium channel blockers may aggravate edema. [51]

In patients not responding to loop diuretics and ARB/ACE-I therapy, blood pressure can be controlled with addiction of potassium-sparing diuretics, such as spironolactone or eneplerone in low dosage, but treatment should be applied with caution because of a high incidence of hyperkaliemia. [52] An essential part of the treatment is lifestyle modification, with sodium intake restriction, smoking cessation and weight normalization.

ii. Treatment of Proteinuria and Hypoalbuminemia

Management of proteinuria and hypoalbuminemia in patients presenting nephrotic syndrome is mandatory, given that reduction of protein excretion to non nephrotic levels, particularly < 500mgh/24h, has been correlated to delay and prevention of progression to ESRD. [53]

Treatment of choice in proteinuria is the combination of ARB and ACE-I. Concomitant administration of ARB and ACE-I, along with sodium intake restriction, can reduce protein excretion up to 60%. [54] Although ACE-Is has an antiproteinuric effect, the ARB/ACE-I combination seems to be more effective than ACE-I monotherapy, even if administered in maximum dosages. [55]

As previously mentioned, ARB/ACE-I combination may reduce GFR, thus renal function should be closely monitored during therapy. Serum creatinine levels generally increase up to 30%, due to alternation of kidney hemodynamics. Withdrawal of treatment should be considered if serum creatinine concentrations continue to rise.

Use of non-steroidal anti-inflammatory drugs (NSAIDs) has also been suggested because of their antiproteinuric properties. However, given their nephrotoxicity, which can be expressed by interstitial nephritis or acute tubular necrosis, a risk-benefit consideration should be made before treatment initiation. [56]

Maintenance of adequate serum protein concentrations is very important, especially in patients with edema. Loop diuretics necessitate proteins to bond with, in order to be delivered to the tubular sites of action. Dietary protein intake, corresponding to urinary losses is important, but often ineffective. Infusion of human serum albumin may transiently resolve the problem in cases of persistent proteinuria.

iii. Treatment of Edema

In mild edema, reduction of dietary salt intake below 3g per day can be effective. If nutritional measures are insufficient, oral thiazide diuretics can be used in patients with normal GFR or loop diuretics such as furosemide (40-80 mg/day) and bumetanide (1-2mg/day) if GFR is reduced. [57] In moderate edema, high doses of oral furosemide (160-480 mg/day) with bumetanide, in dosages 4-8 mg/day, are particularly useful.

Patients with nephrotic syndrome with marked hypoalbuminemia (<2,5g/dL), massive proteinuria >10g/dl, and impaired renal function, can be treated with continuous intravenous infusion of loop diuretics (20mg/h furosemide and 1mg/h bumetanide). Human albumin infusion may enhance loop diuretics.

In nonresponsive patients, despite maximum dosage treatment, slow continuous ultrafiltration sessions are indicated.

iv. Treatment of Hyperlipidemia

High lipidemic levels are noticed in nephrotic syndrome. When the underlying disease is treated, lipidemic levels are restored. Unfortunately, this is not always possible; therefore, measures should be taken.

Dietary restriction of total fat intake is recommended, although its effect on atherogenesis in nephrotic patients remains questionable. Oral administration of bile-acid sequestering agents, such as cholestiramine can reduce total cholesterol but due to gastrointestinal disturbances, it is poorly tolerated.

Statins or HMG-CoA reductase inhibitors are the treatment of choice, although reduction of cardiovascular events in nephrotic syndrome has not been proven yet. It is noteworthy that, use of statins reduces cardiovascular events in patients with CKD. [58]

It has also been suggested that statins could delay progression of CKD in non-diabetic patients, but this still under discussion. [59]

v. Treatment of Hypercoagulability

Nephrotic syndrome with severe hypoalbuminemia <2,5g/dL has been associated with high risk of thromboembolic events. Thus, prophylactic therapy is indicated in patients with nephrotic syndrome, especially if immobilized, obese or having a history of thrombosis.

Low molecular weight heparin has been shown to be efficient even in low dosages (5000 IU subcutaneously) but its usage must be monitored in cases of renal insufficiency because its anticoagulant effect can be excessive. Dose reduction is required in severe renal insufficiency and in ESRD patients.

Use of warfarin is indicated in patients with hypoalbuminemia and heavy proteinuria, but this treatment is also limited. Administration can continue unless the international normalized ratio (INR) reaches the value of 3.0. Values over 3.0 have been associated with marked risk of bleeding, especially in the elderly. The target range of INR is between 2.0 to 2.9. Discontinuation of treatment should be considered after 6 months of therapy and restoration of serum albumin levels.

References

[1] US Renal Data System: Annual Data Report 2013, Reference Tables: ESRD, Vol. 2: 335-358.

[2] Hebert LA. The clearance of immune complexes from the circulation of man and other primates. *Am. J. Kidney Dis*. 1991 Mar;17(3):352-61.

[3] Ohi H, Tamano M, Sudo S, Okada N. Recombinant EPO therapy increases erythrocyte expression of complement regulatory proteins. *Am. J. Kidney Dis*. 2003 Jan;41(1):179-85.

[4] Wynn TA. Cellular and molecular mechanisms of fibrosis. *J. Pathol.* 2008 Jan;214(2):199-210.

[5] Christensen EI, Verroust PJ. Interstitial fibrosis: tubular hypothesis versus glomerular hypothesis. *Kidney Int.* 2008 Nov;74(10):1233-6.

[6] Kang DH, Kanellis J, Hugo C, Truong L, Anderson S, Kerjaschki D, et al. Role of the microvascular endothelium in progressive renal disease. *Am. Soc. Nephrol.* 2002 Mar;13(3):806-16.

[7] Strutz F. How many different roads may a cell walk down in order to become a fibroblast? *J. Am. Soc. Nephrol.* 2008 Dec;19(12):2246-8.

[8] Sakamoto I, Ito Y, Mizuno M, Suzuki Y, Sawai A, Tanaka A, et al. Lymphatic vessels develop during tubulointerstitial fibrosis. *Kidney Int.* 2009 Apr;75(8):828-38.

[9] Pavenstädt H, Kriz W, Kretzler M. Cell biology of the glomerular podocyte. *Physiol. Rev*. 2003 Jan;83(1):253-307.

[10] Chugh SS, Kaw B, Kanwar YS. Molecular structure-function relationship in the slit diaphragm. *Semin. Nephrol*. 2003 Nov;23(6):544-55. Review.

[11] Pollak MR. Inherited podocytopathies: FSGS and nephrotic syndrome from a genetic viewpoint. *J. Am. Soc. Nephrol*. 2002 Dec;13(12):3016-23.

[12] Kestilä M, Lenkkeri U, Männikkö M, Lamerdin J, McCready P, Putaala H, et al. Positionally cloned gene for a novel glomerular protein--nephrin--is mutated in congenital nephrotic syndrome. *Mol. Cell*. 1998 Mar;1(4):575-82.

[13] Philippe A, Nevo F, Esquivel EL, Reklaityte D, Gribouval O, Tête MJ, et al. Nephrin mutations can cause childhood-onset steroid-resistant nephrotic syndrome. *J Am Soc Nephro*l. 2008 Oct;19(10):1871-8. doi: 10.1681/ASN.2008010059. Epub 2008 Jul 9.

[14] Boute N, Gribouval O, Roselli S, Benessy F, Lee H, Fuchshuber A, et al. NPHS2, encoding the glomerular protein podocin, is mutated in autosomal recessive steroid-resistant nephrotic syndrome. *Nat. Genet*. 2000 Apr;24(4):349-54.

[15] Hinkes BG, Mucha B, Vlangos CN, Gbadegesin R, Liu J, Hasselbacher K, et al; Arbeitsgemeinschaft für Paediatrische Nephrologie Study Group. Nephrotic syndrome in the first year of life: two thirds of cases are caused by mutations in 4 genes (NPHS1, NPHS2, WT1, and LAMB2). *Pediatrics*. 2007 Apr;119(4):e907-19.

[16] Machuca E, Hummel A, Nevo F, Dantal J, Martinez F, Al-Sabban E, et al. Clinical and epidemiological assessment of steroid-resistant nephrotic syndrome associated with the NPHS2 R229Q variant. *Kidney Int*. 2009 Apr;75(7):727-35.

[17] Kim JM, Wu H, Green G, Winkler CA, Kopp JB, Miner JH, Unanue ER, Shaw AS. CD2-associated protein haploinsufficiency is linked to glomerular disease susceptibility. *Science*. 2003 May 23;300(5623):1298-300.

[18] Kopp JB, Smith MW, Nelson GW, Johnson RC, Freedman BI, Bowden DW, et al. MYH9 is a major-effect risk gene for focal segmental glomerulosclerosis. *Nat. Genet.* 2008 Oct;40(10):1175-84.

[19] Ashraf S, Gee HY, Woerner S, Xie LX, Vega-Warner V, Lovric S, et al. ADCK4 mutations promote steroid-resistant nephrotic syndrome through CoQ10 biosynthesis disruption. *J. Clin. Invest.* 2013 Dec 2;123(12):5179-89.

[20] Hussain N, Zello JA, Vasilevska-Ristovska J, Banh TM, Patel VP, Patel P, et al. The rationale and design of Insight into Nephrotic Syndrome: Investigating Genes, Health and Therapeutics (INSIGHT): a prospective cohort study of childhood nephrotic syndrome. *BMC Nephrol.* 2013 Jan 26;14:25. doi: 10.1186/1471-2369-14-25.

[21] Cameron JS. Nephrotic syndrome in the elderly. *Semin. Nephrol.* 1996 Jul;16(4):319-29. Review.

[22] Haas M, Meehan SM, Karrison TG, Spargo BH. Changing etiologies of unexplained adult nephrotic syndrome: a comparison of renal biopsy findings from 1976-1979 and 1995-1997. *Am. J. Kidney Dis.* 1997 Nov;30(5):621-31.

[23] Russo LM, Sandoval RM, McKee M, Osicka TM, Collins AB, Brown D, et al. The normal kidney filters nephrotic levels of albumin retrieved by proximal tubule cells: retrieval is disrupted in nephrotic states. *Kidney Int.* 2007 Mar;71(6):504-13.

[24] Birn H, Fyfe JC, Jacobsen C, Mounier F, Verroust PJ, Orskov H, et al. Cubilin is an albumin binding protein important for renal tubular albumin reabsorption. *J. Clin. Invest.* 2000 May;105(10):1353-61.

[25] Birn H, Christensen EI. Renal albumin absorption in physiology and pathology. *Kidney Int.* 2006 Feb;69(3):440-9.

[26] Hurtado-Lorenzo A, Skinner M, El Annan J, Futai M, Sun-Wada GH, Bourgoin S, et al. V-ATPase interacts with ARNO and Arf6 in early endosomes and regulates the protein degradative pathway. *Nat. Cell Biol.* 2006 Feb;8(2):124-36.

[27] Cattran DC, Reich HN, Beanlands HJ, Miller JA, Scholey JW, Troyanov S; Genes, Gender and Glomerulonephritis Group. The impact of sex in primary glomerulonephritis. *Nephrol. Dial. Transplant.* 2008 Jul;23(7):2247-53.

[28] Amsellem S, Gburek J, Hamard G, Nielsen R, Willnow TE, Devuyst O, et al. Cubilin is essential for albumin reabsorption in the renal proximal tubule. *J. Am. Soc. Nephrol.* 2010 Nov;21(11):1859-67.

[29] Doucet A, Favre G, Deschênes G. Molecular mechanism of edema formation in nephrotic syndrome: therapeutic implications. *Pediatr. Nephrol.* 2007 Dec;22(12):1983-90.

[30] Svenningsen P, Bistrup C, Friis UG, Bertog M, Haerteis S, Krueger B, et al. Plasmin in nephrotic urine activates the epithelial sodium channel. *J. Am. Soc. Nephrol.* 2009 Feb;20(2):299-310.

[31] Vaziri ND. Molecular mechanisms of lipid disorders in nephrotic syndrome. *Kidney Int.* 2003 May;63(5):1964-76.

[32] Keane WF. Lipids and the kidney. *Kidney Int.* 1994 Sep;46(3):910-20.

[33] Strippoli GF, Navaneethan SD, Johnson DW, Perkovic V, Pellegrini F, Nicolucci A, et al. Effects of statins in patients with chronic kidney disease: meta-analysis and meta-regression of randomised controlled trials. *BMJ.* 2008 Mar 22;336(7645):645-51.

[34] Glassock RJ. Prophylactic anticoagulation in nephrotic syndrome: a clinical conundrum. *J. Am. Soc. Nephrol.* 2007 Aug;18(8):2221-5.

[35] Cameron JS. Coagulation and thromboembolic complications in the nephrotic syndrome. *Adv. Nephrol. Necker Hosp*. 1984;13:75-114.

[36] Tang J, Liu N, Zhuang S. Role of epidermal growth factor receptor in acute and chronic kidney injury. *Kidney Int.* 2013 May;83(5):804-10.

[37] Sasaki K, Anderson E, Shankland SJ, Nicosia RF. Diffuse proliferative glomerulonephritis associated with cetuximab, an epidermal growth factor receptor inhibitor. *Am. J. Kidney Dis*. 2013 Jun;61(6):988-91.

[38] Mariani AJ, Mariani MC, Macchioni C, Stams UK, Hariharan A, et al. The significance of adult hematuria: 1,000 hematuria evaluations including a risk-benefit and cost-effectiveness analysis. *J. Urol*. 1989 Feb;141(2):350-5.

[39] Froom P, Ribak J, Benbassat J. Significance of microhaematuria in young adults. *Br. Med. J.* (Clin Res Ed). 1984 Jan 7;288(6410):20-2.

[40] Fogazzi GB, Ponticelli C. Microscopic hematuria diagnosis and management. *Nephron.* 1996;72(2):125-34.

[41] Topham PS, Harper SJ, Furness PN, Harris KP, Walls J, Feehally J. Glomerular disease as a cause of isolated microscopic haematuria. *Q. J. Med*. 1994 Jun;87(6):329-35.

[42] Kveder R, Lindic J, Ales A, Kovac D, Vizjak A, Ferluga D. Acute kidney injury in immunoglobulin A nephropathy: potential role of macroscopic hematuria and acute tubulointerstitial injury. *Ther. Apher. Dial*. 2009 Aug;13(4):273-7.

[43] Gutiérrez E, González E, Hernández E, Morales E, Martínez MA, Usera G, et al. Factors that determine an incomplete recovery of renal function in macrohematuria-induced acute renal failure of IgA nephropathy. *Clin. J. Am. Soc. Nephrol.* 2007 Jan;2(1):51-7.

[44] Feith GW, Assmann KJ, Wetzels JF. Acute renal failure in patients with glomerular diseases: a consequence of tubular cell damage caused by haematuria? *Neth J Med.* 2003 Apr;61(4):146-50.

[45] Upadhyay A, Earley A, Haynes SM, Uhlig K. Systematic review: blood pressure target in chronic kidney disease and proteinuria as an effect modifier. *Ann. Intern. Med.* 2011 Apr 19;154(8):541-8.

[46] Kidney Disease: Improving Global Outcomes (KDIGO) Glomerulonephritis Work Group. KDIGO Clinical Practice Guideline for Glomerulonephritis. Kidney inter., *Suppl*. 2012; 2: 139–274.

[47] Agarwal A, Haddad N, Hebert LA. Progression of kidney disease: diagnosis and management. In: Molony DA, Craig JC (eds). Evidence based Nephrology, 1st edn. John Wiley & Sons: Hoboken, NJ, 2008, pp 311–322.

[48] Jafar TH, Schmid CH, Landa M, Giatras I, Toto R, Remuzzi G, et al. Angiotensin-converting enzyme inhibitors and progression of nondiabetic renal disease. A meta-analysis of patient-level data. *Ann. Intern. Med.* 2001 Jul 17;135(2):73-87.

[49] Cravedi P, Ruggenenti P, Remuzzi G. Intensified inhibition of renin-angiotensin system: a way to improve renal protection? *Curr. Hypertens. Rep*. 2007 Nov;9(5):430-6.

[50] Ruggenenti P, Perticucci E, Cravedi P, Gambara V, Costantini M, Sharma SK, et al. Role of remission clinics in the longitudinal treatment of CKD. *J. Am. Soc. Nephrol.* 2008 Jun;19(6):1213-24.

[51] Gansevoort RT, Sluiter WJ, Hemmelder MH, de Zeeuw D, de Jong PE. Antiproteinuric effect of blood-pressure-lowering agents: a meta-analysis of comparative trials. *Nephrol. Dial. Transplant.* 1995 Nov;10(11):1963-74.

[52] Schjoedt KJ, Rossing K, Juhl TR, Boomsma F, Tarnow L, Rossing P, Parving HH. Beneficial impact of spironolactone on nephrotic range albuminuria in diabetic nephropathy. *Kidney Int*. 2006 Aug;70(3):536-42.

[53] Reich HN, Troyanov S, Scholey JW, Cattran DC; Toronto Glomerulonephritis Registry. Remission of proteinuria improves prognosis in IgA nephropathy. *J. Am. Soc. Nephrol*. 2007 Dec;18(12):3177-83.

[54] Pisoni R, Ruggenenti P, Sangalli F, Lepre MS, Remuzzi A, Remuzzi G. Effect of high dose ramipril with or without indomethacin on glomerular selectivity. *Kidney Int*. 2002 Sep;62(3):1010-9.

[55] Kunz R, Friedrich C, Wolbers M, Mann JF. Meta-analysis: effect of monotherapy and combination therapy with inhibitors of the renin angiotensin system on proteinuria in renal disease. *Ann. Intern. Med.* 2008 Jan 1;148(1):30-48.

[56] Pisoni R, Ruggenenti P, Remuzzi G. Renoprotective therapy in patients with nondiabetic nephropathies. *Drugs*. 2001;61(6):733-45.

[57] Ellison DH, Wilcox C.Diuretics. In B Brener (ed), The kidney, 8th edn, Saunders Elsevier, Philadelphia , PA, 2008, pp 1646-78.

[58] Tonelli M, Wiebe N, Culleton B, House A, Rabbat C, Fok M, et al. Chronic kidney disease and mortality risk: a systematic review. *J. Am. Soc. Nephrol.* 2006 Jul;17(7):2034-47.

[59] Tonelli M. Statins for slowing kidney disease progression: as yet unproven indication. *Am. J. Kidney Dis*. 2008 Sep;52(3):391-4.

Section B. Primary Glomerulonephritis

Chapter II

Primary Non-Proliferative Glomerulonephritis

Abstract

Primary non-proliferative glomerulonephritis include different glomerular diseases with common characteristics such as the absence of mesangial, endothelial, and epithelial proliferating alternations.

Minimal change disease is the most common glomerular disease presenting with almost normal histology on light microscopy. In focal segmental glomerulosclerosis, sclerosing non-proliferative lesions are *focal*, involving a minority of glomeruli and *segmental*, involving only a part of the glomerular tuft, defined by accumulation of extracellular matrix, occluding the glomerular capillary lumen.

Membranous glomerulonephritis is characterized by thickening and protrusions of the GBM between immune deposits, giving GBM a characteristic spike-like configuration. In this chapter, these common non-proliferative glomerular diseases will be discussed, focusing on etiopathogenesis, clinical manifestations and treatment options.

1. Minimal Change Disease

Minimal change disease (MCD), also known as lipoid nephrosis or Nil's disease, is the most common cause of nephrotic syndrome in children, characterized by the absence of significant histologic abnormalities on light microscopy examination of kidney biopsy specimen, whereas electron microscopy reveals fusion and effacement of epithelial cell foot processes.

Incidence and Prevalence

MCD accounts for 85-95% of nephrotic syndrome cases in preadolescents, 50% in adolescents and young adults, and 15% in adults. Two to seven new cases per 100,000 children are reported annually, with ages ranging between 2 and 7, and incidence peak at 2 years of age. Males seem to be more susceptible to MCD compared to females, and this incidence difference is expressed by a male-female ratio 2:1.

MCD occurs frequently to Asian and Caucasians, but is rare in African-Americans. The last ones, if affected, present a more severe clinical picture and a worse outcome.

Etiology and Pathogenesis

MCD has been associated to abnormalities of the immune system, mostly regarding T cell function and cell mediated immunity. Immune nature of MCD was first proposed by Shalhoub in 1974. [1] According to Shalhoub hypothesis, abnormal expansion of T cell clones could induce production of certain lymphokines capable of alternating glomerular permeability by acting directly on the glomerular basement membrane or by activating mesangial cells. This hypothesis was based on observations of how MCD responded in different conditions. Shalhoub noticed that MCD remits during measles infection, probably by suppressing cell-mediated immunity, that remission can be obtained with corticosteroid therapy and maintained with cyclophosphamide, and that similar abnormalities can be seen in Hodgkin's disease. [1] Later, in 1990, Clark et al., reinforced Shalhoub's notion on the immune nature of MCD, who after investigating the presence of genes encoding for HLA, concluded that MCD has an immunogenetic background that involves beta-chain HLA-DR7 and HLA-DQw2 genes. [2]

In 2002, Sahali et al., findings also supported Shalhoub's hypothesis. [3] Sahali et al., created a subtractive cDNA library from T cell-enriched peripheral blood mononuclear cells obtained from patients during relapse and remission periods of minimal-change nephrotic syndrome (MCNS). Differential screening of this library demonstrated that at least 18 clones encoding parts of genes involved in T cell activation and that T cell response was related to down regulation of IL-12 receptor (IL-12R) β2 mRNA levels, suggesting that a Th2 phenotype develops early in the course of MCNS. [3]

More recently Audard et al, reported that nuclear factor-related kappa B, a member of chromatin remodeling complex was upregulated in MCNS relapse, mainly in CD4+ T cells and B cells, and restricted to cytoplasm during remission, suggesting T cell involvement and providing additional support to Shalhoub and Sahali's suggestions. [4]

MCD is also related to increased expression of CD80 on the podocytes. CD80 is a cell surface glycoprotein found on activated B cells, which stimulates T activation and survival. Urinary excretion of CD80 in patients with MCD is elevated, in contrast to FSGS. [5] Moreover, cytotoxic T-lymphocyte antigen-4 (CTLA-4), also known as cluster of differentiation 152 (CD152), a protein receptor expressed on regulatory T cells capable of binding and inhibiting CD80, is altered in MCD, reinforcing the hypothesis of T cell involvement on the development of MCD and suggesting that persistent CD80 expression can possibly be on the basis of MCD. [6]

Active MCD is related to both cell-mediated and humoral immunity, [7] and several factors affecting the glomerular filtration barrier have been reported, including cytokines or structural proteins. For instance, expression of IL-13, a cytokine implicated in allergic inflammatory processes, released from T cells, especially T helper type 2 (Th2), has been found to be increased in animal subjects with MCNS. In this animal model, IL-13 seemed to act directly on the podocyte, causing fusion of the foot processes. [8] IL-13 is also over expressed in patients with steroid-resistant nephrotic syndrome (SRNS). [9] Knowledge of the pathway of action of IL-13 in humans remains rudimentary; however, genetic polymorphisms of the IL-13 gene have been correlated to persistence of MCNS with relapses even 5 years after initial remission. [10] Levels of IL-12, a cytokine that induces Th1-mediated immunity, were increased during the acute phase of MCNS and normalized during remission. [11] Polymorphisms of Il-4 related genes have also been associated with predisposition to MCNS. [12] Reduction or lack of expression of structural proteins of the GFB interfering with the normal filtration and proteinuria is well documented. Regarding MCD, decreased expression on the podocytes and granular redistribution of nephrin from the slit diaphragm to the podocyte plasma membrane has been reported. [13, 14]

Decreased hemopexin levels have been observed in MCNS relapse patients compared to MCD patients in remission. Of note, an active isoform of hemopexin, showing enhanced protease activity, was presented exclusively in MCNS relapse patients. [15]

Finally, it is also worth mentioning the widely recognized association of MCN with atopy and allergies. [16] IgE levels have been observed in MCD patients as well as in IgM nephropathy, FSGS and membranous glomerulonephritis. Higher levels of IgE were related to more frequent relapses of MCD, and in steroid-resistant patients, alluding to an important role of allergic processes to the pathogenesis of MCD. [17] Researchers believe that IgE levels can be useful in predicting MCD before biopsy, but further investigation is required for confirmation. [18]

Pathology

In MCD, glomeruli typically appear normal in size and architecture on light microscopy. Electron microscopy reveals fusion and effacement of the podocyte foot processes, while GBM is unremarkable. Immunofluorescence is negative for immunoglobulin or complements deposition, although small amounts of IgM deposits have been seen in some patients often associated with mild mesangial hypercellularity. Mesangial cellularity is usually seen in steroid-resistant patients. [19] Some of the steroid-resistant MCD patients, in a second reappraising biopsy present FSGS. These two findings suggest that mesangial hypercellularity is a bridge between MCD and its progression to FSGS. Whether this variant represents a transitional form between MCD and FSGS or a distinct clinicopathologic entity has created controversy for a long time. However, researchers, based on the different response to corticosteroids and the less favorable prognosis of IgM compared to MCD, consider this as a distinct primary glomerulonephritis. [20] Tubulointerstitial lesions are not usually observed but may occur occasionally, in middle aged or alder adults. In patients treated with cyclosporine, tubular atrophy may result, but is independent and non-proportional to the patients' age.

Clinical Manifestations

MCD is characterized by the common clinical features of nephrotic syndrome. The onset is often abrupt, particularly in children. In fact, patients are often capable of referring the exact day that the symptoms started.

Edema develops rapidly, within days from the onset, initially facial and periorbital, but often the fluid retention exceeds 3% of the body weight, leading to anasarca with impressive edema of legs and external genitals. Excessive edema predisposes for skin lacerations, ulcerations, and infections. Edema of intestinal walls may cause diarrhea. Pleural effusions and ascites are also common. Pericardial effusions may rarely occur, while pulmonary edema is more frequent, especially in patients with underlying cardiac conditions.

Patients with excessively abrupt onset of nephritic syndrome may present marked hypovolemia, particularly in children, with consecutive postural hypotension and shock. Blood pressure is usually within normal range, but children with familiar history of essential hypertension [21] and Afro-American children who have thicker renal arteriole walls and smaller renal arteriole lumens present higher blood pressure in the edematous phase of nephritic syndrome. [22] Hypertension may be related to expansion of intravascular volume due to water retention and edema, but in case of hypovolemia, is a result of the rennin-angiotensin system activation.

Hypoproteinemia, often disproportional to the urinary protein excretion is common. Microscopic hematuria is rare. Renal function is typically preserved, although in adults, oliguric acute renal failure and edema are often initial signs of the syndrome. [23] In relapses of the disease, Muehrcke's nails or leuchonychia striata may be present.

Natural History

MCD shows a tendency of relapses. Relapses are more common in children, and are usually related to reduction or cessation of corticosteroid therapy. Early spontaneous remissions are rare and may occur after 1-2 years of observation. Remarkably, treatment-induced remissions show a higher tendency to relapsing compared to spontaneous remissions and patients who present MCD at a younger age are more predisposed to relapses. [24, 25] However, almost 50% of the children treated with steroids respond to the treatment within 2 weeks and almost 90%, within 8 weeks, whereas adults respond more slowly, [26] usually within 8 weeks, but it could take 3-4 months of steroid treatment to induce remission. [23]

Also, relapses within 6 months from the first remission are predictive of a worse clinical course. Intervals between relapses and remissions can vary from months to years, depending on the responsiveness of the patient to the treatment. Definitive remission is to be expected several years after the onset of the disease. In fact, relapses can be seen in 40% of adults with MCD since childhood. [27]

Renal function is usually preserved in patients responding to treatment. Only less than 5% of the patients progress to ESRD. [23] Fatal events are rare, usually caused by infection or acute hypovolemia in children while adult patients are related to cardiovascular and thrombotic complications of nephritic syndrome. In a recent study considering 138 children with steroid-sensitive nephritic syndrome (SSNS) for the years 1970 to 2003, only one death has been reported. [28]

Treatment

The aim of treating MCD is the complete remission of nephritic syndrome as soon as possible in order to avoid complications and progression to renal failure and minimize or avoid relapses. Responsiveness of the patients to the treatment is classified according to their answer to steroid therapy, achievement of remission, and frequency of relapses. Definitions used in this chapter are adapted from the According KDIGO clinical practice guideline for glomerulonephritis, published in 2012. Patients are considered steroid-resistant (SS) when they fail to achieve remission after more than 16 weeks of steroid therapy, steroid dependent if they present two relapses during steroid therapy or within 2 weeks after treatment is discontinued and frequent relapsers (FR) when they present two or more relapses in 6 months or 4 relapses within 12 months of initial remission. [29] Definition of frequent relapsers is valid only for pediatric patients since a consensus definition for adults is not yet available. [29]

i. Corticosteroids

Corticosteroids are universally recognized as the treatment of choice for the initial episode of MCD in both children and adults. For the first episode of steroid-sensitive nephrotic children, KDIGO guidelines recommend at least 12 months of therapy, divided into two periods with oral prednisone or prednisolone, as a single daily dose of 2mg/kg/day or 60 mg/m^2/day, up to a maximum dose of 60mg/day for 4-6 weeks followed by altered day administration of a single dose of 40mg/m^2 or 1,5mg/kg up to a maximum of 40mg for 8 weeks and then, tapering for 2 to 5 months. Others disapprove of tapering because of the effects of chronic corticosteroid use on growth retardation. Approximately 93% of MCD children respond to corticosteroid therapy, [30] and complete remission is obtained in 80-90% of the cases. [31] In most of the cases, complete remission is achieved within 4 weeks. [26] Children who fail to respond to treatment after 8 weeks are considered initial non-responders or steroid resistant.

Optimal duration of treatment, however, is hard to define; therefore, numerous considerations have been made in the years. Hodson, et al., reported that 6 months of prednisone showed considerably higher effectiveness compared to 3-month treatments. [32] Of great importance, longer treatment periods have been associated with reduced risk of relapses at 6, 12 and 24 months after initial remission. [32] There is no data examining if different initial doses or if dosing according to body weight or surface area is of clinical relevance, so both methods of dosing may be used. [33]

Dividing doses of steroids is usually not recommended, given that once-a-day or alternate-day dosage is better tolerated and that no significant effect on the mean time to remission has been noticed. [32]

Relapse is defined as 3 or more positive dipstick measurements for 3 consecutive days. Relapses are characterized as infrequent if they occur once within 6 months or up to 3 times within 12 months from the initial remission, and frequently, if two or more relapses occur within 6 months, or 4 or more in 12 months.

Almost 90% of the steroid sensitive children with nephrotic syndrome (SSNS) relapse and in 50% of these cases infrequent relapses are observed. Observational data reports that in infrequent relapses, children usually respond to steroids as in the first episode. Therefore, some authors suggest application of the same treatment used for the initial episode for these patients. However, the latest KDIGO guidelines suggest a single daily oral administration of prednisone in doses of 60mg/m^2 or 2mg/kg up to a maximum of 60mg/day for at least 3 consecutive days until achievement of complete remission for at least 3 consecutive days. Once remission is reached, children should continue treatment with prednisone 40mg/m^2 or 1,5mg/kg up to 40mg on an alternate day regimen, for at least 4 weeks. Tapering in this case is not necessary. Others suggest waiting for 3-10 days before initiating treatment because in some patients, relapses remit spontaneously. Approximately 40% of the children SSNS present frequent relapses or belong to the class of steroid-dependent patients. [34]

Higher risk of developing relapses or becoming steroid-dependent (SD) has been associated to younger age at the onset of nephrotic syndrome, male gender, smaller quiescent period between initial episode and first relapse, prolonged time to achieve first remission and microscopic hematuria accompanying the first episode of nephrotic syndrome. [35-37] Different treatment strategies have been reported for frequently relapsing children and they all seem to agree to moderate dosage or in any case the lowest dose in which adverse effect are minimal. [38] Administration of 0.1 to 0.5mg/kg on alternate days for 3 to 6 months and then tapering, and 0.25mg/kg every day are two of the most proposed strategies, based on their effectiveness on maintaining remission. [38]

Frequent relapses in children can be challenging to confront, because of the toxicity and the potential growth retardation due to continuous use of steroids. Thus corticosteroid-sparing agents such us alkylating agents (cyclophosphamide, chlorambucil), calcineurin inhibitors (cyclosporine, tacrolimus) and inhibitors of purine synthesis (azathioprine) and other newer agents have been proposed as alternative treatments for SSNS children (see later discussion).

About 5-7% of children and 10-12% of adults with MCN do not respond to corticosteroid therapy. In case conventional doses of corticosteroids are administered and the patient doesn't respond within 4 weeks, treatment should be continued for at least 8 weeks, in order to define steroid resistance or not. Commonly, the initial treatment is 2mg/kg/day or 60mg/m^2/day for 4 weeks followed by 1,5mg/kg or 40mg/m^2 every other day for 4 weeks.

At this point, if the patient doesn't respond, steroid-resistance is defined, and requires reappraisal of the patient with a second kidney biopsy to determine secondary causes of nephrotic syndrome. Kidney function, estimation of GFR, and quantification of proteinuria are also mandatory.

KDIGO guidelines suggest use of calcineurin inhibitors (CNI) as initial therapy for steroid-resistant children.

Treatment should be continued for at least 6 months. [29] Withdrawal of the treatment should be considered if partial or complete remission is not achieved within these months. If remission, partial or complete, is obtained, treatment with CNI should be continued for a minimum of 12 months. Low corticosteroid therapy and ACE-I or ARBs should be combined to CNI, to reduce proteinuria.

Failure to achieve remission requires use of other agents, such as mycophenolate mofetil (MMF), often combined with corticosteroids. Cyclophosphamide (alkylating agent) is not recommended in children.

In adults with MCD, corticosteroids are also considered the treatment of choice for the initial episode of nephrotic syndrome. Suggested initial therapy consists of a daily dose of 1mg/kg of prednisone, up to a maximum of 80mg per day, or 2mg/kg every other day, up to

120mg, for 4 to 16 weeks, followed by tapering for 6 or more months after complete remission.

The overall responsiveness to steroid therapy among adult MCD patients reaches up to 80% for treatment duration of 13 to 16 weeks. [23, 39, 40] Therefore, adults are not considered steroid-resistant unless 16 weeks of treatment are concluded. Interestingly adult patients respond slower than children, remitting after 3-4 months, whereas 50% of the children achieve complete remission within 2 to 8 weeks. [26, 41] This difference of responsiveness may be due to lower sensitivity of adults to corticosteroids or because adults are often treated with doses lower than the real effective required dose. In some of these patients, misdiagnosed FSGS at the initial biopsy is the cause of steroid-resistance. Whether use of daily or alternate day therapy offers any clinical advantage is not well documented and studies in this regard fail to prove it. [23, 42]

Other observational studies though, have shown similar efficacy and remission rates in comparing daily to alternate-day dosing. [23, 43] No significant differences in time to remission, time of the first relapse, or adverse effects have been noticed between treatment groups. [23]

Relapses are common in adult patients, with reported rates of 56 to 76%. [23, 41, 44] Furthermore, 40% of adults that presents MCD in childhood frequently relapse. [27, 45]

Similar to childhood MCD, age of onset is related to the frequency of relapses in adult patients. In a cohort study, patients having their first episode of nephrotic syndrome before the age of 40, present relapses more frequently compared to those who were older than 40 at the onset. [23, 41]

Steroid resistant, steroid-dependent, and frequent relapsers can be difficult to treat. So far, optimal therapy for these patients remains unclear, although limited evidence indicates cyclophosphamide or cyclosporine as a therapeutic option for frequent relapses. Experience with tacrolimus and MMF is restricted but they are considered a reasonable alternative treatment for frequent relapsers and steroid-dependent patients. [23]

ii. Alkylating Agents

Alkylating agents used in clinical nephrology belong to the group of nitrogen mustards, over which activated metabolites exert a marked cytotoxic effect. Cytotoxic effects are related to the total concentration of active metabolites but not to their generation rate.

The two more used alkylating agents in the treatment of primary glomerulonephritis are cyclophosphamide and clorambucil, although these drugs have not received approved indication for glomerular diseases treatment.

Alkylating agents show high efficacy in treating relapses in frequent relapsing (FR) and in steroid-dependent nephrotic syndrome (SD SSNS), with remission rates of two-year quiescent periods reaching up to 72%, and 36% for a 5-year relapse-free period. [46] There is evidence confirming alkylating agents', and mostly cyclophosphamide's superiority, compared to steroids treatment in preventing relapses. [47] In SD SSNS patients, remission rates are lower after 2 and 5 years, ranging up to 40% and 24% respectively. [46]

For the treatment of FR and SD SSNS children, dose and duration recommended by KDIGO guidelines is 2mg/kg/day for 8 to 12 weeks up to a maximum cumulative dose of 168mg/kg of cyclophosphamide. [29] Chlorambucil can be administered in dose 0.1 to 0.2mg/kg/day for 8 weeks up to a maximum cumulative dose of 11.2 mg/kg. Initiation of treatment should take place, where possible, when remission is achieved.

Duration of treatment is associated with the effectiveness in reducing risk of relapse. Regarding cyclophosphamide, 8 weeks of treatment was significantly more effective compared to two-weeks of therapy in frequently relapsing patients, and 12 weeks of cyclophosphamide had better remission rates in comparison to 8 week treatments in SD SSNS patients. [47]

Ages younger than 3,8 years at cyclophosphamide initiation was associated with lower remission rates, while optimal efficiency can be obtained if cyclophosphamide administration begins in children aged over 7.5 years. [107] On the contrary, gender, age at the onset and levels of steroid-dependence doesn't seem to influence long-term remission rates in cyclophasphamide treated children.

Similar to cyclophosphamide, chlorambucil significantly reduces risk of relapses at 6 to 12 months compared to monotherapy with prednisone and comparison of long-term results between cyclophosphamide and chlorambucil showed no differences. [47]

In adults, cyclophosphamide is suggested to patients who present intolerance to high-dose corticosteroids or for medical conditions such as uncontrolled diabetes or osteoporosis where steroids are contraindicated, and for FR or SD SSNS patients. The indicated dose for oral administration is 2 to 2.5mg/kg/day for 8 weeks. [29]

In treating patients with alkylating agents, limitations due to numerous adverse effects should always be kept in mind and strict monitoring of the patients is mandatory. The most common side effect of cyclophosphamide is bladder toxicity due to accumulation of its metabolite acrolein, in the uroepithelial cells. Bladder toxicity presents as hemorrhagic cystitis with macroscopic hematuria. Bladder fibrosis and transitional cell carcinoma are rare.

Hemorragic cystitis develops after prolonged therapy therefore use of sodium 2 mercaptoethanesulphonate (MESNA), an agent capable of binding acrolein, is indicated in order to prevent bladder toxicity. Patients treated with cyclophosphamide and MESNA should be controlled periodically with urine cytology, and occasionally with cystoscopy. Chlorambucil, on the other hand, doesn't present bladder toxicity and is preferable in adult patients.

Another common side effect of both cyclophosphamide and chlorambucil is gonadal toxicity. In males, both drugs induce aplasia of the germinal epithelium of the testis, with consecutive oligospermia or azoospermia. This complication is dose and age dependent, therefore reduction or withdrawal of the treatment should be considered in patients who wish to maintain fertility. Semen storage is advisable before initiation of the treatment. Chlorambucil shows higher gonadal toxicity than cyclophosphamide. [46]

A "safe" dosage of cyclophosphamide in males has not yet been determined, but studies indicate that 168mg/kg or 2mg/kg/day for 12 weeks are associated with azoosperimia. [46,49] In case that chlorambucil is used, doses should be maintained below 10mg/kg in order to maintain fertility, given that studies reported development of azoospermia in doses between 9,6 and 17mg/kg. [46, 50] Females seem to be less susceptible in gonadal toxicity, but amenorrhea and ovarian failure has been reported in patients receiving cyclophosphamide for 6 to 48 months. Lower doses have been associated with a reduced number of premature ovarian failures. [51] In pregnancy, both drugs are contraindicated due to mutagenic and teratogenic effects.

Knowledge on the effects of chlorambucil on females' fertility is limited. Usually females present regular menstruation and normal pubertal development, [109] although rare cases of amenorrhea have been reported.

Dose dependent myelosuppressive effects on both cyclophosphamide and chlorambucil are well recognized. Leucopenia is the most common finding due to particular susceptibility of leucocytes on the toxic effect of the drugs. White blood cells (WBC) count should be checked regularly, every 7 to 14 days, and administration should be discontinued if the count decreases below 3000 per mm^2. For WBC counts around 5000/mm^2, reduction of the dose is advised. Thrombocytopenia and agranulocytosis are less common. In patients with impaired renal function (GFR<40 ml/min) and in the elderly, it is advisable to halve the dose.

Other side effects often referred are anorexia, nausea, and vomiting, and more rarely drug induced hepatitis. Dermatological effects including alopecia, increased skin pigmentation, and mucosal ulcerations are well known.

The choice between these two agents can be challenging but the characteristics and the individual variability or response to each one of them is often indicative or conclusive. Despite the multitude of side effect, the superiority of these agents compared to steroids and the proven effectiveness in frequent relapsing and steroid-dependent patients puts them in a high position among steroid-sparing treatment of glomerulonephritis.

iii. Calcineurin Inhibitors

Calcineurin inhibitors include cyclosporine A and tacrolimus, two agents widely used for the treatment of MCD, FSGS and membranous nephropathy, despite that no formal indications for their use in the treatment of primary glomerulonephritis exist.

Cyclosporine A or CsA exerts its action by inhibiting dephosphorylation of the nuclear factor of activated T cells (NF-AT), with consequent inability of encoding and synthesizing IL-2 and other cytokines that in turn result in inhibition of proliferation and differentiation of T cells. Moreover, lack of IL-2 secretion inhibits activation of B cells, reducing the humoral immune response. Synthesis of IFNγ, macrophage-activating factor is also inhibited, thus macrophages and monocytes are deactivated, blocking inflammatory processes.

In children with frequent relapses and SD, SSNS cyclosporine can be a second choice treatment in cases where standard steroid therapy fails to achieve remission, or when steroids are not tolerated or contraindicated.

The suggested cyclosporine dose for these patients is 4-5mg/kg/day in two divided doses, for at least 12 months. Target cyclosporine blood levels are <150ng/ml for C_0 (trough) and 400 to 600ng/ml for C_2 (2 hours after administration). If partial remission is obtained, with reduction of proteinuria by 50% within 6 months, CsA administration should be continued for an additional 1-2 years period in full dose, always maintaining non-toxic levels. Prolongation of treatment can be applied in patients with normal or stable renal function. Otherwise, slow tapering for 2-3 years is recommended, with increase of dosage if relapses occur. In complete remission, tapering for 3-4 months is indicated.

Interruption or reduction of the treatment is usually followed by early relapses, and in order to minimize the rate of relapses, prolonged therapy and tapering protocols should be adopted. Rarely, some patients succeed in maintaining remission after cessation of cyclosporine or when given very low doses of CsA (1-2mg/kg/day). [52]

In a randomized control trial (RCT), sustained remission rates in children under CsA therapy were higher, when C_0 (trough) levels were maintained between 60-80mg with a mean dose of 4,7mg/kg/day, compared to children receiving 2.5mg/kg/day. [53] The results of this RCT confirm the dose dependency of CsA effects and the importance of maintaining certain levels of C_0, although limited data suggest that C_2 levels should be used for monitoring in nephrotic syndrome. [54] However, usefulness of C_2 in nephrotic syndrome needs to be evaluated, given that formal target C_2 have not been established yet.

Although no significant differences in the risk of relapsing were noticed in comparing CsA to alkylating agent-treatment, [55, 56] CsA seem to be more effective in SD SSNS children who relapsed after alkylating agent therapy. [57]

Controversially, in a RCT performed by Ponticelli et al., with 73 patients, both children and adults, achieving and maintaining remission at two years rates were significantly higher in patients treated with cyclophosphamide (63%) compared to CsA assigned patients (25%). [56]

In adult FR and SD MCD patients, where cyclophospamide was ineffective or in patients who wish to preserve fertility, CsA treatment is indicated in doses ranging from 3 to 5mg/kg/day for 1 to 2 years, although optimal dose and treatment duration remain questionable. Adult remission rates with CsA vary from 70 to 90%. [23, 58]

Administration of CsA may be limited due to side effects, and dose-related toxicity. A frequent complication of Cs A treatment is hypertension. Cyclosporine increases sympathetic nervous activity, activates the rennin-angiotensin system (RAS), and reduces production of vasodilating factors. RAS blockade with ACE-I and calcium-channel blockers are effective for treating CsA-induced hypertension. ACE-I presents the two-in-one convenience of decreasing blood pressure and reducing proteinuria in SRNS. [59] This effect is dose dependent and it has been reported that o.2mg/kg of ACE-I decreases proteinuria levels up to 33%, while with a 0.6mg/kg dose a 52% reduction can be observed. [59]

Nephrotoxicity is also common and dose dependent, but can be affected by risk factors and the individual sensitivity to the drug of each patient. CsA promotes vascular resistance with decrease of renal blood flow and consecutive histological changes, often irreversible. CsA toxicity affects renal tubules and afferent arterioles. Proximal tubule cells present giant mitochondria and microcalcifications. Afferent arterioles present nodular protein deposits with thickening of the intima and reduction of the lumen diameter. Vasoconstriction and ischemia lead to interstitial fibrosis with tubular atrophy. This condition, also called CsA nephropathy, may deteriorate into renal failure and ESRD. Reduction of the dose is indicated when CsA nephrotoxicity is suspected. A single morning dose instead of the standard double daily administration has been proved efficient, with lower toxicity. [60]

Monitoring renal function regularly is advisable in suspicion of CsA nephrotoxicity. Limited data suggest periodical renal biopsies in patients receiving CsA therapy for more than 2 years. [61]

Other disturbing side effects are gingival hyperplasia that usually occurs after 3 months of CsA therapy, hypertrichosis, and rarely alopecia. Skin hyperpigmentation has also been reported. Gastrointestinal complications are also frequent. Neurological complications include headache, confusion, and more rarely seizures.

Gonadal toxicity has not been reported, therefore CsA can be used as an alternative to cyclofosfamide in patients who wish to preserve fertility, but administration in pregnancy has been associated with risk of premature births and rarely malformations.

Tacrolimus is a macrolide immunosuppressant with similar properties and mechanism of action of CsA. After entering the cell, tacrolimus binds to FK binding protein forming a complex, which allows binding to calcineurin. Once calcineurin is bound, it is deactivated, inhibiting T cell activation and humoral responses.

In FR and SSNS children, suggested treatment consists in administration of an initial dose of 0.1mg/kg/day, given in 2 divided doses, for at least 12 months. [29] It is advisable for 12-hour trough levels (C_0) to be maintained in the range of 5-10ng/ml. These target levels regard kidney transplant but clinicians also use them for monitoring glomerulonephritis. No formal C_0 and C_2 target levels are currently available.

In adults, initial doses may range from 0.05 to 0.1 mg/kg/day, also administered in 2 divided doses but duration of the treatment should be 1 to 2 years, especially in SD MCD patients who relapse despite cyclophosphamide treatment or those who wish to preserve fertility.

The choice between cyclosporine and tacrolimus is mainly based in the intensity of clinical side effects, which seem to be lower in the case of tacrolimus. A reason for preferring tacrolimus to CsA is the CsA dependent hypertrichosis and gingival hyperplasia, not observed with tacrolimus. Comparison of the two, showed no significant difference in efficiency and in proteinuria control. [62, 63]

Finally, in SRNS children, CNIs treatment should be continued for 12 months, combined with low-dose steroid therapy, if partial remission is achieved. If partial or complete remission doesn't occur within 6 months, CNIs administration should be discontinued, and other treating agents should be considered. In adult SRNS MCD patients who fail to achieve remission, other causes of nephrotic syndrome should be taken into consideration.

iv. Nucleotide Synthesis Inhibitors

Nucleotide synthesis inhibitors or inhibitors of purine synthesis include azathioprine and the salts of mycophenolic acids, mycophenolate mofetil (MMF) and sodium mycophenolate.

Azathioprine forms active intracellular nucleotides, which after incorporation to the DNA inhibits de novo purine synthesis with consequent inhibition of proliferation. The immunosuppressive effects of azathioprine can be seen mostly on T cells, but B cells are also affected.

Clinical use of azathioprine regards mostly transplant and autoimmune diseases. Results of its application on MCD nephrotic patients are limited. However, in a small study of 13 patients receiving azathioprine for 4 years, complete remission was observed in all patients after 1 to 3 years of treatment, and follow up of these patients, up to 13 years showed no relapses. [64]

Although several attempts to treat various types of primary glomerulonephritis with azathioprine have been made, results were generally disappointing, and azathioprine has almost been abandoned.

Bone marrow inhibition with leucopenia, thrombocytopenia, and megaloblastic anemia is a common complication. Increased risk of malignancy, hepatic toxicity and teratogenesis are other side effects that limit its administration. Therefore, in the case of MCD, azathioprine use should be preserved only for patients who do not respond in conventional therapies.

Mycophenolate mofetil (MMF) is a reversible inhibitor of inosine monophosphate dehydrogenase (IMPDH) that inhibits the *de novo* synthesis of guanosine, without incorporation to DNA, contrary to azathioprine. This way, MMF exerts a potent cytostatic effect on T- and B- lymphocytes. Reduction of fibroblast contractility and motility has also been reported. Studies have shown that MMF is effective in different types of glomerulonephritis where conventional agents have failed. [65, 66]

In MCD patients, frequently relapsing or presenting steroid-dependence, MMF can be used as a steroid-sparing agent, starting with 1200mg/m^2/day or 30mg/kg/day divided in two doses for at least 12 months, because of the tendency of children to relapse immediately after MMF withdrawal. Results of MMF on steroid sensitive and steroid dependent MCD patients have been encouraging. [67]

In most studies, MMF has been used in doses of 1200mg/m^2/day or 30mg/kg/day. It can be used as an adjunctive agent to cyclosporine in children with severe SD SSNS, with the advantage of reducing cyclosporine dose. [68] In other patients showing severe steroid-dependency, MMF was accompanied by low tapering prednisolone doses. In this study, MMF acted as an effective steroid-sparing agent, obtaining dose halving of prednisolone. [69] However, treatment with MMF in FR MCD patients and SDSSNS children should be initiated with a daily dose of 30mg/kg until complete remission and then tapered to 20-35mg/kg/day for two months and finally 15mg/kg/day. If the treatment is well tolerated, it may be continued for more than 2 years. In fact, a well-tolerated 45-month duration of MMF treatment has been reported. [70]

In SRSN MCD children, MMF should be administered in high doses often accompanied by high-dose steroids. Also, combination with ACE-I had beneficial effects. [71] However, results on SR patients are more disappointing compared to those achieved in FR and SD SSNS patients. [72]

In MCD FR and SD adults, the suggested initial dose of MMF is 500-1000mg twice a day for 1-2 years, reserved for patients intolerant to corticosteroids, cyclophosphamide, or cyclosporine. This dose should be continued until complete remission, followed by 1500g daily for two months and then 1000mg until two years of treatment are concluded. Combination of MMF to dexamethasone showed no significant difference on remission rates compared to cyclosporine treatment. [73]

Withdrawal of MMF therapy in both adults and children should be considered if no remission is observed or if side effects are intolerable. Common side effects are anemia, thrombocytopenia, nausea, vomiting, and diarrhea. Rarely, dry cough, dyspnea, pulmonary fibrosis, and acute respiratory failure may occur. In pregnancy, MMF should be avoided because of its association to pregnancy loss and congenital malformations.

v. Biological Immunomodulators

Rituximab

Rituximab is a chimeric monoclonal antibody that targets CD20 antigen expressed on B-lymphocytes and pre-B-cells, inhibiting CD20-mediated B-cell proliferation and differentiation. Stem cells and plasma cells are spared because of lack of CD20 antigen. It has been successfully used in Non-Hodgkin lymphoma, rheumatoid arthritis, SLE, and glomerulonephritis such as MCD, FSFS and membranous nephropathy.

Accumulating data suggest that B-lymphocytes play an important role in the pathogenesis of MCNS. It has been stipulated that permeability factors responsible for nephrotic syndrome may be produced directly by B-cells or by T-cells under control or stimulation by B-cells. Also, specific B-cell abnormalities have been described in SSNS. [74]

Rituximab induces B-cell depletion by multiple pathways, including complement activation and complement-dependent toxicity, induction of apoptosis, and sensibilization to other chemotherapeutic agents. [75] Depletion of memory cells, increased number of regulatory T-cells and abolition of antigen presentation by B-cells have also been suggested as possible mechanism of rituximab's action. Some properties of rituximab, including prolonged circulation and capacity of interacting with human effector cells, favor its action.

Rituximab can only be considered for SD SSNS children who present frequent relapses despite long-term administration of steroids and steroid-sparing agents, or when the last ones are not tolerated.

There is no formal therapeutic protocol for rituximab in children. In studies, good results with a single dose of 375mg/m^2 has been reposted, [76] but in other studies, complete remission was achieved with repeated weekly doses of 375mg/m^2 up to 4 weeks. [75, 77]

There is no indication for rituximab on SD SSNS adults nevertheless numerous studies advocate its efficiency in adults with SD MCD. [78-80] In one study, 17 MCD adult patients were treated with 1 to 4 weekly doses of 375mg/m^2 or with two fixed doses of 1000mg every 15 days. Eleven of these patients (65%) responded to the treatment and obtained a long-term relapse-free period (>2 years).

Almost all patients developed SDNS during childhood, but they were treated with rituximab after at least 18 years from the onset, suggesting that rituximab can be as safe and efficient in adults as in children. [78] Researchers noticed that in relapsing patients, reappearance of NS occurred months after completing rituximab treatment, where CD19 B-cell numbers where back to normal or increased. [78]

Other authors have also noticed association of relapses with increased CD19 B-cells. [81-83] No correlation was found between doses and number of infusions to relapses. Also, relapsing rates were lower in patients who received rituximab after steroid-induced remission compared to patients who were treated during relapse. [78]

In a one-year prospective study, patients presented nephrotic range proteinuria, although B-cell counts remained subnormal 12 months after conclusion of rituximab therapy. [84] This finding suggests that pharmacokinetics of rituximab in nephrotic patients may be different, given that a part of this monoclonal antibody is excreted with urine.

Adverse effects of rituximab include severe leucopenia, anemia and thrombocytopenia, susceptibility to infections, allergic reactions, and rarely anaphylaxis. The first dose of rituximab can induce lysis syndrome with massive lysis of B-cells and release of cytokines that presents with fever, rigor, hypotention, arrhythmias, and bronchospasm. Therefore, infusion of steroids or antihistamines before rituximab administration is advisable.

Although no association to teratogenesis has been reported, still, it can't be excluded, thus rituximab should be avoided during pregnancy. Rituximab can pass the placenta, and reach the fetus, inhibiting B-lymphocytes' development for many months after birth. [85]

In conclusion, even though rituximab seems to efficient in MCD SD patients, further investigations and prospective randomized trials are needed to confirm these data, and risk-benefit ratio considerations should always be made before treatment initiation.

vi. Miscellaneous Immunomodulating agents

Levamisole

Levamisole is a synthetic imidazothiazole that stimulates differentiation of T-cells and restores their function, increases macrophages activity ad neutrophils motility, thus amplifying the cell-mediated immunity.

Immunoregolatory properties of levamisole have been successful in immunologically mediated diseases such as rheumatoid arthritis. Although the exact mechanism of action of levamisole on the kidney is poorly understood, results of its use on MCD children seem promising. Application on MCD was based on the hypothesis that levamisole could restore T-cell function.

The recommended dose in frequently relapsing SD SSNS children is 2,5mg/kg on alternate days for at least 12 months. Most children relapse when levamisole is withdrawn, therefore prolonged administration is required. Long-term administration, of 12 to 24 months, has been associated with lower relapse rates. [86, 87]

Effectiveness of levamisole has been found to be higher in reducing relapses than steroids alone, at 6 and 12-month treatment regimens, but long-term effects are unknown. [47]

Common adverse effects of levamisole are fatigue, fever, nausea, diarrhea, and metallic taste and are usually associated with high doses. Neutropenia may occur in 10% of the patients. Allergic reactions are common and often cause discontinuation of the therapy. Neurologic complications are rare and include confusion, tremors, and seizures. An also rare complication is leukocytoplastic vasculitis. [88]

In pregnancy, levamisole is to be avoided due to lack of knowledge of the effect on the fetus, although teratogenesis has not been reported.

Optimal doses and duration of the treatment, and its application on adult MCD patients need further investigation. Of note, the drug is not available in many countries.

2. Focal Segmental Glomerulosclerosis

Focal and segmental glomerulosclerosis (FSGS) is a histologic pattern of glomerular injury, first described by Fahr in 1925, as lipoid *nephrosis with degeneration* notifying the association of FSGS with MCD. [89] Later, in 1957 Rich postulated that FSGS was a result of progression to kidney failure in nephrotic patients and that sclerosis is initially present at the corticomedullary junction before affecting other parts of the renal cortex. [90] Nowadays, FSGS is considered a distinct clinicopathologic entity.

At the onset of the disease, sclerosing lesions are *focal*, involving a minority of glomeruli and *segmental*, involving only a part of the glomerular tuft. Although the term FSGS is used to refer to this condition as a glomerular disease, it actually corresponds to a pattern of glomerular injury, existing in a primary or idiopathic form, without any known associated cause, and a secondary form, associated to a variety of factors.

Incidence and Prevalence

Primary or idiopathic FSGS accounts for 7-10% of NS in children, while in nephrotic adults, incidence rates from 20 to 40%. In childhood it is more frequent in females, while in adults there is a predominance of males. [91]

Racial differences in incidence of FSGS have been widely reported; African Americans present an incidence 3 to 7 times higher than Caucasians. [92] This difference has been attributed to different expression of podocyte function proteins among the two races.[93,94] Moreover, there is different prevalence of histologic variants among races; Caucasians present tip lesions more frequently while in African Americans the collapsing variant prevails. [95]

Even though risk of ESRD attributed to idiopathic FSGS is higher in African Americans, idiopathic FSGS is the glomerular disease that most frequently leads to ESRD in all races. [96]

When high proteinuria levels accompany FSGS, progression to ESRD takes place within 3 to 8 years. FSGS accounts for 4% of all ESRD causes. [97]

In the past decades, an increased prevalence of FSGS in both adults and children has been noticed in different countries. [98] Secondary FSGS is more prevalent among heroin addicts and HIV adult patients. Incidence of HIV associated FSGS has almost disappeared due to serologic screening of pregnant mothers and use of antriretroviral drugs during pregnancy and the perinatal period.

Etiology and Pathogenesis

Etiologic agents and mechanisms in 80% of FSGS patients are unknown and far from being explained. In the remaining 20% of the cases, FSGS develops as progression of other underlying glomerular diseases. However, it is widely accepted that all forms of FSGS originate from a direct or inherited injury to podocytes, categorizing FSGS as a podocytopathy. [99, 100]

Injured podocytes promote altered signaling and reorganization of the cytoskeleton with resulting podocyte detachment from the GBM, effacement of the foot processes and adhesions or synechia of GBM to the parietal layer to Bowman's capsule. In this way, integrity of glomerular architecture can no longer be maintained.

It has also been suggested that injury of podocytes activates a "domino effect" with progression of the damage to adjacent podocytes by interfering to nephrin signaling or by mechanical strain on the remaining podocytes with progression of glomerular sclerosis. Moreover, recurrence of FSGS after renal transplantation has demonstrated that podocytes are the first to be involved. In order to explain this observation, speculations about the existence of a circulating permeability factor were made. [101]

According to this hypothesis, a circulating factor affects the permeability of the glomerular capillary wall, alternating the charge barrier with consequent loss of negatively charged proteins, including albumin, into Bowman's space. This hypothesis has been confirmed by animal studies where rats were injected with serum of patients with biopsy-proven FSGS presented transient albuminuria and proteinuria, especially if the serum derived from patients with the collapsing FSGS variant. [102, 103] In humans, several authors have confirmed the presence of permeability factor. [104, 105]

Furthermore, a recent case report of retransplantation reinforces this hypothesis. [106] In this case, a patient with primary FSGS, developed marked proteinuria on the second postoperative day after receiving a kidney transplant. Plasmapheresis was performed, followed by biopsy that demonstrated recurrence of FSGS. The allograft was removed and retransplanted into a patient with diabetic nephropathy. A new biopsy was performed that surprisingly revealed reversal of the histologic lesions.

Presence of transient nephrotic syndrome in neonates belonging to women with FSGS also supports this hypothesis. [107]

Good results of plasmapheresis on recurrent FSGS after transplant, suggest that the circulating permeability factors are confined in the plasma. [106,108] In an animal model of two groups, Spargue-Dawley rats were exposed to serum obtained from patients with recurrent FSGS that have submitted plasmapheresis and to the plasmapheresis fluid. The group exposed to plasmapheresis fluid developed increased protenuria whereas the other group presented low levels of proteinuria. This finding proved that the circulating permeability factor is confined in the plasma and that its synthesis doesn't take place rapidly after plasmapheresis. [109]

Nature and biochemical properties of the circulating factor are not clear. It has been suggested that its molecular weight is between 30 to 100 kDa and that it could be a part of a complex with immunoglobulins. [110]. Several plasma factors were proposed as circulating permeability factors, but urokinase-type plasminogen activator-receptor (suPAR) and cardiotrophin-like cytokine-1 (CLC1) are most likely the responsible circulating factors.

Significantly elevated levels of the soluble form of suPAR were found in two-thirds of patients with primary or recurrent FSGS. High levels of suPAR activate β3 integrin, alternating the anchoring of podocytes to GBM with resulting foot processes effacement and proteinuria. [111]

Cardiotrophin-like cytokine-1, a member of IL-6 family has also been proposed as a candidate. Podocytes present receptors for CLC1, who are overexpressed in human recurrent FSGS and concentration of CLC1 may be up to 100 times higher than normal. [112]

In the past years, several genes responsible for FSGS have been identified. Genetic defects account for 8% of FSGS cases [113]. These mutations or polymorphisms regard mainly proteins of the podocyte cytoskeleton and determine steroid resistant FSGS. Genetic forms of FSGS may be renal-limited or make part of a syndrome.

Mutation of NPHS1 encoding for nephrin, an important protein for the slit diaphragm structure, first identified as a cause of Finnish congenital nephrotic syndrome, results in diffuse mesangial sclerosis, manifesting as severe nephrotic syndrome and leading to ESRD within a year from the onset. NPHS2 gene, encoding for podocin was identified later. Podocin is also a protein taking part at the formation of slit diaphragm. Recessive mutation of NPHS2 has been identified in familial and sporadic steroid resistant nephrotic syndrome, in African Americans. A bigenic mutation of NPHS1 and NPHS2 was associated to a modified phenotype of Finnish nephropathy, similar to FSGS. [114]

α-actinin-4 (ACTN4) is an actin-binding protein, taking part in the maintenance of the morphology and function of the podocytes. Mutation of ACTN4 gene causes a rare dominant form of FSGS, characterized by subnephrotic proteinuria in adolescents, progressing slowly to ESRD in adulthood.

Transient receptor potential cation channel 6 (TRPC6) is a calcium channel that permits calcium entry into the cell, effecting actin cytoskeleton through the RhoA, a GTPase that modulates actin cytoskeleton. TRPC6 mutation increases intracellular calcium flux into the podocyte, damaging the podocyte and leading to FSGS. It manifests as severe nephrotic syndrome in adults, with progression to ESRD within 10 years, in more than 50% of these patients. Tacrolimus seem to block TRPC6 channels. [115]

Phospholipase Cε1 (PLCε1) is an isoform of phospholipase C, important in intracellular signaling for the development and dedifferentiation of the podocytes. Homozygous mutation of PLCε1 determines early-onset nephrotic syndrome and rapid progression to ESRD.

Mutation of Wilms' tumor type 1 (WT1) gene has been associated to FSGS presented as isolated nephrotic proteinuria. This mutation, as well as familial cases of WT1 mutations, is very rare.

Inverted informin 2 (INF2), an actin-regulating protein, inhibits actin polymerization through the Rho/mDia pathway. Autosomal dominant mutations of inverted informin are a common cause of familial FSGS, accounting for up to 17% of the cases. [116] It typically presents in the second to fourth decade of life, with nephrotic syndrome progressing to renal failure within 10 years.

Deficiency of intrinsic lysosomal protein human scavenger receptor class B (SCARB2 or LIMP2) causes collapsing FSGS with nephrotic range proteinuria and progressive kidney failure. [117]

Finally, autosomal dominant mutation of CD2AP provokes steroid resistant FSGS. CD2AP is a crucial protein for the slit diaphragm structure and function.

In addition, some gene mutations and polymorphisms have been associated to elevated susceptibility to FSGS. For example, mutations of myosin heavy chain 9 (MYH9) and Apolipoprotein 1 (APOL1) genes were identified as a risk factor for FSGS in African patients. [93] APOL1 showed a stronger association to FSGS compared to MYH9 and it is believed to be the main susceptibility gene for FSGS. [118] The main cause of primary or idiopathic FSGS is the circulating permeability factor, while etiopathogenesis of secondary FSGS includes [119]:

- Mutations in: α-actinin4 (ACTN4), nephrin (NPHS1), podocin (NPHS2), transient receptor potential cation 6 channel (TRPC6), transient receptor potential cation 6 channel (TRPC6), WT-1 (Wilms' Tumor), informin-2 (INF2), CD2 associated protein (CD2AP), phospholipase Cε1 (NPHS3)
- Viral Infections: HIV associated, HCV, Parvovirus B19, HBV, CMV, SV-40
- Toxins, Medication or Drugs: heroin, interferon-α, lithium, pamidronate/alendronate, cyclosporine, tacrolimus, sirolimus, andriamycin, puromycin, anabolic steroids
- adaptive structural-functional responses mediated by glomerular hypertrophy or hyperfiltration with reduced kidney mass: oligomeganephronia, unilateral renal agenesis, renal dysplasia, cortical necrosis, surgical renal ablation, chronic allograft nephropathy, reflux nephropathy, partial nephrectomy, very low birth weight
- adaptive structural-functional responses mediated by glomerular hypertrophy or hyperfiltration with initially normal renal mass: diabetes mellitus, hypertension, massive obesity, cyanotic congenital heart disease, sickle cell anemia, obstructive sleep apnea

- Malignancies: lymphomas, melanoma, sarcoma, esophageal cancer, lung cancer, eenal cell carcinoma
- Other causes: focal proliferative glomerulonephritis, thrombotic microangiopathy Alport Syndrome, membranous glomerulopathy

Pathology

Pathology of FSGS is quite heterogeneous, presenting a number of morphologic subtypes that have different prognostic and therapeutic indications. Recently these morphologic variants were defined by Columbia classification that recognizes 5 histologic variants. [120]

This classification was based on light microscopy observations, can be applied in both primary and secondary FSGS and includes the *classic* or *not otherwise specified (NOS)* FSGS, the *perihilar* variant, characterized by segmental perihilar hyalinosis in more than 50% of the glomeruli, the *cellular* variant with segmental endocapillary hypercellularity, the *tip* variant characterized by segmental lesions on the tubular pole and the *collapsing* variant, with global collapse of the glomeruli and podocyte hyperplasia and hypertrophy.

i. Classic or NOS FSGS

Classic or NOS, is the common form of FSGS, defined by segmental accumulation of extracellular matrix, occluding the glomerular capillary lumen. This lesion may affect the perihilar regions, but peripheral lesions are more common.

On light microscopy, insudation of amorphous material beneath GBM (hyalinosis) may also be observed, along with endocapillary foam cells and wrinkling of GBM. Hyalinosis of a glomerulus may be in continuity with the hyalinosis on the contiguous afferent arteriole. Adhesions or synechiae to Bowmans' capsule are common. Visceral epithelial cells are often swollen and form a cellular cap over the sclerosing segment.

Mesangial hypercellularity is common, especially in children. Tubular atrophy and interstitial fibrosis is present in advanced FSGS. Interstitial foam cells may be present, isolated or in aggregates.

On immunofluorescence, focal and segmental deposition o IgM and C3 and rarely C1 may be present in the distribution of glomerular sclerosis and hyalinosis. IgA and IgM may be found within the podocytes.

On electron microscopy, segmental sclerotic lesions display accumulation of intramembranous matrix (hyalinosis) with wrinkling and retraction of the GBM and occlusion of the glomerular capillary lumen. Hyaline deposits contain lipid granules and membranous particles.

Over the segmental sclerotic lesions, there is usually complete podocyte effacement. Podocytes are hypertrophic and transformed in microvillus.

Diagnosis requires exclusion of the perihilar, cellular, tip and collapsing variants.

ii. Perihilar Variant

The perihilar variant, is defined by perililar hyalinosis and sclerosis in more that 50% of segmental sclerotic glomeruli. Podocyte hyperplasia and hypertrophy may be present.

Immunofluorescence reveals deposits of IgM and C3 in the sclerotic regions. On electron microscopy, there is variable foot processes effacement.

The perihilar variant is more often noticed in secondary forms of FSGS, in oligonephrotic states, such as renal agenesis, renal dysplasia, and oligomeganephronia.

Diagnosis requires exclusion of the cellular, tip and collapsing variants.

iii. Cellular Variant

The cellular variant is characterized by segmental endocapillary hypercellularity, which occludes the capillary lumen, in at least one glomerulus. Usually, more than 25% of the capillary tuft is involved, in perihilar or peripheral regions. The endocapillary hypercellularity is often confused with focal proliferative glomerulonephritis. [121]

Endocapillary cells include endothelial cells, foam cells, infiltrating leucocytes as monocytes, macrophages, lymphocytes and neutrophils, often accompanied by hyaline material and fibrin, reassembling necrotizing lesions.

Extracapillary hypercellularity may be present due to hyperplasia of the podocytes, often forming preudocrescents, not attached to Bowmans' capsule, on the contrary to real crescents. Bowmans' capsule is intact.

On immunofluorescence, there is segmental glomerular deposition of IgM and C3. On electron microscopy severe foot processes effacement can be noticed.

Diagnosis requires exclusion of the tip and collapsing variants.

iv. Tip Variant

The tip variant is characterized by at least one glomerulus with segmental lesion involving the peripheral 25% of the glomerular tuft next to the origin of the proximal tubule (tip domain). There may be confluence of the podocytes with the tubular epithelial cells giving the impression that the affected segment herniates into the tubular lumen. There also may be adhesion of the tuft to the Bowmans' capsule. The affected lobule may present endocapillary hypercellularity.

On immunofluorescence, there is deposition of IgM and C3. Electron microscopy reveals foot processes effacement.

Diagnosis requires exclusion of the collapsing variant.

v. Collapsing Variant

The collapsing variant is defined by at least one glomerulus with segmental or global collapse of the glomerular lumen accompanied by wrinkling and collapse of the GBM and podocyte hypertrophy.

Hypertrophic podocytes loose their differentiation and cytoarchitecture by disruption of their cytoskeleton. Podocytes may detach and fill the urinary space forming pseudocrescents.

Collapsing glomeruli lack hyalinosis, endocapillary hypercellularity, and adhesion to Bowmans' capsule, characteristics that distinguishes this variant from the classic FSGS. Also, there is no mesangial hypercellularity.

Tubular atrophy and interstitial fibrosis with interstitial edema and inflammation is usually prominent and widespread. Presence of tubular microcysts containing proteinaceous casts is also common.

On immunofluorescence there are segmental to global deposits of IgM and C3 and in some cases C1.

On electron microscopy, podocytes are hypertrophic with severe foot processes effacement, detached and dedifferentiated. Even non-affected glomeruli present foot processes effacement. GBM is wrinkled but with no thickening.

The collapsing variant may occur as a primary form of FSGS but is more common in secondary forms due to HIV infection or drug-induced nephropathy.

Because of its particular characteristics, it doesn't require exclusion of the other variants, but differential diagnosis from crescentic glomerulonephritis, distinguished from FSGS by the presence of necrotizing lesions and brakes in the GBM.

Natural History and Prognosis

Natural history of FSGS is quite variable, with outcomes depending on the magnitude of proteinuria, kidney function level, and responsiveness to corticosteroids and immune-suppressive therapy.

Not treated or unresponsive patients with primary FSGS present progressive increase of proteinuria, progression of renal failure and eventually development of ESRD, usually within 10-15 years from the onset. 50% of the patients reach ESRD within 10 years. In some cases the disease progresses rapidly, especially the collapsing variant, manifesting severe proteinuria, severe hypertension, marked hyperlipidemia, and thrombotic complications, noticed more frequently in younger patients. [122] Spontaneous remissions are exceptional, accounting 1.5 to 3% of untreated patients. [123]

Prognosis may be influenced by a number of clinical and histological factors. Severity and persistence of proteinuria predicts prognosis in patients with idiopathic FSGS. Patients with persisting nephrotic range proteinuria despite therapy have poor prognosis compared to patients with non nephrotic proteinuria, who show kidney survival rates higher than 95% after a mean follow up of 6.5 to 9.3 years. [124] Proteinuria may directly injure renal tubules and promote interstitial fibrosis, worsening the kidney damage and decreasing its functionality [125].

Also, responsiveness to treatment has been found to be lower in African Americans compared to Caucasians with FSGS. [126]

Different histologic variants of FSGS have important differences in renal survival. The collapsing variant shows a 3-year renal survival of 33% compared to 67% of other variants. The tip variant is more likely the most treatment-responsive, achieving complete remission more often than other variants. [122]

FSGS patients with diffuse interstitial fibrosis and tubular atrophy in biopsy had poor renal outcome. Glomerular hypertrophy and mesangial proliferation has been associated with higher risk of progression to renal failure in primary FSGS. [127]

Finally, age, arterial hypertension and hyperlipidemia have been associated to worse renal and long term survival in FSGS patients.

Clinical Presentation

Clinical manifestations are common in adults and childhood, consisting in nephrotic range proteinuria, hypoalbuminemia, hyperlipidemia, and edema, thus nephrotic syndrome. The onset is usually insidious, taking a few years to reach full-blown nephrotic syndrome, but it can also be abrupt.

About 70% of the patients present nephrotic syndrome. Patients presenting asymptomatic proteinuria will show nephrotic syndrome with the progression of the disease. Proteinuria ranges from less than 1 to more than 30 g/day and is typically non selective. In 50% of the cases, microscopic hematuria is found, while macrohematuria is rare.

Edema is the most common clinical symptom of FSGS. Pleural effusion, ascites, or pericardial effusions are quite rare.

Hypertension is present at the onset in 30 to 40% of the patients, in some cases severe, especially in African Americans with renal insufficiency. [92] Rarely, xantomas may be present due to severe hyperlipidemia.

Diagnosis and Differential Diagnosis

Although clinical manifestations may be suggestive, diagnosis of FSGS can be established only by biopsy. Diagnosis may be dismissed because of the lesions being focal and segmental.

In order to avoid this inconvenience and be able to establish diagnosis and distinguish FSGS variants, a large sample of 10 to 20 glomeruli should be examined. Serologic tests and complement levels should be evaluated to exclude glomerular diseases with positive serologic tests.

In children with FSGS and NS, differential diagnosis should be made to exclude MCD and other causes of steroid resistant NS. In adults, membranous nephropathy and MCD should be considered.

Also, sclerosing lesions and segmental scaring due to other glomerular diseases should be excluded. In patients younger than 25 years old, genetic scanning for eventual mutations may be useful.

Treatment

Treating patients with FSGS may present challenging results because of the morphological and pathogenic heterogeneity of the disease that often renders distinction of primary and secondary forms difficult, even after biopsy.

Lack of randomized control trials (RCTs) and long term prospective studies, despite the variety of therapeutic agents proposed and used over the years, complicate evaluation of the effectiveness of these agents.

However, the goal of specific treatment of FSGS is to delay or halt progression of the disease, to achieve partial or complete remission and by that, prevent complications of NS.

The decision of the therapeutic agent to use should always be based on estimation of the risk/benefit ratio.

i. Corticosteroids

Before 1985, primary FSGS was considered as a steroid resistant disease, but studies conducted through the years in patients receiving higher doses of corticosteroids and for longer periods, have reported better outcomes. Responsiveness to steroid treatment depends on initial renal function, the level of podocyte effacement, and the magnitude of interstitial fibrosis. [128,129]

Treatment for the initial episode consists in administration of a daily dose of 1mg/kg of prednisone or prednisolone, up to a maximum of 80mg or a single alternate-day dose of 2mg/kg up to maximum of 120mg, for at least 4 weeks if complete remission is achieved or for 16 weeks if no remission is obtained, followed by tapering for a maximum of 6 months. [29]

Patients with FSGS usually respond to treatment and achieve complete remission in an average time of 3 to 4 months, but in most cases, response is noticed within 6 months. Initial response rates vary from 30 to 80%, but only 25% of the patients maintain remission. 50% of the cases will develop steroid-resistance after the initial treatment or after several relapses.

Use of high doses of steroids is associated with various dose- and time-related adverse effects.

To reduce this risk, steroids should be administered early in the morning, in order to mimic the circadian rhythm of cortisol secretion. Salt intake should be limited or abolished for the entire treatment period. Menopausal women with osteoporosis should receive biphosphonates.

ii. Calcineurin Inhibitors (CNIs)

In steroid–resistant patients, frequent relapsers, and in patients where steroids are not well-tolerated or contraindicated, calcineurin inhibitors (cyclosporine, tacrolimus) can be used as second line treatment.

Indication for calcineurin inhibitors in FSGS is based on the hypothesis that podocyte lesions are mediated by activation of immune responses. Also, calcineurin inhibitors directly affect podocytes by interfering with the architecture of their cytoskeleton.

Suggested doses of cyclosporine A (CsA) are 3 to 5 mg/kg/day in two divided doses for at least 4 to 6 months. Trough levels (C_0) should be maintained between 150 and 200ng/ml. Levels higher than 150ng/ml have been associated to nephrotixicity and other adverse effects. If remission is achieved, partial, or complete, treatment should continue for at least 12 months, followed by tapering. Association of CsA to low dosed of steroids may ameliorate probabilities of remission. Patients, who have not remitted after 6 months of treatment with CNIs with or without concomitant low-dose steroid treatment, should be considered as resistant to these drugs. Of note, patients who are resistant to steroids are resistant to CSA at the beginning of the treatment.

Remission rates vary from 60 to 70% in FSGS patients with SRNS, [130] but in most of the cases, relapses are noticed soon after CsA withdrawal (60-80%). In that case, even though precise guidelines do not exist, relapsing patients should be administered the initial dose of CNIs that allow them to obtain remission. [29]

Almost 20% of these patients develop dependence and require continuous treatment with CsA, but caution is recommended in prolonged therapy due to nephrotoxicity. Deterioration of kidney function is usually noticed with administration of high-dose CsA, more than 5.5mg/kg/day, when is given to patients with impaired renal function with GFR lower than 60ml/min per 1.73m^2, and if the initial renal biopsy revealed numerous sclerotic glomeruli and interstitial fibrosis. [52, 61]

Periodic monitoring of renal function by GFR measurement is recommended, and in cases of prolonged CsA treatment, repeating renal biopsy after 2-3 years is suggested, although some authors are contrary to this strategy because they believe that this risky procedure may not benefit the patients as it is very difficult to distinguish if the interstitial fibsosis and the glomerular scaring are a result of drug toxicity or the natural progression of the disease.

Patients, who do not tolerate or do not respond CsA, should be treated with mycophenolate mofetil (MMF) and high doses of steroids.

Although no RCTs exist and experience with tacrolimus is limited, observational studies suggest that tacrolimus has similar efficacy to CsA and it has been considered as a valuable alternative to CsA. [131-133]

Suggested doses are 0.1 to 0.2 mg/kg/day in two divided doses for at least 6 months. Target trough levels (C_0) are 5 to 10ng/ml, but some authors suggest 7 to 15ng/ml as target C_0. [134].

The treatment strategy is similar to CsA. If remission is obtained, partial, or complete, treatment should be continued for at least 12 months.

In one study, 25 CsA-resistant and CsA-dependent FSGS patients were treated with tacrolimus 0.15mg/kg/day, dose adjusted in order to maintain C_0 through levels between 5-10ng/ml. All patients showed 100% remission. Additionally, a 62% remission rate was recorded in patients who presented resistance at the initial treatment with CsA. These data suggest that tacrolimus may be an alternative treatment for patients intolerant of CsA. [133]

Tacrolimus may induce similar adverse effects to CsA although in the case of tacrolimus intensity seems to be lower than CsA. However, the same precautions should be adopted if administration of tacrolimus is decided. Careful monitoring of renal function and in some cases repeat renal biopsy is suggested.

In cases of non-response to tacrolimus, administration of mycophenolate mofetil (MMF) and high dose steroids is indicated.

iii. Inhibitors of Purine Synthesis

Azathioprine (AZA) and mycophenolate mofetil (MMF) had been suggested as treatment in steroid and CNIs resistant patients, but there are no RCTs confirming their efficacy and evaluating their effect on proteinuria, on glomerular scaring and interstitial fibrosis. There are RCTs going on but their results are still inconclusive.

Azathioprine has been used in adults with FSGS in association with prednisone. [127] Remission rates were satisfying, but the small number of patients limits the value of this study. Given the insufficiency of evidence to support its use, azathioprine is not indicated for FSGS patients.

Results of MMF on SR and CNIs resistant FSGS patients have been disappointing. Although reduction of proteinuria varies between 30 and 50%, total or partial remissions were limited. [67] A recent multi-centered trial, confronting the efficacy of MMF and dexamethasone treatment, versus CsA in SR FSGS patients, showed no significant difference between the two groups suggesting that MMF could be used as an alternative to CsA in SR FSGS patients. [73]

Suggested initial dose of MMF is 1000mg twice a day for 6 months, accompanied by high doses of dexamethasone, until complete remission, followed by 1000mg/day for 18 to 24 months until a total of two years treatment is completed.

iv. mTor Inhibitors

Sirolimus has been administered in FSGS patients but results were controversial. In one study, results were favorable with important reduction of proteinuria and partial or total remission of NS. [135] Other trials had to be interrupted because of adverse effects, often severe, including increased proteinuria and deterioration of renal function. [136,137]

Remarkably, it has been suggested that sirolimus could cause a *de novo* FSGS [137]

The available data are not sufficient to support the use of sirolimus in FSGS. [29]

v. Biological Immunomodulators

Rituximab has been used in only a few FSGS patients and reported results are conflicting, in both proteinuria and renal function. Use of rituximab in SR FSGS patients has been based on the hypothesis that podocyte lesions were immune-mediated, a hypothesis powered by evidence suggesting that rituximab reduces proteinuria by acting directly on the podocyte. [138]

Complete or partial remission in SR patients has been reported, [139] while in another study remission has not been obtained. [140] Results seemed to be more promising when rituximab was associated to plasmapheresis. However, according to KDIGO guidelines, use of rituximab in SR FSGS patients is not indicated. [29]

vi. Other Treatments

Alkylating agents, chlorambucil and cyclophosphamide, have been used in SR FSGS patients with discouraging results. A metanalysis, comparing use of prednisone versus use of cyclophosphamide combined with prednisone, reported no difference in rates of complete remissions. [141]

Chlorambucil, on the other hand, showed no superiority compared to CsA. Additionally, patients undergoing chlorambucil treatment had increased creatinine levels while levels of proteinuria were not significantly improved. [142]

Also, use of alkylating agents has been associated to a vast number of adverse effects, including bone marrow toxicity, gonadal toxicity, and neoplasia, limiting their use.

There is no formal indication for the use of alkylating agents in SR FSGS, but it may be considered as an alternative for patients who cannot be treated with CNIs or MMF due to risk of renal toxicity or intolerance to these drugs.

vii. Plasmapheresis

Application of plasmapheresis and immunoabsorption with protein A in SR FSGS has been based on the hypothesis of the circulating permeability factor. In fact, in post-transplant recurrence of FSGS, good results have been obtained with plasmapheresis, probably by removing the circulating permeability factor. [143]

Recently suPAR, a soluble urokinase receptor has been identified as a possible circulating permeability factor. Levels of suPAR were decreased after plasmapheresis and remission was obtained in recurrent post-transplated FSGS. [111]

In some cases plasmapheresis has been combined with steroids, rituximab, CsA and MMF with good results, but data are too limited to support the use of this combined treatment.

3. Membranous Glomerulonephritis

Membranous glomerulonephritis (MGN), also called membranous nephropathy is an immunologically mediated glomerular disease, defined histopathologically by the presence of immunoglobulin-containing and complement-component deposits on the extracapillary side or the subepithelial surface of the glomerular basement membrane (GBM), predominantly beneath podocytes. The term “membranous” refers to the pathognomonic uniform thickening of the GBM due to the granular subepithelial immune complex deposits, observed in light microscopy.

Most cases of MGN are idiopathic, of unknown etiology. Secondary forms are also frequent, associated with a wide spectrum of autoimmune diseases, tumors, infections, or exposure to drugs or toxic agents. [144]

In 70% of the cases, it manifests as nephrotic syndrome, with non-selective proteinuria. Microscopic hematuria with dysmorphic red cells is observed in 50% of the cases, although red cell casts are rare. Other patients may be asymptomatic, with subnephrotic range proteinuria. Hypertension and impaired renal function are rarely present on the onset of the disease and are more likely to occur during the disease progression.

Etiology and Pathogenesis

Both idiopathic and secondary forms of MGN are considered immune mediated. In idiopathic forms, no obvious etiology has been identified, but frequent occurrence of MGN in autoimmune disorders points out the autoimmune nature of the disease. In the secondary forms, a vast number of etiological factors have been recognized as responsible, although the pathogenic mechanisms have not been clarified completely [144]:

- Immune Diseases: systemic lupus erythematous, rheumatoid arthritis, ankylosing spondylitis, Graves’ disease, Crohn’s disease, Hashimoto’s disease, spondylitis, Graves’ disease, Crohn’s disease, Hashimoto’s disease, Sjögren's syndrome, Guillain Barrè syndrome, multiple sclerosis, myasthenia gravis, mixed-connective tissue disease, graft-versus-host disease
- Infections: Hepatitis B, hepatitis C, HIV, Enterococcal endocarditis, tuberculosis, filariasis, leprosy, quartan malaria, hydatid cysts, schistosomiasis, syphilis, streptococcal infections

- Malignancies: lung carcinoma, prostate carcinoma, colon carcinoma, kidney carcinoma (Wilm's tumor), hepatic adenoma, chronic lymphocytic leukemia, lymphomas, melanoma, mesothelioma, neuroblastoma
- Drugs and Toxins: captopril, clopidogrel, heavy metals (gold, mercury), hydrocarbons, formaldehyde, NSAIDs, lithium, probenecib, sulindac, bucillamine agents, penicillamine, trimetadione
- Others: Kimura disease, sarcoidosis, sickle cell disease, systemic mastocytosis, diabetes mellitus, polycystic kidney disease

Independently from the triggering factor or event, a Th2 immune response seems to be the basis of MGN pathogenesis, more likely due to an imbalance between Th1/Th2 immune response, with Th2 predominance, increased $CD4^+/CD8^+$ ratio and increased expression of IL-10, IL-13, IL-4 and other cytokines. [145,146] In presence of Il-4 and other cytokines, B cells produce IgG4, a human homologue of murine Th2-type subclass IgG1, which predominates and is overexpressed in circulating immune complexes in idiopathic MGN. [147,148] The Th2 dependent humoral response leads to immune complexes formation and complement activation.

Immune complexes can form in 3 different ways. First, antibodies can bind to exogenous antigens present on the subepithelial surface; second, immune complexes can arrive with the circulation on the glomerulus, dissociate, and reform in the subepithelial surface; third constituents of the podocyte may be recognized from the antibodies as an endogenous antigen and form complexes in situ.

Experimental models suggest that MGN pertains in the third case of immune complex formation. In the Heymann nephritis model of MGN, rats were immunized against antigens derived from rat proximal tubular brush border, with consequent formation of subepithelial deposits. The antigenic target was a large transmembrane glycoproteic endocytic receptor (516kD), called megalin, located in the proximal tubule and glomerular podocytes, which binds to a smaller receptor-associated protein (RAP) to be transported to the cell surface.

Antibodies (IgGs) bind to megalin forming immune complexes in situ that detach from the podocytes and attach to the GBM, accumulating beneath the slit pore membrane, persisting for months as immune deposits detectable by immunofluorescence and electron microscopy.

Experimental studies have shown that immune complexes formed in situ are unable, per se, to produce proteinuria. Thus, it has been hypothesized that immune complexes activate complement, with generation of C5b-9 pore-forming complex, called also membrane attack complex (MAC). Activated MAC inserts into the podocyte cell membrane, inducing production of oxidants, proteases and cytokines, and promote cytoskeletal modifications. These events lead to podocyte apoptosis and detachment, degradation of the GBM and slit diaphragm, with consequent proteinuria. Urinary excretion of C5b-9 is increased in MGN, and measurement of its levels has been suggested as a diagnostic method and indicator of therapy responsiveness.

In humans, a similar pathogenic mechanism is thought to take place, although the target antigens of IgGs have not yet been identified. The only confirmation of this hypothesis was provided by an antenatal form of MGN, in which the target antigen was represented by a neutral endopeptidase (NEP), expressed on the podocyte membrane. [149] Women with hereditary lack of NEP epitopes, due to homozygous mutation after the first pregnancy, become sensitized and develop circulating anti-NEP IgGs. In a consecutive pregnancy, the IgGs are transferred through the placenta to the fetus, which develops severe congenital nephrotic syndrome. NEP has also been identified in transplanted patients with post-transplantation recurrence of MGN. In adult patients with idiopathic MGN, NEP has not been found. [149]

Recently, phospholipase A2 receptor (PLA2R), an enzyme expressed on the foot processes has been identified as an antigen. Anti-PLA2R IgGs were found in patients with active idiopathic MGN but not in secondary forms, and their levels were associated with the disease activity and responsiveness to therapy. [150] Levels of circulating anti-PLA2R are decreased or disappear before a partial or complete remission of proteinuria and reappear with recurrence of nephrotic syndrome. Circulating anti-PLA2R antibodies are not detected in approximately 30% of patients with idiopathic MGN, indicating the heterogeneity of the pathogenic processes in the basis of the disease. [151]

In the secondary forms of MGN, etiological factors are variable (reported in Table 2.2) but it is believed that the pathogenic mechanism is similar to the primary forms. However, antigens provided from infections, tumor antigens, and auto-antibodies, in case of autoimmune disease, are not necessarily involved in the pathogenic course. It is possible though that immune disorders, provoked by these conditions, make patients more susceptible to developing immune mediated nephropathy.

In summary, despite the confirmed immune mediated nature of MGN, pathogenic mechanisms are far from being elucidated and further studies are required.

Epidemiology

Idiopathic MGN (iMGN) accounts for about 25% of the cases of nephrotic syndrome in adults, while it is quite uncommon in children accounting for less than 3%. It most commonly occurs in patients between the ages of 30 and 60 years with a peak incidence at about 55 years of age. MGN has a predilection for men, prevailing with a 2 to 1 ratio over women. [152]

It is characterized by a tendency to spontaneous remission and slow progression to ESRD. According to USRD 2012, the incidence of ESRD due to MGN from 2007 to 2011 is about 0.4% of the total ESRD population, corresponding to 2406 patients. The mean age of the patients is 59 years and Caucasians prevail with a 66.9% over 28.3% of African Americans. [153] Increased incidence in Caucasians has been associated with the presence of HLA-DR3, HLA-DR8, and HLA-B18. [154]

MGN recurrence after transplantation occurs within 1 to 2 years, with incidence varying from 10 to 30%. De novo MGN in renal allografts ranges from 2 to 9% and occurs within 2 to 3 years post-transplantation. It seems to be related to donor-specific alloantibody rejection. [155]

Mortality is associated with extra-renal complications of nephrotic syndrome in non-treated or non-responding patients, mainly due to cardiovascular events. According to USRD 2012, 11.4% of patients die within the first year after reaching ESRD. [153]

Pathology

Pathologic features of MGN in the earliest stages are related to the formation of immune complexes at the subepithelial surface of GBM, beneath podocytes. On light microscopy, affected glomeruli and interstitium appear normal, or thickening of the GBM may be the only finding, resembling MCD and leading to misdiagnosis. At these stages, diagnosis may be established with immunohistology and electron microscopy.

As the disease advances, thickening of the GBM appears homogeneous and more pronounced compared to the earliest stages. Later, protrusions of the GBM seem to herniate between the immune deposits, giving GBM a characteristic spike-like configuration. In more advanced stages, immune complexes are enriched by the GBM matrix, with resulting double-contour appearance of the GBM.

In some cases, glomeruli exhibit areas with sclerotic lesions, similar to focal segmental glomerulosclerosis. Interstitial fibrosis, tubular atrophy, and segmental sclerosis are usually seen in very advanced stages or in rapidly progressive MGN and are related to worse prognosis. Rarely, crescents may be found in advanced iMGN, but they are more commonly seen in secondary forms of MGN.

MGN is characterized only by changes on the GBM and podocytes, without glomerular hypercellularity. This is probably because podocytes are highly differentiated and rarely proliferate. [150]

On immunofluorescence, performed early in the course of the disease, subepithelial deposits are visualized as finely granular formations and coarsely granular in more advanced stages. The predominant IgG subclass in iMGN is IgG4, followed by IgM or IgA and rarely C1q. C3 is present in around 50% of the cases, indicating an ongoing process of immune deposit formation. Noteworthy, presence of C5b-9 noted in most of the cases, confirm its' importance on the pathogenic processes of iMGN.

If Ig G1, Ig A, IgM and C1q are present along with mesangial deposits on immunofluorescence, secondary MGN due to systemic lupus erythematosus (SLE) should be considered. When IgG1 and IgG2 deposits predominate over IgG4, an underlying malignancy should be suspected.

By electron microscopy, the immune complexes are visualized as granular electron-dense deposits with subepithelial or intramembranous distribution. Different locations of the deposits in the course of the disease reflect a sequence of changes in the GBM, diffused or global, fueled by the initial deposition of immune complexes and complement component activation.

Ehrenreich and Churg have classified glomerular lesions in the course of the disease into 4 stages. [156] In the early stage 1, subepithelial deposits are small and often confluent with no surrounding GBM. GBM is normal without thickening or protrusions, lacking spikes.

In stage 2, projections of the GBM matrix protrude between the deposits forming the spikes.

In stage 3, deposits are surrounded by the GBM matrix, giving GBM an irregular thickening appearance.

In stage 4, deposits become electron lucent and are reabsorbed into the GBM, leaving behind lucent areas that assume a Swiss cheese appearance.

At all stages, changes of the GBM are associated with foot processes effacement, and in advanced stages (3, 4) interstitial fibrosis, tubular atrophy, and segmental sclerosis may also be present.

Clinical Manifestations

Idiopathic MGN manifests in 60-70% of the patients with full-blown nephrotic syndrome, thus proteinuria higher than 3.5g/24h can be accompanied by hypoalbuminemia, hypercholesterolemia and edema. In the remaining 30-40% of the cases, subnephrotic range proteinuria lower than 3.5g/24h is observed, often in asymptomatic patients that discover the urinary disorder and the disease in routine check-up. [157] Of note, 60% of the patients with subnephrotic proteinuria will progress to full-blown nephrotic syndrome (NS) within 1 to 2 years from the onset of the disease.

Proteinuria is non-selective, often associated with microscopic hematuria (30-40% of the cases). Macroscopic hematuria and red cell casts are rare, but if present, differential diagnosis with other glomerular diseases is advised.

At presentation, most of the patients are normotensive, with only 10 to 20% of cases presenting hypertension. [157] Renal function is usually normal at the onset, but in elderly patients and in cases of delayed diagnosis, renal impairment with decline of GFR may be established.

In secondary forms of MGN, the clinical picture is correlated to the underlying disease. In malignancies, proteinuria may appear long before the underlying tumor manifests its clinical symptoms and signs; therefore an extensive work-up is indicated in order to exclude malignancy.

If proteinuria is triggered by drug assumption, withdrawal is usually accompanied by reduction or disappearing proteinuria, but this process may take a long time, proportional to the time of exposure. In case of MGN secondary to infection, treatment of the infection itself often resolves proteinuria and eventually MGN.

Natural History and Prognosis

Clinical course of MGN is characterized by a tendency to spontaneous remissions, occurring in up to 30% of untreated patients, usually within 2 years from the onset.

Female patients and patients with non-nephrotic range proteinuria at the onset seem to be more predisposed to spontaneous remissions, contrary to patients with high levels of proteinuria, particularly those exceeding 8gr/24h. [158]

Even in untreated patients, studies on long-term renal survivals, reported percentages up to 70% for 10-year survival, therefore iMGN has been considered for long time as benign renal disease. Given that more than 50% of patients with iMGN and nephrotic syndrome develop ESRD within 8 to 15 years from the onset, iMGN remains the fourth leading cause of ESRD among primary glomerulonephritis and it is quite incorrect to consider it as a benign disease. [153]

However, predicting the clinical course of a patient with iMGN at the onset is quite difficult or even impossible, given the variety of factors that influence both the course and the long-term outcome. In a general and oversimplified appreciation of iMGN course, the "one-third" model has been suggested, according which one third of the patients will spontaneously remit, another third will remain proteinuric without renal impairment, and the final third will progress to ESRD.

In an attempt to evaluate risk for chronic renal failure in iMGN patients, Cattran et al., proposed a predicting model, based on the degree of renal impairment, levels of proteinuria along with variation of creatinine clearance during a 6-month observation period. [159,160] Recruited patients belong in two different geographically iMGN populations, Italian and Finnish. According to this model, patients with normal serum creatinin, normal renal function and proteinuria lower than 4g/24h have excellent prognosis, with less than 6% probability of progressing to renal failure and they constitute a low risk group.

Patients with stable creatinine clearance over the 6-month period but with proteinuria ranging from 4 to 8g/24h have a 55% probability of developing chronic renal failure (CRF) and they are considered a moderate risk group. Patients with persistent proteinuria and reduced renal function at the onset of the disease or with deterioration of renal function over 6 months, show a 75% risk of further deterioration and are considered the group of patients with the highest risk.

Of note, patients with proteinuria more than 8g/24h, independent from the degree of renal impairment, present a 66 to 80% probability of progression to CRF within 10 years.

Patients with non-nephrotic proteinuria, or patients who achieve remission, have excellent prognosis for complete remissions or even partial remissions with significantly slow progression to CRF. [161]

Several factors have been proposed as predictor of iMGN progression including gender, age, histologic modification, and urinary excretion of microglobulins and other biomarkers. Older age and male gender are associated with a higher risk of developing renal failure. Younger patients and children have a better prognosis, although a recent study reported that 25% of iMGN children with nephrotic syndrome, treated or not, developed CRF. [162]

The degree of glomerular lesions and the severity of histologic changes seen on biopsy at the time of MGN presentation, such as tubule interstitial fibrosis and glomerular sclerosis, have been related to poor prognosis and worse long term outcome, probably because these alternations reflect an already progressed renal disease, with low GFR and possibly higher proteinuria. [163]

Other than the quantity, the quality of proteinuria may provide further prognostic information. Elevation of α1-microglobulin, β2-microglobulin, IgM, and IgG in urine excretion, independently from the total proteinuria levels, has been correlated with progression of the disease. [164] Presence of C5b-9 in the urine indicates an active iMGN, and it has been associated with poor outcome. However, its use as a prognostic factor is limited because in advanced stages of the disease, its levels are minimal to null and it is non-MGN specific, but it may be present in other glomerulonephritis.

Finally, even in patients who do not progress to ESRD, outcome may be poor due to complications of nephrotic syndrome, often life-threatening such us thromboembolic phenomena and cardiovascular events. Prevention of these events may ameliorate outcome, but in these cases, long-term outcome is usually unpredictable.

Diagnosis and Differential Diagnosis

Diagnosis of iMGN requires renal biopsy, indicated for nephrotic patients older than 30 years of age and is established when the characteristic spikes of the GBM are observed. Histopathologic diagnosis should be complemented by laboratory work-up in order to investigate presence of underlying diseases and evaluate the extension of renal impairment.

Quantitative evaluation of proteinuria with 24-hour urine collection is mandatory. In 80% of the cases, proteinuria is higher than 3,5g/24h and non-selective.

Urine sediment is not pathognomonic because it is nephrotic with oval fat bodies and fatty casts, similar to other glomerular diseases. Urinary levels of C5b-9 indicate an active glomerular disease, but it can be noticed in other glomerulonephritis.

Blood tests should include complement component levels, antinuclear antibodies, anti-GBM antibodies, and cryoglobulins. C3 is normal in iMGN. If C3 levels are reduced, a systemic underlying disease should be suspected, such as SLE or Hepatitis C, and Hepatitis B if low C3 levels are accompanied by cryoglobulinemia.

IgGs are usually reduced while IgM are increased. Antinuclear-antibody testing is usually positive, but in rare cases of iMGN may result negative. If results from antinuclear-antibody testing are positive, anti-double strand DNA testing should be performed. Anti-ss-DNA usually tests negative, with the exception of SLE as the underlying disease.

HLA-DRW3 and HLA-B8 antibodies are increased especially in patients with rapid progression of renal impairment. HLA-DRW3 is also increased in cases of exposure to gold or penicillamine. Anti-GBM antibodies rarely test positive.

Differential diagnosis aims on distinguishing MGN from other similar nephrotic glomerulonephritis such as MCD, FSGS, membranoproliferative glomerulonephritis type 1 (MPGN1), dense deposits disease (DDD), and in the distinction of idiopathic and secondary forms of FSGS.

MGN symptoms may precede malignancies and SLE symptoms, for a long time, even for years. If suspicions of malignancy are raised, laboratory and imagine studies should include chest radiography, mammography in women, sigmoidoscopy, PSA testing in men, and tumor specific markers.

Treatment

Treating iMGN goals are the prevention of renal function loss and avoidance of complications of nephrotic syndrome. Treating regimens are based on predicting algorithms previously described, according to which patients are assigned to conservative or immunosuppressive therapy. In this context, only treatment of iMGN will be discussed.

It is mandatory to perform adequate investigation, including laboratory and imaging studies along with renal biopsy in order to exclude secondary causes of MGN, given that recognition of the underlying disorder responsible for secondary MGN has important implications on prognosis and therapy. Secondary causes of MGN should be excluded before specific immunosuppressive therapy is initiated. In all cases supportive or conservative treatment including antihypertensive agents, diuretics and lipid-lowering drugs should be.

The optimal timing for specific treatment initiation has, for a long time, been a controversial subject among nephrologists. In case of subnephrotic iMGN, there is a general "wait and see" policy, given that non-nephrotic iMGN patients rarely develop renal failure, unless the disease progresses, manifesting in full-blown nephrotic syndrome. For these patients, conservative treatment is indicated. Yet, a periodic follow up is mandatory, because sooner or later nephrotic syndrome develops. The same "wait and see" policy has been proposed for nephrotic iMGN patients, from some authors who believe that specific treatment should be delayed until a predictive risk factor of poor outcome presents. Others advocate for early initiation of therapy, as they think that a treatment delay leaves patients exposed to the negative consequences of the nephrotic state.

According to KDIGO guidelines for iMGN, specific immunosuppressive treatment should be for patients with nephrotic syndrome that present persistent proteinuria in levels higher than 4g/24h, with no progressive decline shown even under antihypertensive and antiproteinuric treatment for an observational period of at least 6-months; in nephrotic patients with a 30% increase of serum creatinine within 6 to 12 months from onset, not attributed to underlying conditions, that maintain eGFR higher than 25-30 ml/min; in patients who present life-threatening adverse events of nephrotic syndrome. [29]

Immunosuppressive therapy should be avoided in patients with serum creatinine levels higher than 3.5mg/dl, GFR lower than 30ml/min per $1.73m^3$, reduction of kidney's dimension on ultrasound in less than 8cm of length or severe infections. [29] The limit on proteinuria and GFR levels, lays on the common but unofficial agreement that these levels reflect an advanced renal impairment with interstitial fibrosis, tubular atrophy and glomerular sclerosis, defining a point that once crossed, immunosuppressive therapy becomes ineffective and futile. However, all currently available treatment regimens should be applied after extensive evaluation of selected patients, taking into consideration potential toxicity and adverse effects, in order to maximize results and minimize treatment-related adverse events.

i. Corticosteroids

Over the years, oral administration of corticosteroids for the treatment of iMGN has been examined, with controversial results. In 1989, Cattran et al, [165] compared results of steroid therapy to symptomatic therapy assigned to two groups of 158 patients in total, with biopsy-proven iMGN. The first group (n=81) received prednisone at a dose of $45mg/m^2$ on alternating days, and the second group received symptomatic therapy, for a 6-month course of therapy. Outcomes were similar in both groups, with no differences in mean protein excretion, mean creatinine clearance, progression to renal failure and mortality during follow up (mean duration 48 months). This study failed to provide evidence of prednisone superiority over conservative treatment and authors concluded that prednisone treatment is of no benefit in iMGN patients. Similar results were obtained by Cameron, et al., [166] with the Medical Research Council trial, which provided additional evidence of corticosteroids being of no benefit to renal function in iMGN.

Recently an uncontrolled retrospective Japanese study of 1066 patients, reported a higher renal survival rate, exceeding 80%, in patients receiving steroid therapy, with significant reduction of risk for progression of the disease, compared to the control group. [167]

These controversial results provide no evidence of consistent benefit of corticosteroids over symptomatic therapy, probably because of the low doses. High doses and prolonged treatment periods may be of help, but potential severe side effects limit their use. Therefore, as long as no significant benefit of the use of steroids as monotherapy is proven, this treatment regimen is not recommended as a first-line therapy for iMGN.

ii. Alkylating Agents

In the past, oral administration of alkylating agents, cyclophosphamide, and chlorambucil in high doses, has been suggested as monotherapy to iMGN, but results were quite confounding.

Although decline of proteinuria and improvement on remission rates have been observed, outcomes showed no significant difference to supportive therapy. Additionally, one could not neglect the risk of adverse effects due to high dose administration of this agent, which in some cases were considerably severe, requiring withdrawal of the treatment and discontinuation of the studies.

Intravenous administration of low doses of cyclophosphamide, in monthly pulses, has also been considered, but no efficacy was proven, as patients showed significant increase of serum creatinine or reached ESRD. [168] Thus, there is no evidence supporting the use of alkylating agents as a monotherapy in iMGN.

iii. Cyclical Corticosteroid/Alkylating Agents Therapy - The Ponticelli's Regimen

Given that monotherapy with alternate day administration of steroids or alkylating agents presented no benefit on treating iMGN, but the possibility of obtaining better outcomes with a more aggressive therapy, consisting of high doses of these drugs, couldn't be excluded. Ponticelli et al., hypothesized that a combination of the two could be effective. [169]

So, in 1984 Ponticelli et al, [169] randomly assigned symptomatic therapy to 30 patients, with methylprednisolone alternated with chlorambucil every other month in 32 patients, for a 6-month course of treatment. Patients were followed for 1 to 7 years. Twelve patients of the treated group were in complete remission while only 2 patients of the control group remitted. During follow up, the treated group presented stable renal function whereas in the control group creatinine clearance decreased significantly.

More recently, in 2007 Jha et al, [170] reported results of comparing the effect of a 6-month cyclic combined therapy of prednisolone and oral cyclophosphamide to conservative treatment. 93 patients with biopsy proven iMGN and nephrotic syndrome were recruited. Group 1 received supportive therapy, consisting of dietary sodium restriction, diuretics, and antihypertensive agents. Group 2 (control group) received a 6-month course of 3 cycles of treatment consisting in iv methyloprednisolone, 1g daily for 3 consecutive days, followed by oral prednisolone 0.5mg/kg daily for 27 days, and then a month of oral cyclophosphamide administered at doses of 2mh/kg daily. The follow up duration ranged from 10.5 to 12 years with a median of 11 years.

Results were favorable for the cyclophosphamide group, with remission rates reaching up to 72%, prevailing over 35% of the control group. Renal survival rates at 10 years were 89% and 65% for the treated and control group, respectively.

In 1992, Ponticelli et al, [171] based on the results of their first study, [169] compared the effects of the combined therapy with methylprednisolone and chlorambucil to those of methylprednisolone monotherapy. They recruited 92 patients divided into two groups. The first group consisted of 45 patients, who received 3 cycles of the combined therapy, with 1g of IV methylprednisolone for 3 consecutive days, followed by 0.4mg/kg of oral methylprednisolone for 27 days and then 30 days treatment with oral chlorambucil in daily doses of 0.2/kg. The second group included 47 patients treated with 1g of IV methylprednisolone for 3 consecutive days, followed by 0.4mg/kg methylprednisolone every other day. The IV pulses were repeated two and 4 months later.

Patients were followed for an average time of 54 months. Clinical response was evaluated at 1 year, 2 years, and 3 years for the patients in combined therapy. The number of complete or partial remissions was higher in the combined therapy group with rates varying from 58 to 66%. Differences in remission rates after 4 years were not statistically significant. Patients of the combined therapy group remained in remission for longer periods compared to the steroid-treatment group.

In 1995 Ponticelli et al, [172] updated at 10 years the results of this trial, in order to evaluate remission rates and renal survival, randomly assigning 81 iMGN patients with nephrotic syndrome to symptomatic (n=39) or combined therapy (n=42) with methylprednisolone and chlorambucil. The treated group presented higher remission rates (83% versus 38% of the control group) and higher renal survival rates at 10 years (92% versus 60%).

Later, in 1998, Ponticelli et al, [173] trying to establish if the alkylating agents clorambucil and cyclophosphamide had similar effects when combined with steroids in iMGN, organized a multicenter, controlled trial in which results of 6 months combined therapy of methylprednisolone with oral chlorambucil were compared to the combined therapy of prednisolone and cyclophosphamide. The chlorambucil group (n=44) received 3 cycles of treatment in dose as previously described while the cylophosphamide group (n=43) received the same 3 cycles of prednisolone but chlorambucil was replaced with oral cyclophosphamide at doses of 2.5mg/kg daily. Total duration of treatment was 6 months for both groups and the follow up period was an average of 36 months in the chlorambucil group and 42 months for the cyclophosphamide group.

Of the 87 patients followed in the first year, 36 of 44 of the chlorambucil group entered remission, complete or partial (82%) versus 40 to 43 of the cyclophosphamide group (93%). Relapses occurred between the sixth and the thirtieth month, with rates higher in the chlorambucil group (31 over 25% of cyclophosphamide group).

Although the difference of remission and relapsing rates between the two groups was not significant, these findings still provided low quality evidence that cyclophosphamide can lead to more frequent and longer remission periods than chlorambucil.

Results obtained from all these trials suggest that a combination of corticosteroids to alkylating agents is effective on iMGN patients with nephrotic syndrome, especially if renal function is preserved at the time of treatment initiation. This combined treatment, also known as Ponticelli's regimen, has been supported by KDIGO foundation, which recommends a 6-month course of 3 alternating monthly cycles of oral and IV corticosteroids and oral alkylating agents. [29]

In the first month, methylprednisolone should be administered intravenously for 3 consecutive days at doses of 1g/daily and the following 27 days orally, at doses of 0.5mg/kg daily. In the second month, oral chlorambucil, if chosen, should be administered at doses 0.15 to 0.20mg/kg daily. In case of cyclophosphamide, the suggested dose is 20mg/kg daily.

Nevertheless, doses should be adjusted according to the age and renal function (eGFR) of the patient in order to avoid bone toxicity and other adverse effects. During treatment, monitoring every 2 weeks for 2 months, and then every month for 6 months, of serum creatinine, urinary protein excretion, serum albumin, and white blood cells count is advisable.

If total leukocyte count falls below 3500/mm^3, administration of alkylating agents should be held until the white blood cell count recovers to more than 4000/mm^3. If kidney function deteriorates rapidly within 1 to 2 months, a repeat kidney biopsy is indicated, in order to identify superimposed drug related toxicity, and if this is the case, changes treatment approach.

In relapses, a single cycle of Ponticelli's regimen is indicated, or the use of the same therapy with remission was initially obtained. In case of resistance to Ponticelli's regimen, use of CNIs should be considered.

iv. Calcineurin Iinhibitors

Available data provides low to moderate quality evidence supporting the use of CNIs as an alternative to Ponticelli's regimen.

According to KDIGO guidelines, cyclosporine A (CsA) could be used in iMGN patients who present persistent proteinuria higher than 4g/day but with stable renal function with GFR not lower than 25 to 30 ml/min per 1.73m^3 and with serum creatinine levels that haven't increased more than 30% within 6 to 10 months from diagnosis, in case Ponticelli's regimen is contraindicated or patients choose not to receive it. Suggested dosage is 3.5 to 5mg/kg per day in two equally divided doses, associated with prednisone at doses of 0.15mg/kg daily for at least 6 months.

It is advisable that treatment initiates with low doses and increases gradually in order to avoid acute nephrotoxicity. Treatment should be continued for at least 6 to 12 months if remission, partial or complete, is achieved, tapering the doses by about 50% every 4 to 8 weeks.

Official indications on optimal CsA blood levels are not available to date, but acceptable non-toxic levels are considered C_0 trough levels 125-175ng/ml or 400-600ng/dl C_2 (2 hours post dose levels). If an unexplained rise of serum creatinine of 20% is noticed, treatment should be discontinued. Cyclosporine blood levels should be monitored regularly during treatment.

Although early-uncontrolled studies support the use of CsA in iMGN, RCTS reinforcing this notion are limited. In a single blind RCT, 51 steroid-resistant patients with biopsy proven iMGN were recruited and divided in 2 groups; the first group (n=23) was treated with placebo plus low dose prednisone and the second one received CsA at doses of 2 to 5 mg/kg daily plus low dose prednisone. Remission, complete or partial, was obtained in 755 members of the cyclosporine group versus 22 members of the placebo group, but relapsing rates were elevated, approximately 45% within a year after treatment discontinuation. [174] Therefore, up to date recommendation is to continue CsA treatment for at least a year, if patients respond and tolerate the treatment. [61]

Despite current guidelines, which suggest CsA treatment is only for patients with preserved renal function, in one small RCT, CsA was used in patients with high-grade proteinuria and progressive renal failure. [175] Recruited patients (n=17) presented mean creatinine clearance of 55ml/min and mean proteinuria of 11mg/24h. After 12 months of treatment with CsA, in treated patients (n=9), both proteinuria and rate of renal function loss decreased compared to the control group (n=8). Twenty months after CsA withdrawal, creatinine clearance remained stable in six of the 8 treated patients although a number of transient rises in serum creatinine were noted.

In summary, CsA may obtain remission in iMGN patients with both stable or impaired renal function but significant adverse events, often dose dependent, such us nephrotoxicity, limit their use. Additionally, high relapsing rates require prolonged treatment periods, which have been associated with dose or duration dependent adverse events.

Tacrolimus (TAC) is also considered as a promising therapeutic option for iMGN patients who refuse or have contraindications to Ponticelli's regimen. KDIGO guidelines' suggest doses of 0.05 to 0.075mg/kg per day, given in two divided doses with a 12-hour interval between them.

As in CsA treatment, TAC should be administered at low initial doses, in order to avoid acute nephrotoxicity, which will gradually increase if necessary. Treatment duration is at least 12 months if remission is maintained and no nephrotoxicity occurs.

Studies showed that remission rates achieved with TAC are similar to those reported with CsA. In a RCT evaluating TAC monotherapy results in biopsy proven iMGN, 25 patients received 0.05mg/kg of TAC daily for 12 months, with a 6 month taper, and compared to 23 conservatively treated controls. Remission rates after 12 months were 72% in the TAC group versus 22% of the control group and the possibility of remission after 18 months was significantly higher in the treated group with a 94% overall remission rate versus 35% in the control group. [176] Half of the TAC patients relapsed after withdrawal of treatment, showing relapsing rates similar to CsA. Median time of relapse was 4.2 months after TAC discontinuation. [176] Praga et al., also noticed that during the tapering period, in spite of the low doses of TAC, no relapses were observed. This observation could suggest that very low doses of TAC for prolonged periods could be useful in maintaining a sustained remission of nephrotic syndrome in iMGN patients, but safety of this approach is uncertain, considering the adverse effects of CNIs and in particular nephrotoxicity. [176]

Given that the overall remission rates achieved with TAC are higher than those reported with CsA, [174, 176] TAC is considered more efficient than CsA for the treatment of iMGN. In addition, proteinuria seems to be twice as high after tapering or withdrawal of CsA compared to TAC, suggesting a more potent effect of TAC on controlling proteinuria. [177]

v. Comparison of CNIs to Ponticelli's Regimen

The effectiveness of CNIs versus the Ponticelli's regimen has been evaluated by several investigators, taking into consideration potential toxicity and adverse effects, but results have long been inconclusive. In a recent multi-centered RCT, 39 patients who received TAC plus prednisolone were compared to 34 patients treated with cyclophosphamide plus prednisolone, for 6 to 9 months. [178] Results indicated higher remission rates (85% versus 65%) and a greater effect on proteinuria in the TAC group, providing evidence of a better short-term efficacy with TAC plus corticosteroids.

More recently, in a metanalysis including 17 studies and involving 696 Chinese adults with iMGN, CNIs prevailed over alkylating agents to both overall responsiveness and remission rates, with fewer side effects. Remarkably, TAC has shown statistical significance in inducing more remissions. [179]

These data support that CNIs are more effective than Ponticelli's regimen in remission achievement, in proteinuria reduction and with side effects that are more acceptable. Nevertheless, more RCTs are needed to evaluate and confirm superiority on long-term efficacy.

vi. Inhibitors of Purine Synthesis

Mycophenolate mofetil (MMF) seems to have a role in the treatment of iMGN but results to date are conflicting. Although current guidelines discourage use of MMF as initial therapy for iMGN, a number of studies evaluated efficacy of this treating regimen.

In 2008, Dussol et al, [180] in a 1-year RCT including 36 patients with biopsy proven iMGN and nephrotic syndrome, compared MMF monotherapy to conservative treatment. Treated patients (n=19) received 2g per day of MMF for 12 months. In the control group (n=17), conservative treatment consisted in ACEIs, diuretics, statins, and salt and protein dietary restrictions.

After 1 year of follow up, researchers concluded that MMF has no benefit on proteinuria and remission rates, or superiority over conservative treatment.

On the other hand, two recent case reports of an adult and of 4 children respectively, with iMGN, receiving MMF monotherapy, reported favorable results. [181,182]

Comparison of MMF plus steroids to Ponticelli's regimen also provided conflicting results. In a small RCT, 21 patients with iMGN, receiving MMF plus steroids, showed no difference in remission rates, frequency of relapse and severity of adverse effects compared to those receiving Ponticelli's regimen. [183]

By contrast, Chan et al, [184] in a small prospective study found that more than 60% of iMGN patients with nephrotic syndrome remitted, suggesting potential benefit of MMF as an alternative to cytotoxic agents.

Based on data available, it is cautious to advise against MMF monotherapy in iMGN and preserve this regimen only for those who are resistant or intolerant to other more conventional treatments.

Azathioprine has also been proposed as an alternative to alkylating agents, but results were disappointing. There is no evidence justified from RCTs regarding efficacy of azathioprine, therefore, its use is not indicated in iMGN. [185]

vii. Rituximab

As mentioned, rituximab is a mouse/human IgG_1k chimeric monoclonal antibody against the CD20 cells surface receptor of B cells. Given that a Th2 dependent humoral response mediated by B cells, with autoantibody formation and immune complex deposition is on the basis of the iMGN pathogenesis, the use of rituximab seems more than reasonable.

Rituximab as first-line therapy for iMGN was proposed for the first time in 2002 by Remuzzi et al, [186] who administered 4 weekly doses of $375mg/m^2$ of rituximab in 8 nephrotic iMGN patients. Proteinuria started to decrease at week 4 and by week 20, a 70% of proteinuria reduction was achieved, with no major adverse events, providing a favorable short-term profile of the drug.

Subsequently, in order to evaluate long-term effects, these 8 patients were followed for 1 year by Ruggenenti et al, [84] who reported a reduction of proteinuria and albumin fractional clearance of 66% and 76% respectively at month 12, with mild adverse events, pointing out the beneficial long term effects and safety of this regimen.

Later, in 2008 Ruggenenti et al, [187] studied the morphological and functional changes due to rituximab, in 7 iMGN patients who consent to repeat biopsies. Immunofluorescence showed significant decrease of IgG4 staining score, whereas C3 staining was no longer detectable in 2 biopsies. On electron microscopy, electron-dense deposits almost completely disappeared and podocyte changes were remarkably less severe. Electron-dense deposits were reabsorbed and replaced by electron-lucent material, similar to stage 4 of iMGN. Functional changes included reduction of the albumin and sodium fractional clearance. These findings strongly suggest interference of rituximab with the pathogenic processes of iMGN.

A recent meta-analysis, summarizing rituximab results in 85 iMGN patients, reported rates of 15 to 20% and 35 to 40% for complete and partial remission respectively, similar to the response rates of alkylating agents and CNIs, but better tolerated. [188] Plasmapheresis combined with rituximab has also been suggested for refractory iMGN but effectiveness is still to be proved. [189]

Despite excellent tolerability and quite promising treatment effect, this regimen is still in its infant stage and well-designed RCTs are needed to confirm these encouraging results. Yet, there is not enough data supporting use of rituximab as initial treatment of iMGN, and it is recommended to apply this regimen only in selected patients who have contraindications or intolerance to conventional immunosuppressive regimens.

vii. Synthetic Adrenocorticotropic Hormone (ACTH)

A synthetic ACTH analog has been widely used, with some success for the treatment of nephrotic syndrome in patients with MCD, iMGN, FSGS and MPGN.

Favorable results were first obtained by Berg et al, [190] who intramuscularly synthetic ACTH at the maximal dose of 1 mg in 5 patients, twice a week for one year, with follow-up time after discontinuing treatment of 18 months. Urine albumin excretion decreased by 90% and GFR increased by 25%. Deterioration was observed in all cases when ACTH was discontinued. In a further study, Berg and Arnadottir, [191] administered ACTH analog in 23 patients with various etiologies of nephrotic range proteinuria, including iMGN, mesangioproliferative glomerulonephritis, MCD, FSGS, MPGN type 1, and hereditary nephropathy. In this study of 10 patients presenting iMGN, 4 obtained complete remission and 6, partial remission. Only one of these patients relapsed after treatment withdrawal.

Based on these results, Ponticelli et al, [192] conducted a small RCT, comparing Ponticelli's regimen to im synthetic ACTH. In this study, although both groups responded to either treatment, no significant differences between them were observed.

In a more recent study, 21 patients with nephrotic syndrome of various etiologies were treated with synthetic ACTH analog in gel formulation. [193] Of the 11 patients with iMN, 3 (27%) achieved complete remission and 6 (55%) achieved partial remission. Only 2 of these patients didn't respond to the treatment.

Available data do not provide any clarification on the mechanisms of action of ACTH analog in iMGN. It is believed that ACTH analog is more efficient in iMGN than in other glomerulonephritis and that it could be a viable treatment option to resistant nephrotic syndrome. To date, no large RCTs have been conducted and knowledge on ACTH analog is still rudimentary. Therefore, their use is not recommended for initial treatment of iMGN.

REFERENCES

[1] Shalhoub RJ. Pathogenesis of lipoid nephrosis: a disorder of T-cell function. *Lancet.* 1974 Sep 7;2(7880):556-60.

[2] Clark AG, Vaughan RW, Stephens HA, Chantler C, Williams DG, Welsh KI. Genes encoding the beta-chains of HLA-DR7 and HLA-DQw2 define major susceptibility determinants for idiopathic nephrotic syndrome. *Clin. Sci.* (Lond). 1990 Apr;78(4): 391-7.

[3] Sahali D, Pawlak A, Valanciuté A, Grimbert P, Lang P, Remy P, et al. A novel approach to investigation of the pathogenesis of active minimal-change nephrotic syndrome using subtracted cDNA library screening. *J. Am. Soc. Nephrol.* 2002 May;13(5):1238-47.

[4] Audard V, Pawlak A, Candelier M, Lang P, Sahali D. Upregulation of nuclear factor-related kappa B suggests a disorder of transcriptional regulation in minimal change nephrotic syndrome. *PLoS One.* 2012;7(1):e30523. doi: 10.1371/journal.pone.0030523.

[5] Garin EH, Diaz LN, Mu W, Wasserfall C, Araya C, Segal M, et al. Urinary CD80 excretion increases in idiopathic minimal-change disease. *J. Am. Soc. Nephrol.* 2009 Feb;20(2):260-6.

[6] Ishimoto T, Shimada M, Araya CE, Huskey J, Garin EH, Johnson RJ. Minimal change disease: a CD80 podocytopathy? *Semin. Nephrol.* 2011 Jul;31(4):320-5.

[7] Mathieson PW. Immune dysregulation in minimal change nephropathy. *Nephrol. Dial. Transplant.* 2003 Aug;18 Suppl 6:vi26-9.

[8] Lai KW, Wei CL, Tan LK, Tan PH, Chiang GS, Lee CG, et al. Overexpression of interleukin-13 induces minimal-change-like nephropathy in rats. *J. Am. Soc. Nephrol.* 2007 May;18(5):1476-85.

[9] Yap HK, Cheung W, Murugasu B, Sim SK, Seah CC, Jordan SC. Th1 and Th2 cytokine mRNA profiles in childhood nephrotic syndrome: evidence for increased IL-13 mRNA expression in relapse. *J. Am. Soc. Nephrol.* 1999 Mar;10(3):529-37.

[10] Wei CL, Cheung W, Heng CK, Arty N, Chong SS, Lee BW, et al. Interleukin-13 genetic polymorphisms in Singapore Chinese children correlate with long-term outcome of minimal-change disease. *Nephrol. Dial. Transplant.* 2005 Apr;20(4):728-34.

[11] Lin CY, Chien JW. Increased interleukin-12 release from peripheral blood mononuclear cells in nephrotic phase of minimal change nephrotic syndrome. *Acta Paediatr Taiwan.* 2004 Mar-Apr;45(2):77-80.

[12] Ikeuchi Y, Kobayashi Y, Arakawa H, Suzuki M, Tamra K, Morikawa A. Polymorphisms in interleukin-4-related genes in patients with minimal change nephrotic syndrome. *Pediatr Nephrol.* 2009 Mar;24(3):489-95.

[13] Doublier S, Ruotsalainen V, Salvidio G, Lupia E, Biancone L, Conaldi PG, et al. Nephrin redistribution on podocytes is a potential mechanism for proteinuria in patients with primary acquired nephrotic syndrome. *Am. J. Pathol.* 2001 May;158(5):1723-31.

[14] Kim BK, Hong HK, Kim JH, Lee HS. Differential expression of nephrin in acquired human proteinuric diseases. *Am. J. Kidney Dis.* 2002 Nov;40(5):964-73.

[15] Bakker WW, van Dael CM, Pierik LJ, van Wijk JA, Nauta J, Borghuis T, et al. Altered activity of plasma hemopexin in patients with minimal change disease in relapse. *Pediatr Nephrol.* 2005 Oct;20(10):1410-5.

[16] Meadow SR, Sarsfield JK, Scott DG, Rajah SM. Steroid-responsive nephrotic syndrome and allergy: immunological studies. *Arch Dis Child.* 1981 Jul;56(7):517-24.

[17] Shu KH, Lian JD, Lu YS, Chen CH, Tsai DY, Chao KS, et al. Immunoglobulin-E-specific suppressor factors in primary glomerulonephritis with nephrotic syndrome. *Nephron.* 1992;60(4):432-5.

[18] Shao YN, Chen YC, Jenq CC, Hsu HH, Chang MY, Tian YC, et al. Serum immunoglobulin E can predict minimal change disease before renal biopsy. *Am. J. Med. Sci.* 2009 Oct;338(4):264-7.

[19] Border WA. Distinguishing minimal-change disease from mesangial disorders. *Kidney Int.* 1988 Sep;34(3):419-34.

[20] Mokhtar GA. IgM nephropathy: clinical picture and pathological findings in 36 patients. *Saudi J. Kidney Dis. Transpl.* 2011 Sep;22(5):969-75.

[21] Kontchou LM, Liccioli G, Pela I. Blood pressure in children with minimal change nephrotic syndrome during oedema and after steroid therapy: the influence of familial essential hypertension. *Kidney Blood Press Res.* 2009;32(4):258-62.

[22] Rostand SG, Cross SK, Kirk KA, Lee JY, Kuhlmann A, Amann K. Racial differences in renal arteriolar structure in children with minimal change nephropathy. *Kidney Int.* 2005 Sep;68(3):1154-60.

[23] Waldman M, Crew RJ, Valeri A, Busch J, Stokes B, Markowitz G, et al. Adult minimal-change disease: clinical characteristics, treatment, and outcomes. *Clin. J. Am. Soc Nephrol.* 2007 May;2(3):445-53.

[24] Trompeter RS, Lloyd BW, Hicks J, White RH, Cameron JS. Long-term outcome for children with minimal-change nephrotic syndrome. *Lancet.* 1985 Feb 16;1(8425):368-70.

[25] Hoyer PF, Brodeh J. Initial treatment of idiopathic nephrotic syndrome in children: prednisone versus prednisone plus cyclosporine A: a prospective, randomized trial. *J. Am. Soc. Nephrol.* 2006 Apr;17(4):1151-7.

[26] The primary nephrotic syndrome in children. Identification of patients with minimal change nephrotic syndrome from initial response to prednisone. A report of the International Study of Kidney Disease in Children. *J. Pediatr.* 1981 Apr;98(4):561-4.

[27] Fakhouri F, Bocquet N, Taupin P, Presne C, Gagnadoux MF, Landais P, et al. Steroid-sensitive nephrotic syndrome: from childhood to adulthood. *Am. J. Kidney Dis.* 2003 Mar;41(3):550-7.

[28] Rüth EM, Kemper MJ, Leumann EP, Laube GF, Neuhaus TJ. Children with steroid-sensitive nephrotic syndrome come of age: long-term outcome. *J. Pediatr.* 2005 Aug;147(2):202-7.

[29] Kidney Disease: Improving Global Outcomes (KDIGO) Glomerulonephritis Work Group. KDIGO Clinical Practice Guideline for Glomerulonephritis. *Kidney inter.*, Suppl. 2012; 2: 139–274.

[30] Primary nephrotic syndrome in children: clinical significance of histopathologic variants of minimal change and of diffuse mesangial hypercellularity. A Report of the International Study of Kidney Disease in Children. *Kidney Int.* 1981 Dec;20(6):765-71.

[31] McKinney PA, Feltbower RG, Brocklebank JT, Fitzpatrick MM. Time trends and ethnic patterns of childhood nephrotic syndrome in Yorkshire, UK. Pediatr Nephrol. 2001 Dec;16(12):1040-4.

[32] Hodson EM, Knight JF, Willis NS, Craig JC. Corticosteroid therapy for nephrotic syndrome in children. *Cochrane Database Syst. Rev.* 2005 Jan 25;(1):CD001533.

[33] Feber J, Al-Matrafi J, Farhadi E, Vaillancourt R, Wolfish N. Prednisone dosing per body weight or body surface area in children with nephrotic syndrome: is it equivalent? *Pediatr. Nephrol.* 2009 May;24(5):1027-31.

[34] Tarshish P, Tobin JN, Bernstein J, Edelmann CM Jr. Prognostic significance of the early course of minimal change nephrotic syndrome: report of the International Study of Kidney Disease in Children. *J. Am. Soc. Nephrol.* 1997 May;8(5):769-76.

[35] Andersen RF, Thrane N, Noergaard K, Rytter L, Jespersen B, Rittig S. Early age at debut is a predictor of steroid-dependent and frequent relapsing nephrotic syndrome. *Pediatr. Nephrol.* 2010 Jul;25(7):1299-304.

[36] Noer MS. Predictors of relapse in steroid-sensitive nephrotic syndrome. *Southeast Asian J. Trop. Med. Public Health.* 2005 Sep;36(5):1313-20.

[37] Constantinescu AR, Shah HB, Foote EF, Weiss LS. Predicting first-year relapses in children with nephrotic syndrome. *Pediatrics.* 2000 Mar;105(3 Pt 1):492-5.

[38] Indian Pediatric Nephrology Group, Indian Academy of Pediatrics, Bagga A, Ali U, Banerjee S, Kanitkar M, Phadke KD, Senguttuvan P, et al. Management of steroid sensitive nephrotic syndrome: revised guidelines. *Indian Pediatr.* 2008 Mar;45(3): 203-14.

[39] Nolasco F, Cameron JS, Heywood EF, Hicks J, Ogg C, Williams DG. Adult-onset minimal change nephrotic syndrome: a long-term follow-up. *Kidney Int.* 1986 Jun;29(6):1215-23.

[40] Korbet SM, Schwartz MM, Lewis EJ. Minimal-change glomerulopathy of adulthood. *Am. J. Nephrol.* 1988;8(4):291-7.

[41] Nakayama M, Katafuchi R, Yanase T, Ikeda K, Tanaka H, Fujimi S. Steroid responsiveness, and frequency of relapse in adult-onset minimal change nephrotic syndrome. Am. *J. Kidney Dis.* 2002 Mar;39(3):503-12.

[42] Mak SK, Short CD, Mallick NP. Long-term outcome of adult-onset minimal-change nephropathy. *Nephrol. Dial Transplant.* 1996 Nov;11(11):2192-201.

[43] Nair RB, Date A, Kirubakaran MG, Shastry JC. Minimal-change nephrotic syndrome in adults treated with alternate-day steroids. *Nephron.* 1987;47(3):209-10.

[44] Tse KC, Lam MF, Yip PS, Li FK, Choy BY, Lai KN, et al. Idiopathic minimal change nephrotic syndrome in older adults: steroid responsiveness and pattern of relapses. *Nephrol. Dial Transplant.* 2003 Jul;18(7):1316-20.

[45] Philibert D, Cattran D. Remission of proteinuria in primary glomerulonephritis: we know the goal but do we know the price? *Nat. Clin. Pract. Nephrol.* 2008 Oct;4(10):550-9.

[46] Latta K, von Schnakenburg C, Ehrich JH. A meta-analysis of cytotoxic treatment for frequently relapsing nephrotic syndrome in children. *Pediatr. Nephrol.* 2001 Mar;16(3):271-82.

[47] Hodson EM, Willis NS, Craig JC. Non-corticosteroid treatment for nephrotic syndrome in children. *Cochrane Database Syst. Rev.* 2008 Jan 23;(1):CD002290.

[48] Azib S, Macher MA, Kwon T, Dechartres A, Alberti C, Loirat C, et al. Cyclophosphamide in steroid-dependent nephrotic syndrome. *Pediatr. Nephrol.* 2011 Jun;26(6):927-32.

[49] Wetzels JF. Cyclophosphamide-induced gonadal toxicity: a treatment dilemma in patients with lupus nephritis? *Neth. J. Med.* 2004 Nov;62(10):347-52.

[50] Callis L, Nieto J, Vila A, Rende J. Chlorambucil treatment in minimal lesion nephrotic syndrome: a reappraisal of its gonadal toxicity. *J. Pediatr.* 1980 Oct;97(4):653-6.

[51] Appenzeller S, Blatyta PF, Costallat LT. Ovarian failure in SLE patients using pulse cyclophosphamide: comparison of different regimes. *Rheumatol. Int.* 2008 Apr;28(6):567-71.

[52] Meyrier A, Noël LH, Auriche P, Callard P. Long-term renal tolerance of cyclosporin A treatment in adult idiopathic nephrotic syndrome. Collaborative Group of the Société de Néphrologie. *Kidney Int.* 1994 May;45(5):1446-56.

[53] Niaudet P, Broyer M, Habib R. Treatment of idiopathic nephrotic syndrome with cyclosporin A in children. *Clin. Nephrol.* 1991;35 Suppl 1:S31-6.

[54] Filler G. How should microemulsified Cyclosporine A (Neoral) therapy in patients with nephrotic syndrome be monitored? *Nephrol. Dial Transplant.* 2005 Jun;20(6):1032-4.

[55] Niaudet P. Comparison of cyclosporin and chlorambucil in the treatment of steroid-dependent idiopathic nephrotic syndrome: a multicentre randomized controlled trial. The French Society of Paediatric Nephrology. *Pediatr. Nephrol.* 1992 Jan;6(1):1-3.

[56] Ponticelli C, Edefonti A, Ghio L, Rizzoni G, Rinaldi S, Gusmano R, et al., Cyclosporin versus cyclophosphamide for patients with steroid-dependent and frequently relapsing idiopathic nephrotic syndrome: a multicentre randomized controlled trial. *Nephrol. Dial Transplant.* 1993;8(12):1326-32.

[57] El-Husseini A, El-Basuony F, Mahmoud I, Sheashaa H, Sabry A, Hassan R, et al. Long-term effects of cyclosporine in children with idiopathic nephrotic syndrome: a single-centre experience. *Nephrol. Dial Transplant.* 2005 Nov;20(11):2433-8.

[58] Meyrier A, Condamin MC, Broneer D. Treatment of adult idiopathic nephrotic syndrome with cyclosporin A: minimal-change disease and focal-segmental glomerulosclerosis. Collaborative Group of the French Society of Nephrology. *Clin. Nephrol.* 1991;35 Suppl 1:S37-42.

[59] Bagga A, Mudigoudar BD, Hari P, Vasudev V. Enalapril dosage in steroid-resistant nephrotic syndrome. *Pediatr. Nephrol.* 2004 Jan;19(1):45-50.

[60] Chishti AS, Sorof JM, Brewer ED, Kale AS. Long-term treatment of focal segmental glomerulosclerosis in children with cyclosporine given as a single daily dose. *Am. J. Kidney Dis.* 2001 Oct;38(4):754-60.

[61] Cattran DC, Alexopoulos E, Heering P, Hoyer PF, Johnston A, Meyrier A, et al. Cyclosporin in idiopathic glomerular disease associated with the nephrotic syndrome: workshop recommendations. *Kidney Int.* 2007 Dec;72(12):1429-47.

[62] Sinha MD, MacLeod R, Rigby E, Clark AG. Treatment of severe steroid-dependent nephrotic syndrome (SDNS) in children with tacrolimus. Nephrol. Dial Transplant. 2006 Jul;21(7):1848-54.

[63] Choudhry S, Bagga A, Hari P, Sharma S, Kalaivani M, Dinda A. Efficacy and safety of tacrolimus versus cyclosporine in children with steroid-resistant nephrotic syndrome: a randomized controlled trial. *Am. J. Kidney Dis.* 2009 May;53(5):760-9.

[64] Cade R, Mars D, Privette M, Thompson R, Croker B, Peterson J, et al. Effect of long-term azathioprine administration in adults with minimal-change glomerulonephritis and nephrotic syndrome resistant to corticosteroids. *Arch. Intern. Med.* 1986 Apr;146(4):737-41.

[65] Choi MJ, Eustace JA, Gimenez LF, Atta MG, Scheel PJ, Sothinathan R, et al. Mycophenolate mofetil treatment for primary glomerular diseases. *Kidney Int.* 2002 Mar;61(3):1098-114.

[66] Fu YF, Liu GL. Mycophenolate mofetil therapy for children with lupus nephritis refractory to both intravenous cyclosphosphamide and cyclosporine. *Clin. Nephrol.* 2001 Apr;55(4):318-21.

[67] Sepe V, Libetta C, Giuliano MG, Adamo G, Dal Canton A., Mycophenolate mofetil in primary glomerulopathies. *Kidney Int.* 2008 Jan;73(2):154-62.

[68] Barletta GM, Smoyer WE, Bunchman TE, Flynn JT, Kershaw DB. Use of mycophenolate mofetil in steroid-dependent and -resistant nephrotic syndrome. *Pediatr. Nephrol.* 2003 Aug;18(8):833-7.

[69] Bagga A, Hari P, Moudgil A, Jordan SC. Mycophenolate mofetil and prednisolone therapy in children with steroid-dependent nephrotic syndrome. *Am. J. Kidney Dis.* 2003 Dec;42(6):1114-20.

[70] Afzal K, Bagga A, Menon S, Hari P, Jordan SC. Treatment with mycophenolate mofetil and prednisolone for steroid-dependent nephrotic syndrome. *Pediatr. Nephrol.* 2007 Dec;22(12):2059-65.

[71] Moudgil A, Bagga A, Jordan SC. Mycophenolate mofetil therapy in frequently relapsing steroid-dependent and steroid-resistant nephrotic syndrome of childhood: current status and future directions. *Pediatr. Nephrol.* 2005 Oct;20(10):1376-81.

[72] Mendizábal S, Zamora I, Berbel O, Sanahuja MJ, Fuentes J, Simon J. Mycophenolate mofetil in steroid/cyclosporine-dependent/resistant nephrotic syndrome. *Pediatr. Nephrol.* 2005 Jul;20(7):914-9.

[73] Gipson DS, Trachtman H, Kaskel FJ, Greene TH, Radeva MK, Gassman JJ, et al. Clinical trial of focal segmental glomerulosclerosis in children and young adults. *Kidney Int.* 2011 Oct;80(8):868-78.

[74] Kemper MJ, Meyer-Jark T, Lilova M, Müller-Wiefel DE. Combined T- and B-cell activation in childhood steroid-sensitive nephrotic syndrome. *Clin. Nephrol.* 2003 Oct;60(4):242-7.

[75] Benz K, Dötsch J, Rascher W, Stachel D. Change of the course of steroid-dependent nephrotic syndrome after rituximab therapy. *Pediatr Nephrol.* 2004 Jul;19(7):794-7.

[76] Smith GC. Is there a role for rituximab in the treatment of idiopathic childhood nephrotic syndrome? *Pediatr. Nephrol.* 2007 Jun;22(6):893-8.

[77] Gilbert RD, Hulse E, Rigden S. Rituximab therapy for steroid-dependent minimal change nephrotic syndrome. *Pediatr. Nephrol.* 2006 Nov;21(11):1698-700.

[78] Munyentwali H, Bouachi K, Audard V, Remy P, Lang P, Mojaat R, et al. Rituximab is an efficient and safe treatment in adults with steroid-dependent minimal change disease. *Kidney Int.* 2013 Mar;83(3):511-6.

[79] Beco A, Castro-Ferreira I, Coentrao L, Neto R, Sampaio S, Pestana M. Rituximab for steroid-dependent nephrotic syndrome. *Clin. Nephrol.* 2010 Oct;74(4):308-10.

[80] Hoxha E, Stahl RA, Harendza S. Rituximab in adult patients with immunosuppressive-dependent minimal change disease. *Clin. Nephrol.* 2011 Aug;76(2):151-8.

[81] Guigonis V, Dallocchio A, Baudouin V, Dehennault M, Hachon-Le Camus C, Afanetti M, et al. Rituximab treatment for severe steroid- or cyclosporine-dependent nephrotic syndrome: a multicentric series of 22 cases. *Pediatr. Nephrol.* 2008 Aug;23(8):1269-79.

[82] Sellier-Leclerc AL, Macher MA, Loirat C, Guérin V, Watier H, Peuchmaur M, et al. Rituximab efficiency in children with steroid-dependent nephrotic syndrome. *Pediatr. Nephrol.* 2010 Jun;25(6):1109-15.

[83] Fujinaga S, Hirano D, Nishizaki N, Kamei K, Ito S, Ohtomo Y, et al. Single infusion of rituximab for persistent steroid-dependent minimal-change nephrotic syndrome after long-term cyclosporine. *Pediatr. Nephrol.* 2010 Mar;25(3):539-44.

[84] Ruggenenti P, Chiurchiu C, Brusegan V, Abbate M, Perna A, Filippi C, et al. Rituximab in idiopathic membranous nephropathy: a one-year prospective study. *J. Am. Soc. Nephrol.* 2003 Jul;14(7):1851-7.

[85] Klink DT, van Elburg RM, Schreurs MW, van Well GT. Rituximab administration in third trimester of pregnancy suppresses neonatal B-cell development. *Clin. Dev. Immunol.* 2008;2008:271363.

[86] Fu LS, Shien CY, Chi CS. Levamisole in steroid-sensitive nephrotic syndrome children with frequent relapses and/or steroid dependency: comparison of daily and every-other-day usage. *Nephron Clin Pract.* 2004;97(4):c137-41.

[87] Hafeez F, Ahmed TM, Samina U. Levamisole in steroid dependent and frequently relapsing nephrotic syndrome. *J. Coll. Physicians Surg. Pak.* 2006 Jan;16(1):35-7.

[88] Palcoux JB, Niaudet P, Goumy P. Side effects of levamisole in children with nephrosis. *Pediatr. Nephrol.* 1994 Apr;8(2):263-4.

[89] Fahr T. Pathologische anatomie des morbus brightii, in Henke F, Lubarsch O (eds): Handbuch der speziellen pathologischen anatomie und histologie (vol 6). Berlin, Springer, 1925, p 156.

[90] Rich Ar. A hitherto undescribed vulnerability of the juxtamedullary glomeruli in lipoid nephrosis. *Bull Johns Hopkins Hosp.* 1957 Apr;100(4):173-86.

[91] Boyer O, Moulder JK, Somers MJ. Focal and segmental glomerulosclerosis in children: a longitudinal assessment. *Pediatr. Nephrol.* 2007 Aug;22(8):1159-66.

[92] Freedman BI, Hicks PJ, Bostrom MA, Cunningham ME, Liu Y, Divers J, et al. Polymorphisms in the non-muscle myosin heavy chain 9 gene (MYH9) are strongly associated with end-stage renal disease historically attributed to hypertension in African Americans. *Kidney Int.* 2009 Apr;75(7):736-45.

[93] Kopp JB, Smith MW, Nelson GW, Johnson RC, Freedman BI, Bowden DW, et al. MYH9 is a major-effect risk gene for focal segmental glomerulosclerosis. *Nat. Genet.* 2008 Oct;40(10):1175-84.

[94] Kopp JB, Nelson GW, Sampath K, Johnson RC, Genovese G, An P, et al. APOL1 genetic variants in focal segmental glomerulosclerosis and HIV-associated nephropathy. *J. Am. Soc. Nephrol.* 2011 Nov;22(11):2129-37.

[95] Stokes MB, Markowitz GS, Lin J, Valeri AM, D'Agati VD. Glomerular tip lesion: a distinct entity within the minimal change disease/focal segmental glomerulosclerosis spectrum. *Kidney Int.* 2004 May;65(5):1690-702.

[96] Kitiyakara C, Eggers P, Kopp JB. Twenty-one-year trend in ESRD due to focal segmental glomerulosclerosis in the United States. *Am. J. Kidney Dis.* 2004 Nov;44(5):815-25.

[97] D'Agati VD, Kaskel FJ, Falk RJ. Focal segmental glomerulosclerosis. *N. Engl. J. Med.* 2011 Dec 22;365(25):2398-411.

[98] Haas M, Meehan SM, Karrison TG, Spargo BH. Changing etiologies of unexplained adult nephrotic syndrome: a comparison of renal biopsy findings from 1976-1979 and 1995-1997. *Am. J. Kidney Dis.* 1997 Nov;30(5):621-31.

[99] Meyrier A. Mechanisms of disease: focal segmental glomerulosclerosis. *Nat Clin Pract Nephrol.* 2005 Nov;1(1):44-54.

[100] D'Agati VD. Podocyte injury in focal segmental glomerulosclerosis: Lessons from animal models (a play in five acts). *Kidney Int.* 2008 Feb;73(4):399-406.

[101] Hoyer JR, Vernier RL, Najarian JS, Raij L, Simmons RL, Michael AF. Recurrence of idiopathic nephrotic syndrome after renal transplantation. *J. Am. Soc. Nephrol.* 2001 Sep;12(9):1994-2002.

[102] Avila-Casado Mdel C, Perez-Torres I, Auron A, Soto V, Fortoul TI, Herrera-Acosta J. Proteinuria in rats induced by serum from patients with collapsing glomerulopathy. *Kidney Int.* 2004 Jul;66(1):133-43.

[103] Sharma M, Sharma R, Reddy SR, McCarthy ET, Savin VJ. Proteinuria after injection of human focal segmental glomerulosclerosis factor. *Transplantation.* 2002 Feb 15;73(3):366-72.

[104] Savin VJ, McCarthy ET, Sharma R, Charba D, Sharma M. Galactose binds to focal segmental glomerulosclerosis permeability factor and inhibits its activity. *Transl. Res.* 2008 Jun;151(6):288-92.

[105] Sharma M, Sharma R, McCarthy ET, Savin VJ. The focal segmental glomerulosclerosis permeability factor: biochemical characteristics and biological effects. *Exp. Biol. Med.* (Maywood). 2004 Jan;229(1):85-98.

[106] Gallon L, Leventhal J, Skaro A, Kanwar Y, Alvarado A. Resolution of recurrent focal segmental glomerulosclerosis after retransplantation. *N. Engl. J. Med.* 2012 Apr 26;366(17):1648-9.

[107] Lagrue G, Branellec A, Niaudet P, Heslan JM, Guillot F, Lang P. [Transmission of nephrotic syndrome to two neonates. Spontaneous regression]. *Presse Med.* 1991 Feb 16;20(6):255-7. [Article in French

[108] Matalon A, Markowitz GS, Joseph RE, Cohen DJ, Saal SD, Kaplan B, et al. Plasmapheresis treatment of recurrent FSGS in adult renal transplant recipients. *Clin. Nephrol.* 2001 Oct;56(4):271-8.

[109] Savin VJ, Sharma R, Sharma M, McCarthy ET, Swan SK, Ellis E, et al. Circulating factor associated with increased glomerular permeability to albumin in recurrent focal segmental glomerulosclerosis. *N. Engl. J. Med.* 1996 Apr 4;334(14):878-83.

[110] Dantal J, Godfrin Y, Koll R, Perretto S, Naulet J, Bouhours JF, et al. Antihuman immunoglobulin affinity immunoadsorption strongly decreases proteinuria in patients with relapsing nephrotic syndrome. *J. Am. Soc. Nephrol.* 1998 Sep;9(9):1709-15.

[111] Wei C, El Hindi S, Li J, Fornoni A, Goes N, Sageshima J, et al. Circulating urokinase receptor as a cause of focal segmental glomerulosclerosis. *Nat. Med.* 2011 Jul 31;17(8):952-60.

[112] Savin VJ, Sharma M, McCarthy ET, et al: Cardiotrophin like cytokine-1: Candidate for the focal glomerular sclerosis permeability factor. *J. Am. Soc. Nephrol* 2008; 19:59A.

[113] Büscher AK, Konrad M, Nagel M, Witzke O, Kribben A, Hoyer PF, et al. Mutations in podocyte genes are a rare cause of primary FSGS associated with ESRD in adult patients. *Clin Nephrol.* 2012 Jul;78(1):47-53.

[114] Niaudet P. Genetic forms of nephrotic syndrome. *Pediatr Nephrol.* 2004 Dec;19(12):1313-8.

[115] Winn MP. 2007 Young Investigator Award: TRP'ing into a new era for glomerular disease. *J Am Soc Nephrol.* 2008 Jun;19(6):1071-5.

[116] Gbadegesin RA, Lavin PJ, Hall G, Bartkowiak B, Homstad A, Jiang R, et al. Inverted form in 2 mutations with variable expression in patients with sporadic and hereditary focal and segmental glomerulosclerosis. *Kidney Int.* 2012 Jan;81(1):94-9.

[117] Berkovic SF, Dibbens LM, Oshlack A, Silver JD, Katerelos M, Vears DF, et al. Array-based gene discovery with three unrelated subjects shows SCARB2/LIMP-2 deficiency causes myoclonus epilepsy and glomerulosclerosis. *Am. J. Hum. Genet.* 2008 Mar;82(3):673-84.

[118] Genovese G, Friedman DJ, Ross MD, Lecordier L, Uzureau P, Freedman BI, et al. Association of trypanolytic ApoL1 variants with kidney disease in African Americans. *Science.* 2010 Aug 13;329(5993):841-5.

[119] D'Agati V. Pathologic classification of focal segmental glomerulosclerosis. *Semin Nephrol.* 2003 Mar;23(2):117-34.

[120] D'Agati VD, Fogo AB, Bruijn JA, Jennette JC. Pathologic classification of focal segmental glomerulosclerosis: a working proposal. *Am. J. Kidney Dis.* 2004 Feb;43(2):368-82.

[121] Stokes MB, Valeri AM, Markowitz GS, D'Agati VD. Cellular focal segmental glomerulosclerosis: Clinical and pathologic features. *Kidney Int.* 2006 Nov;70(10):1783-92.

[122] Thomas DB, Franceschini N, Hogan SL, Ten Holder S, Jennette CE, Falk RJ, et al. Clinical and pathologic characteristics of focal segmental glomerulosclerosis pathologic variants. *Kidney Int.* 2006 Mar;69(5):920-6.

[123] Korbet SM. Angiotensin antagonists and steroids in the treatment of focal segmental glomerulosclerosis. *Semin. Nephrol.* 2003 Mar;23(2):219-28.

[124] Korbet SM, Schwartz MM, Lewis EJ. Primary focal segmental glomerulosclerosis: clinical course and response to therapy. *Am. J. Kidney Dis.* 1994 Jun;23(6):773-83.

[125] Abbate M, Zoja C, Rottoli D, Corna D, Tomasoni S, Remuzzi G. Proximal tubular cells promote fibrogenesis by TGF-beta1-mediated induction of peritubular myofibroblasts. *Kidney Int.* 2002 Jun;61(6):2066-77.

[126] Crook ED, Habeeb D, Gowdy O, Nimmagadda S, Salem M. Effects of steroids in focal segmental glomerulosclerosis in a predominantly African-American population. *Am. J. Med Sci.* 2005 Jul;330(1):19-24.

[127] Banfi G, Moriggi M, Sabadini E, Fellin G, D'Amico G, Ponticelli C. The impact of prolonged immunosuppression on the outcome of idiopathic focal-segmental glomerulosclerosis with nephrotic syndrome in adults. A collaborative retrospective study. *Clin. Nephrol.* 1991 Aug;36(2):53-9.

[128] Chun MJ, Korbet SM, Schwartz MM, Lewis EJ. Focal segmental glomerulosclerosis in nephrotic adults: presentation, prognosis, and response to therapy of the histologic variants. *J. Am. Soc. Nephrol.* 2004 Aug;15(8):2169-77.

[129] Troyanov S, Wall CA, Miller JA, Scholey JW, Cattran DC; Toronto Glomerulonephritis Registry Group. Focal and segmental glomerulosclerosis: definition and relevance of a partial remission. *Am. Soc. Nephrol.* 2005 Apr;16(4):1061-8.

[130] Braun N, Schmutzler F, Lange C, Perna A, Remuzzi G, Risler T, et al. Immunosuppressive treatment for focal segmental glomerulosclerosis in adults. *Cochrane Database Syst. Rev*. 2008 Jul 16;(3):CD003233.

[131] Duncan N, Dhaygude A, Owen J, Cairns TD, Griffith M, McLean AG, et al. Treatment of focal and segmental glomerulosclerosis in adults with tacrolimus monotherapy. *Nephrol. Dial Transplant*. 2004 Dec;19(12):3062-7.

[132] Li X, Li H, Ye H, Li Q, He X, Zhang X, et al. Tacrolimus therapy in adults with steroid- and cyclophosphamide-resistant nephrotic syndrome and normal or mildly reduced GFR. *Am. J. Kidney Dis*. 2009 Jul;54(1):51-8.

[133] Segarra A, Vila J, Pou L, Majó J, Arbós A, Quiles T, et al. Combined therapy of tacrolimus and corticosteroids in cyclosporin-resistant or -dependent idiopathic focal glomerulosclerosis: a preliminary uncontrolled study with prospective follow-up. *Nephrol Dial Transplant. 2002* Apr;17(4):655-62.

[134] Bhimma R, Adhikari M, Asharam K, Connolly C. Management of steroid-resistant focal segmental glomerulosclerosis in children using tacrolimus. *Am. J. Nephrol*. 2006;26(6):544-51.

[135] Tumlin JA, Miller D, Near M, Selvaraj S, Hennigar R, Guasch A. A prospective, open-label trial of sirolimus in the treatment of focal segmental glomerulosclerosis. *Clin. J. Am. Soc. Nephrol*. 2006 Jan;1(1):109-16.

[136] Kamar N, Frimat L, Blancho G, Wolff P, Delahousse M, Rostaing L. Evaluation of the efficacy and safety of a slow conversion from calcineurin inhibitor- to sirolimus-based therapies in maintenance renal-transplant patients presenting with moderate renal insufficiency. *Transpl Int*. 2007 Feb;20(2):128-34.

[137] Cho ME, Hurley JK, Kopp JB. Sirolimus therapy of focal segmental glomerulosclerosis is associated with nephrotoxicity. *Am. J. Kidney Dis*. 2007 Feb;49(2):310-7.

[138] Fornoni A, Sageshima J, Wei C, Merscher-Gomez S, Aguillon-Prada R, Jauregui AN, Li J, et al. Rituximab targets podocytes in recurrent focal segmental glomerulosclerosis. *Sci. Transl. Med*. 2011 Jun 1;3(85):85ra46.

[139] Kisner T, Burst V, Teschner S, Benzing T, Kurschat CE. Rituximab treatment for adults with refractory nephrotic syndrome: a single-center experience and review of the literature. *Nephron. Clin. Pract*. 2012;120(2):c79-85.

[140] Ochi A, Takei T, Nakayama K, Iwasaki C, Kamei D, Tsuruta Y, et al. Rituximab treatment for adult patients with focal segmental glomerulosclerosis. *Intern. Med*. 2012;51(7):759-62.

[141] Habashy D, Hodson EM, Craig JC. Interventions for steroid-resistant nephrotic syndrome: a systematic review. *Pediatr. Nephrol*. 2003 Sep;18(9):906-12.

[142] Heering P, Braun N, Müllejans R, Ivens K, Zäuner I, Fünfstück R, et al; German Collaborative Glomerulonephritis Study Group. Cyclosporine A and chlorambucil in the treatment of idiopathic focal segmental glomerulosclerosis. *Am. J. Kidney Dis*. 2004 Jan;43(1):10-8.

[143] Ponticelli C. Recurrence of focal segmental glomerular sclerosis (FSGS) after renal transplantation. *Nephrol. Dial Transplant*. 2010 Jan;25(1):25-31.

[144] Passerini P, Ponticelli C. Membranous Nephropathy. In: Ponticelli C, Glassock J, eds. Treatment of Primary Glomerulonephritis, Oxford New York: Oxford University Press 2009: 266-9

[145] Hirayama K, Ebihara I, Yamamoto S, Kai H, Muro K, Yamagata K, et al. Predominance of type-2 immune response in idiopathic membranous nephropathy. Cytoplasmic cytokine analysis. *Nephron.* 2002 Jun;91(2):255-61.

[146] Masutani K, Taniguchi M, Nakashima H, Yotsueda H, Kudoh Y, Tsuruya K, et al. Up-regulated interleukin-4 production by peripheral T-helper cells in idiopathic membranous nephropathy. *Nephrol Dial Transplant.* 2004 Mar;19(3):580-6

[147] Kuroki A, Shibata T, Honda H, Totsuka D, Kobayashi K, Sugisaki T. Glomerular and serum IgG subclasses in diffuse proliferative lupus nephritis, membranous lupus nephritis, and idiopathic membranous nephropathy. *Intern. Med.* 2002 Nov;41(11):936-42.

[148] Ohtani H, Wakui H, Komatsuda A, Okuyama S, Masai R, Maki N, et al. Distribution of glomerular IgG subclass deposits in malignancy-associated membranous nephropathy. *Nephrol. Dial Transplant.* 2004 Mar;19(3):574-9.

[149] Ronco P, Debiec H. New insights into the pathogenesis of membranous glomerulonephritis. *Curr Opin Nephrol Hypertens.* 2006 May;15(3):258-63.

[150] Beck LH Jr, Bonegio RG, Lambeau G, Beck DM, Powell DW, Cummins TD, et al. M-type phospholipase A2 receptor as target antigen in idiopathic membranous nephropathy. *N. Engl. J. Med.* 2009 Jul 2;361(1):11-21.

[151] Ronco P, Debiec H. Antigen identification in membranous nephropathy moves toward targeted monitoring and new therapy. *J. Am. Soc. Nephrol.* 2010 Apr;21(4):564-9.

[152] Hogan SL, Muller KE, Jennette JC, Falk RJ. A review of therapeutic studies of idiopathic membranous glomerulopathy. Am. J. Kidney Dis. 1995 Jun;25(6):862-75.

[153] US Renal Data System: *Annual Data Report* 2013, Reference Tables: ESRD, Vol. 2: 335-358.

[154] Fervenza FC, Sethi S, Specks U. Idiopathic membranous nephropathy: diagnosis and treatment. *Clin. J. Am. Soc. Nephrol.* 2008 May;3(3):905-19.

[155] El Kossi M, Harmer A, Goodwin J, Wagner B, Shortland J, Angel C, et al. De novo membranous nephropathy associated with donor-specific alloantibody. *Clin. Transplant* 2008 Jan-Feb;22(1):124-7.

[156] Ehrenreich T, Churg J. Pathology of membranous nephropathy. In: Sommers SC, ed. Appleton-Century-Crofts, New York: Pathology Annual 1968;3:145.

[157] Cattran DC. Idiopathic membranous glomerulonephritis. *Kidney Int.* 2001 May;59(5):1983-94.

[158] Ponticelli C, Passerini P, Altieri P, Locatelli F, Pappalettera M. Remissions and relapses in idiopathic membranous nephropathy. *Nephrol. Dial Transplant.* 1992;7 Suppl 1:85-90.

[159] Cattran DC, Pei Y, Greenwood CM, Ponticelli C, Passerini P, Honkanen E. Validation of a predictive model of idiopathic membranous nephropathy: its clinical and research implications. Kidney Int. 1997 Mar;51(3):901-7.

[160] Pei Y, Cattran D, Greenwood C. Predicting chronic renal insufficiency in idiopathic membranous glomerulonephritis. *Kidney Int.* 1992 Oct;42(4):960-6.

[161] Troyanov S, Wall CA, Miller JA, Scholey JW, Cattran DC; Toronto Glomerulonephritis Registry Group. Idiopathic membranous nephropathy: definition and relevance of a partial remission. *Kidney Int.* 2004 Sep;66(3):1199-205.

[162] Makker SP. Treatment of membranous nephropathy in children. *Semin. Nephrol.* 2003 Jul;23(4):379-85.

[163] Troyanov S, Roasio L, Pandes M, Herzenberg AM, Cattran DC. Renal pathology in idiopathic membranous nephropathy: a new perspective. *Kidney Int.* 2006 May;69(9):1641-8.

[164] Branten AJ, du Buf-Vereijken PW, Klasen IS, Bosch FH, Feith GW, Hollander DA, et al. Urinary excretion of beta2-microglobulin and IgG predict prognosis in idiopathic membranous nephropathy: a validation study. *J. Am. Soc. Nephrol.* 2005 Jan;16(1):169-74.

[165] Cattran DC, Delmore T, Roscoe J, Cole E, Cardella C, Charron R, et al. A randomized controlled trial of prednisone in patients with idiopathic membranous nephropathy. N Engl. J. Med. 1989 Jan 26;320(4):210-5.

[166] Cameron JS, Healy MJ, Adu D. The Medical Research Council trial of short-term high-dose alternate day prednisolone in idiopathic membranous nephropathy with nephrotic syndrome in adults. The MRC Glomerulonephritis Working Party. *Q. J. Med.* 1990 Feb;74(274):133-56.

[167] Shiiki H, Saito T, Nishitani Y, Mitarai T, Yorioka N, Yoshimura A, et al; Research Group on Progressive Renal Diseases in Japan. Prognosis and risk factors for idiopathic membranous nephropathy with nephrotic syndrome in Japan. *Kidney Int.* 2004 Apr;65(4):1400-7.

[168] Falk RJ, Hogan SL, Muller KE, Jennette JC. Treatment of progressive membranous glomerulopathy. A randomized trial comparing cyclophosphamide and corticosteroids with corticosteroids alone. The Glomerular Disease Collaborative Network. *Ann. Intern. Med.* 1992 Mar 15;116(6):438-45.

[169] Ponticelli C, Zucchelli P, Imbasciati E, Cagnoli L, Pozzi C, Passerini P, et al. Controlled trial of methylprednisolone and chlorambucil in idiopathic membranous nephropathy. *N. Engl. J. Med.* 1984 Apr 12;310(15):946-50.

[170] Jha V, Ganguli A, Saha TK, Kohli HS, Sud K, Gupta KL, et al. A randomized, controlled trial of steroids and cyclophosphamide in adults with nephrotic syndrome caused by idiopathic membranous nephropathy. *J. Am. Soc. Nephrol.* 2007 Jun;18(6):1899-904.

[171] Ponticelli C, Zucchelli P, Passerini P, Cesana B. Methylprednisolone plus chlorambucil as compared with methylprednisolone alone for the treatment of idiopathic membranous nephropathy. The Italian Idiopathic Membranous Nephropathy Treatment Study Group. *N. Engl. J. Med.* 1992 Aug 27;327(9):599-603.

[172] Ponticelli C, Zucchelli P, Passerini P, Cesana B, Locatelli F, Pasquali S, et al. A 10-year follow-up of a randomized study with methylprednisolone and chlorambucil in membranous nephropathy. *Kidney Int.* 1995 Nov;48(5):1600-4.

[173] Ponticelli C, Altieri P, Scolari F, Passerini P, Roccatello D, Cesana B, et al. A randomized study comparing methylprednisolone plus chlorambucil versus methylprednisolone plus cyclophosphamide in idiopathic membranous nephropathy. *J. Am. Soc. Nephrol.* 1998 Mar;9(3):444-50.

[174] Cattran DC, Appel GB, Hebert LA, Hunsicker LG, Pohl MA, Hoy WE, et al; North America Nephrotic Syndrome Study Group. Cyclosporine in patients with steroid-resistant membranous nephropathy: a randomized trial. *Kidney Int.* 2001 Apr;59(4):1484-90.

[175] Cattran DC, Greenwood C, Ritchie S, Bernstein K, Churchill DN, Clark WF, et al. A controlled trial of cyclosporine in patients with progressive membranous nephropathy. Canadian Glomerulonephritis Study Group. *Kidney Int.* 1995 Apr;47(4):1130-5.

[176] Praga M, Barrio V, Juárez GF, Luño J; Grupo Español de Estudio de la Nefropatía Membranosa. Tacrolimus monotherapy in membranous nephropathy: a randomized controlled trial. *Kidney Int.* 2007 May;71(9):924-30.

[177] Matsuura T, Hiramoto N, Iwasa T, Shoji M, Ohashi K. [Complete remission of repeated recurrent membranous nephropathy after non-myeloablative allogeneic peripheral blood stem cell transplantation]. *Nihon Jinzo Gakkai Shi.* 2013;55(7):1327-34. [Article in Japanese]

[178] Chen M, Li H, Li XY, Lu FM, Ni ZH, Xu FF, et al; Chinese Nephropathy Membranous Study Group. Tacrolimus combined with corticosteroids in treatment of nephrotic idiopathic membranous nephropathy: a multicenter randomized controlled trial. *Am. J. Med. Sci.* 2010 Mar;339(3):233-8.

[179] Xie G, Xu J, Ye C, Chen D, Xu C, Yang L, et al. Immunosuppressive treatment for nephrotic idiopathic membranous nephropathy: a meta-analysis based on Chinese adults. *PLoS One.* 2012;7(9):e44330.

[180] Dussol B, Morange S, Burtey S, Indreies M, Cassuto E, Mourad G, et al. Mycophenolate mofetil monotherapy in membranous nephropathy: a 1-year randomized controlled trial. *Am. J. Kidney Dis.* 2008 Oct;52(4):699-705.

[181] Kobayashi M, Kojima C, Sugiura H, Aoki A, Itabashi M, Tsukada M, et al. [Case of MMF monotherapy for membranous nephropathy]. Nihon Jinzo Gakkai Shi. 2010;52(5):572-7. [Article in Japanese]

[182] Bhimma R, Naicker E, Ramdial PK. Mycophenolate mofetil therapy in children with idiopathic membranous nephropathy. *Clin. Nephrol.* 2013 Dec;80(6):441-8.

[183] Senthil Nayagam L, Ganguli A, Rathi M, Kohli HS, Gupta KL, Joshi K, et al. Mycophenolate mofetil or standard therapy for membranous nephropathy and focal segmental glomerulosclerosis: a pilot study. *Nephrol. Dial Transplant.* 2008 Jun;23(6):1926-30.

[184] Chan TM, Lin AW, Tang SC, Qian JQ, Lam MF, Ho YW, et al. Prospective controlled study on mycophenolate mofetil and prednisolone in the treatment of membranous nephropathy with nephrotic syndrome. *Nephrology* (Carlton). 2007 Dec;12(6):576-81.

[185] Goumenos DS, Ahuja M, Davlouros P, El Nahas AM, Brown CB. Prednisolone and azathioprine in membranous nephropathy: a 10-year follow-up study. *Clin. Nephrol.* 2006 May;65(5):317-23.

[186] Remuzzi G, Chiurchiu C, Abbate M, Brusegan V, Bontempelli M, Ruggenenti P. Rituximab for idiopathic membranous nephropathy. *Lancet.* 2002 Sep 21;360(9337):923-4.

[187] Ruggenenti P, Cravedi P, Sghirlanzoni MC, Gagliardini E, Conti S, Gaspari F, et al., Effects of rituximab on morphofunctional abnormalities of membranous glomerulopathy. *Clin. J. Am. Soc. Nephrol.* 2008 Nov;3(6):1652-9.

[188] Bomback AS, Derebail VK, McGregor JG, Kshirsagar AV, Falk RJ, Nachman PH. Rituximab therapy for membranous nephropathy: a systematic review. *Clin. J. Am. Soc. Nephrol.* 2009 Apr;4(4):734-44.

[189] Wen M, Küchle C, Sarkar O, Renders L, Heemann U, Schmaderer C. Plasmapheresis combined with rituximab for refractory idiopathic membranous nephropathy. *Int. Urol. Nephrol. 2014* Mar 1. [Epub ahead of print]

[190] Berg AL, Nilsson-Ehle P, Arnadottir M. Beneficial effects of ACTH on the serum lipoprotein profile and glomerular function in patients with membranous nephropathy. *Kidney Int.* 1999 Oct;56(4):1534-43.

[191] Berg AL, Arnadottir M. ACTH-induced improvement in the nephrotic syndrome in patients with a variety of diagnoses. *Nephrol. Dial Transplant.* 2004 May;19(5):1305-7.

[192] Ponticelli C, Passerini P, Salvadori M, Manno C, Viola BF, Pasquali S, et al., A randomized pilot trial comparing methylprednisolone plus a cytotoxic agent versus synthetic adrenocorticotropic hormone in idiopathic membranous nephropathy. *Am. J. Kidney Dis.* 2006 Feb;47(2):233-40.

[193] Bomback AS, Tumlin JA, Baranski J, Bourdeau JE, Besarab A, Appel AS, et al. Treatment of nephrotic syndrome with adrenocorticotropic hormone (ACTH) gel. *Drug Des. Devel. Ther.* 2011 Mar 14;5:147-53.

Chapter III

Primary Proliferative Glomerulonephritis

Abstract

Primary proliferative glomerulonephritis are characterized by mesangial hypercellularity, proliferation of infiltrating, mesangial, endothelial, and epithelial cells and formation of crescents, a fibrocellular lesion associated with poor prognosis. IgA nephropathy is the most common primary proliferative glomerular disease, followed by post-infectious glomerulonephritis, a disease that occurs mostly in children. Membranoproliferative or mesangiocapillary glomerulonephritis exists in idiopathic and secondary form, which seems to prevail. Rapidly progressive rapidly progressive glomerulonephritis is the primary proliferative glomerular disease with the worse clinical course and outcome, leading to ESRD within 3 months from the onset. This chapter focuses on the pathogenesis, clinical manifestations, prognosis, and therapeutic option for the above mentioned diseases.

1. IgA Nephropathy

IgA nephropathy (IgAN) is the most common glomerular disease worldwide, characterized by dominant or codominant diffuse mesangial deposition of IgA and mesangial proliferation, [1, 2] manifesting with recurrent macro and persistent microhematuria. It was first described by Berger and Hingalis in 1968 in Paris, [3] with the introduction to immunofluorescence techniques in renal biopsy studies therefore it has long been referred to as Berger's disease.

Initial assumptions on the disease advocated for its benign nature, often called *benign recurrent hematuria* but long term follow up studies proved that IgAN is a slowly progressive disease and currently one of the most important causes of ESRD. [4,5] Up to 50% of affected patients develop ESRD 20 to 25 years from the onset. [6]

The histopathological picture at the time of presentation is notoriously variable, rending prediction of progression to ESRD based on histopathological features controversial. [7, 8]

The recent publication of Oxford classification of IgAN is considered a milestone in the prognostic evaluation of the disease but not all morphological features have been considered during the development of this classification, therefore further validation studies are suggested. [9]

Clinical presentation of IgAN ranges from asymptomatic hematuria to chronic kidney disease, but the two major clinical symptoms are recurrent macroscopic hematuria with or without proteinuria, in most of the cases, mild or moderate. Hypertension is rare, but if present, is predictive of worse outcome. [10]

Incidence and Prevalence

As above mentioned, IgAN is the most common primary glomerulonephritis worldwide, affecting 25 to 50 patients per 100,000 people. [2] Distribution varies in different geographic regions, probably because of the different policy on performing renal biopsy in patients with isolated hematuria among different countries. For instance, USA nephrologists are more reluctant to perform biopsies in asymptomatic patients compared to nephrologists in Asia. As a result, IgA nephropathy accounts for 40% of biopsies performed in Asia and only 10% of those performed in USA. Low incidence percentages are to be expected in Europe, where renal biopsies in asymptomatic patients are quite limited. However, IgAN remains the most common renal disease in young adults in the developed countries. [11]

According to USRD 2013, IgAN prevails among Caucasians with 74.2% compared to 17.2% in Asians and 6.5% in African Americans. [12] There is a higher male predilection with reported ratios varying from 2:1 up to 6:1 depending on the geographic regions.

It can affect patients at all ages but it is more common in the second and third decade of life with percentages up to 83%. Most of the patients reach ESRD at a mean age of 45 years. IgAN accounts for 0.9% among all causes of ESRD. 4.4% of ESRD IgAN patients die within the first year of renal replacement treatment initiation. [12]

Pathophysiology

Although the precise etiology of primary IgAN remains unclear, clinical association of macroscopic hematuria with upper respiratory infection in IgAN suggests that exposure to infectious agents; both bacterial and viral may be in the basis of the disease.

Staphylococcus aureus, Campylobacter, Yersinia, mycoplasma, and Haemophilus are some of the bacteria with reported association to IgAN. Viral agents involved in IgAN pathogenesis include Cytomegalovirus, Adenovirus, Coxsackievirus, Epstein-Barr virus, and HIV. Food antigens such as gliadin, gluten, and casein have also been proposed but their involvement in IgAN pathogenesis is still to be proven.

Repeated exposure to antigens, especially the mucosas that seem to be their site of entrance, stimulates the plasma cells of the mucosa-associated lymphoid tissue to secrete abnormal polymeric IgA_1 ($pIgA_1$). These $pIgA_1$, present abnormal O-linked hinge-region sugars with reduced glycosylation. [13] The exact mechanism that leads to alter IgA_1O-glycosylation is unknown but it may be due to defective function of glycosyltransferases that O-glycosylate IgA_1. The same authors believe that the mucosal $pIgA_1$ that reaches circulation have different glycosylation patterns than serum IgA_1. [14] However, the abnormal $pIgA_1$ glycosylation in IgAN is inherited. In patients with familial IgAN by autosomal dominant transmission, levels of abnormal $pIgA_1$ were found to be elevated. [15] It is also possible that hepatic clearance of $pIgA_1$ is impaired by inhibition of their interaction with asialoglycoprotein receptors and Kupfer cell FcA receptors.

IgG autoantibodies against the abnormal $pIgA_1$ are produced, promoting circulating or *in situ* immune complexes formation and their deposition to the mesangium. These bind to and interact with mesangial cells, leading to their activation and proliferation. Activated mesangial cells produce cytokines and growth factors such as platelet derived growth factor (PDGF) and transforming growth factor β (TGF-β), promoting tissue injury and progression of the disease. Complement activation by the alternative pathway has also been documented but its role on the pathogenesis of IgAN remains unclear.

TGF-β_1 and TGF-β_2 gene polymorphisms seem to play an important role in the pathogenesis and progression of IgAN, through regulation of cell proliferation and extracellular matrix (ECM) synthesis. [16] ECM expansion leads to fibrosis and glomerular sclerosis and finally in ESRD. Also, TGF-β_1 may alter the glomerular permeability leading to proteinuria and tubulointerstitial injury in IgAN patients. [17] Finally, C509T and T869C polymorphisms of the TGF-β_1 gene have been associated with higher susceptibility to IgAN in Caucasians. [18]

Given the familial tendency of the disease (10 to 50% of the cases), a genetic background of IgAN has been suggested and confirmed by the identification of the IgAN1 Locus in 6q22 position. [19] Other genetic loci have also been identified but currently there is no genetic test available, capable of predicting or diagnosing IgAN. However, progress on genome mapping may provide more information on polymorphism associated to IgAN.

Genetic associations have been suggested as prognostic factors of progression of IgAN. Patients with DD phenotype of the ACE gene, which results in higher plasma ACE levels, seem to promote progression of the disease. [20] The angiotensinogen gene has also been evaluated but results were conflicting. [21,22] Polymorphisms of the megsine gene, encoding for megsin - a serin protease inhibitor expressed in the mesangium - has been associated with mesangial hypercellularity and higher levels of serum creatinine. [23]

Pathology

Light microscopy appearance is remarkably variable ranging from minimal mesangial expansion to diffuse proliferative lesions, sclerosing or crescentic. The most common findings are mesangial proliferation and mesangial matrix expansion, usually focal and segmental and in some cases diffuse or global.

Endocapillary proliferation may be present with focal segmental or diffuse distribution. Occasionally, focal segmental sclerosis with tubular atrophy and interstitial fibrosis may be present, more often in chronic cases. In severe cases with acute kidney injury, segmental necrosis, crescents, tubular occlusion by red cells and acute tubular epithelial necrosis may also be noticed.

The extension and type of lesion may be of prognostic value, therefore classifications based on light microscopy appearance have been proposed. In the past, the WHO classification for lupus nephritis has been proposed for IgAN, [24] but it has not been widely used because of limitations on the reproducibility of histologic variables.

In 2009, the Oxford classification for IgAN was developed, based on detailed examination of all lesions, as a predicting classification system of the risk of disease progression. [9] Six pathologic variables were identified, including mesangial hypercellularity, segmental glomerulosclerosis or adhesion, cellular or fibrocellular crescents and tubular atrophy/interstitial fibrosis. Four of these pathologic features, along with their scoring, were shown to have independent predicting value for the disease progression, being linked to worse prognosis.

Of note, this classification does not include the prognostic value of crescents, due to their low prevalence. However, it is well recognized that presence of diffuse crescentic formation in IgAN, often referred to as crescentic IgAN, is associated with reduced renal survival, with a rapidly progressive course and a poor prognosis. [25, 26]

The Oxford classification has been validated by different cohorts, [27, 28] but a potential weakness of the classification other than the exclusion of crescents or necrotizing lesions, is that immunofluorescence and electron microscopy findings were not evaluated for their prognostic importance or their correlation to the light microscopic morphologic variables.

Immunofluorscence findings are the hallmark of the disease, revealing dominant or codominant deposits of IgA confined in diffuse granular pattern in the mesangium, or extended to subepithelial sites of the capillary loops. The deposits are mainly represented by pIgA1 but IgG and IgM may be found in minor density than pIgA1. C3 is usually present while C1q is rarely positive.

By electron microscopy, deposits are found in mesangial and paramesangial areas, or may also show a subendothelial and subepithelial distribution in cases of endocapillary proliferation. Foot processes effacement is noticed in areas of sclerosis and occasionally thinning of the GBM. Recently an observational study conducted on 114 IgAN patients found significant association of IgA, IgM, and C3 deposition with the S variable, and IgA and C3 with the E variable of the Oxford classification. [29] Among these deposits, C3 had significant positive association with global sclerosing lesions. This observation is of confirmation to Ohsawa's finding that C3 deposits are associated with worse clinical outcomes, [30] and that only C3 deposits are correlated to higher serum creatinine levels. [29] It has also been suggested that IgM deposition is related to crescent formation. [31] However the significance of these immunostaining findings in relation to Oxford classification of IgAN remains controversial, [29] therefore further validating investigations are needed.

Clinical Manifestations

Primary IgAN typically presents with recurrent episodes of macroscopic hematuria, of glomerular origin (dysmorphic red blood cells) with or without proteinuria, often in concomitance or soon after upper respiratory infection. Other infections associated with IgAN include gastroenteritis, urinary tract infections, mononucleosis, and influenza.

It usually appears within the first 48-72 hours from the onset of the upper respiratory infection, persisting for less than 3 days, often accompanied by loin pain, probably because of renal capsular swelling. The timing of the hematuria presentation differentiated IgAN from post-infectious glomerulonephritis where hematuria presents 2 to 3 weeks after the infection.

Between episodes of macroscopic hematuria, patients present persistent microscopic hematuria with or without proteinuria. Proteinuria is usually less than 2 g/24h. Nephrotic range proteinuria may be seen in more advanced stages of the disease, but full-blown nephrotic syndrome is rarely observed. Patients with proteinura higher than 3g/24h present higher rates of renal function decline compared to those with proteinuria lower than 1g/24h, and are at higher risk of developing ESRD. [32]

Acute kidney failure with edema hypertension and oliguria rarely occurs, and in most of the cases is reversible, through conservative treatment or occasionally after a few sessions of renal replacement therapy.

Hypertension is uncommon at the onset of the disease but becomes more frequent as the disease progresses.

Natural History and Prognosis

Primary IgAN is quite variable and often unpredictable. In most of the cases, progression is slow, with ESRD occurring in up to 20% of the patients within 10 years and in about 30% within 20 years from the onset.

Some patients will present a decrease of renal function that will be stable in abnormal levels for many years without reaching ESRD. Episodes of acute renal failure, in most cases reversible, often take place.

There are multiple factors determining the course and the prognosis of IgA nephropathy. For instance, older age and male gender have been widely correlated to worse prognosis. African American children seem to have worse clinical course and faster development of ESRD although the incidence of the disease is much greater in the Caucasian race.

Impaired renal function with elevated serum creatinine levels and lower GFR at the time of diagnosis is a negative prognostic sign, especially if it is accompanied by blood pressure higher than 140/90 mmHg.

Patients with nephrotic range proteinuria present worse outcomes but remains controversial if obtaining partial remission, defined as proteinuria lower than 1g/24h, affects long-term renal survival. [32]

Persistent microscopic hematuria has been widely associated with poor prognosis especially if accompanied by proteinuria.

Other factors related to worse prognosis in IgAN are obesity, hyperlipidemia, hyperuricemia, [33] elevated C3 serum levels, elevated CRP levels, increased leukocyte count, low serum albumin, and urinary excetion of podocytes, vitamin D binding protein (VDTP), hemopexin, afamin, leucin-rich a2-glycoprotein (A2GL). [34] Urinary excretion of uromodulin and elevated levels of uric acid are indices of tubular atrophy and interstitial fibrosis. [33, 35] Also, zinc deficiency was found to be associated with IgAN progression and zinc supplementation prevented disease aggravation. [36]

Also, as before mentioned, different histologic morphology in renal biopsy corresponds to different severity and prognosis. Given the limitations of the Oxford classification several studies attempted to create predicting scores for IgAN patients. Recently Tanaka et al., proposed a predictive model formed with the combination of Oxford classification and clinical risk factors to evaluate 5-year risk for ESRD. Of the Oxford classification, mesangial hypercellularity, segmental sclerosis, and tubular atrophy/interstitial fibrosis were included, associated to eGFR and 24h proteinuria. [37] These factors were assigned points. Patients with less than 8 points present less than a 1% risk of developing ESRD, while patients with a score higher than 23 points had more than 50% probability of developing ESRD within 5 years. However, the application of these scoring systems is not always of consistent prognostic value. Validation studies and research of more accurate prognostic models are required.

Diagnosis and Differential Diagnosis

Diagnosis of IgAN requires renal biopsy in which presence of mesangial IgA deposits is confirmed. A careful urinanalysis and examination of the urine sediment may be helpful in identifying the origin of RBCs. Glomerular origin hematiuria may occur in other glomerular diseases, therefore, urinary sediment is not pathognomonic.

A 24h measurement of proteinuria and creatinine clearance test should also be performed.

Serum IgA levels are usually elevated. Serum levels of the complement components C3, C4, and C1q are in most cases normal, but complement degradation products may be elevated, indicating activation of the complement cascade, although its role on the pathogenesis of IgAN remains unclear.

IgAN should be differentiated from other conditions presenting with macro or microscopic hematuria. These conditions are thin basement membrane disease (TBMD), Alport's syndrome, membranoproliferative glomerulonephritis (MPGN), post-infectious glomerulonephritis, and Fabry's disease.

Most commonly, acute post-infectious glomerulonephritis can be confused with IgAN. In that case, timing of appearance of hematuria and history of streptococcal or staphylococcal infection could resolve the diagnostic dilemma. However, renal biopsy is the only way to provide accurate differentiation.

Treatment

Despite numerous attempts of different studies to establish a specific treatment for IgAN, currently no such cure exists. This is probably attributed to the limited comprehension of the pathogenic mechanisms of the disease and the heterogeneity of its clinical and pathologic manifestations.

Based on this limited up to date knowledge, many therapeutic regimens targeted the altered immune response of the mucosas. However, most current treatment strategies aim at the delay of the disease progression and in most cases, are symptomatic and non-specific.

i. Antihypertensives

Given that uncontrolled hypertension is associated with more rapid progression to renal failure and higher levels of proteinuria, [38] blood pressure should be maintained lower than 130/80 mmHg in patients with proteinuria higher than 0.3g/24h and lower than 125/75 mmHg when urinary excretion of proteins exceed 1g/24h. [39]

ACEIs and ARBs are the preferred agents, for their beneficial effects on both blood pressure and proteinuria.

Patients with proteinuria higher than 3g/24h lose kidney function up to 25 times faster than those with proteinuria lower than 1g/24h. [32] Therefore, in IgAN patients, target levels of proteinuria are less than 500mg/24h, and treatment with ACEIs or ARBs or a combination of those two agents should be initiated in patients with proteinuria higher than 500mg/24h. [40] Angiotensin inhibition, though, does not seem to be of any help in non-proteinuric patients or those with proteinuria lower than 500mg/24h. [41]

Yet, there is no evidence that reducing proteinuria below 500mg/24h provides any additional benefit to long-term kidney survival in IgAN. There is evidence though that ACEIs and ARBs directly affect podocytes and mesangial cells by interfering with proliferation, fibrosis, and inflammation due to their anti-inflammatory, anti-fibrotic, and anti-proliferative properties.

Preference of ACEIs to ARBS or vice versa remains controversial since there are no data supporting one or the other. Some nephrologists prefer initiating treatment with ACEIs, keeping ARBs only for patients who do not tolerate ACEIs or as a supplementary treatment if results with ACEIs are not satisfying. However, the ARBs–ACEIs combination has shown greater reduction rates of proteinuria. [42]

Patients treated with the ARBs–ACEIs combination should be closely monitored due to the risk of developing hyperkaliemia, and this treatment should be avoided in advanced renal failure.

ii. Fish Oils

The possible role of fish oil treatment in IgAN has not yet been well defined given the conflicting results obtained by various RCTs.

Fish oils's eicosapentanoic acid (EPA) and docosahexanoic acid (DHA) serve as cyclosygenase and liposygenase substrates. Interfering with these pathways leads to limitation of the inflammatory response by limiting cytokine production. [43]

Treatment with 1.8g of EPA and 1.2g of DHA daily for 2 years slowed the progression of IgAN to renal failure. After 6.4 years of follow up, results continued to be favorable for the patients who continued treatment. [43]

A more recent randomized double blind study evaluated the effectiveness of fish oils compared to prednisolone and placebo. Neither treatment showed superiority over the placebo. Additionally, the fish oils treatment group showed a higher urine protein to creatinine ratio. [44]

Whether these discordant results were dose dependent or not remains a question not yet answered. A retrospective trial compared results obtained with high and low doses of fish oil and deduced that there were no differences between the two groups. [45] Currently, there are no data to support whether the dosage of fish oil should be on a weight basis or if higher dosage of fish oil is more efficient in IgAN.

It has been suggested, though, that a combination of fish oils with ACEIs and/or ARBs could provide better results in both reduction of proteinuria and progression of the disease. In a small RCT, combined treatment provided higher reduction rates of proteinuria compared to rennin-angiotensin system blockers (RASB) but no significant changes in renal function or blood pressure were observed.

However, given the benefits of fish oils on cardiovascular disease and the lack of adverse effects, current guidelines suggest the use of 3.3g/day of fish oils in IgAN patients with persistent proteinuria despite 3 to 6 months of RASB treatment. [46]

iii. Corticosteroids

Corticosteroids, alone or in combination with pressure and lipid lowering therapy, have been widely used in the treatment of IgAN as there is evidence that corticosteroids provide additional benefit.

A recent metanalysis of nine RCTs including 536 IgAN patients showed that corticosteroid therapy significantly reduced the incidence of renal events. Association of ACEIs to steroids was of benefit in both proteinuria and renal function. These favorable results were greater when steroids doses were higher and administered for less than 12 months. [47]

Optimal doses and indications for corticosteroids use in IgAN are not well defined yet. Two different RCTs proposed two different regimens. Pozzi et al, [48] in 1999 treated 86 adult IgAN patients with moderate proteinuria with 1g of intravenous methylprednisolone for 3 days at month 1,3 and 5, combined with 0.5mg/kg of oral prednisolone on alternate days for 6 months. Not all patients received ACEIs or ARBS. This regimen demonstrated long-term benefit, continuing for up to 10 years. [49]

In 2009, Manno et al., randomly assigned 97 IgAN patients with proteinuria higher than 1g/day and GFR higher than 50ml/min to prednisone in doses of 0.8 to 1 mg/kg per day combined with ramipril for two months, followed by tapering of 0.2mg/kg per day, or ramipril alone. Patients treated with the combined therapy showed lower decline of eGFR and higher reduction of proteinuria. In addition, the combined treatment showed higher effectiveness in preventing progression of renal disease in these patients. [50]

Based on these RCTs, KDIGO guidelines suggest use of steroid therapy in IgAN patients with persistent proteinuria higher than 1g/day despite a 6-month RASB treatment. [46] Given that data on IgAN patients with GFR lower than 50ml/min under steroid treatment are limited, [50] there is no evidence to suggest use of steroids in these patients.

iv. Immunosuppressive Agents

Nucleotide Synthesis Inhibitors

Cyclophosphamide plus corticosteroids (40mg/day) were used in an RCT in lowered doses of 1mg/kg/day followed by 1.5mg/kg/day of azathioprine in patients with moderately progressive IgAN. They were followed for 2 to 6 years and compared to control groups. [51]

Patients treated with the combined therapy presented a significant reduction of proteinuria and higher renal survival rates. The combined regimen was associated with higher protective effects from declining renal function and ESRD.

On the other hand, the addition of azathioprine to steroid therapy does not seem to provide further benefit compared to steroids.

Pozzi et al., treated 207 IgAN patients with intravenous methylprednisolone of 3/day pulses in months 1, 3, 5 and prednisone 0.5mg/kg everyday with or without azathioprine at

1.5mg/kg per day for 6 months. [52] No difference was noticed in proteinuria and renal survival rates, although proteinuria was reduced in both groups.

Although there is no evidence advocating for azathioprine or cyclophosphamide monotherapy, a combination regimen of cyclophosphamide/azathioprine and steroids could be an effective IgAN with impaired kidney function.

CNIs

Cyclosporin A and Tacrolimus have been proposed for IgAN in various studies. Although these agents had favorable results in proteinuria, the effect on renal survival is limited mostly due to nephrotoxicity. [53]

Mycophenolate Mofetil

Mycophenolate mofetil has been investigated in different RCTs with conflicting results, ranging from no benefit to reduction of proteinuria. [54, 55] Also, a recent study has shown that response to MMF may vary according to race and ethnicity. [56]

These results provide no evidence of use of MMF for IgAN. However, further investigations are required taking into consideration pharnacocinetics, pharmacodynamics and racial variables along with the potential adverse effects of this regimen.

v. Tonsillectomy

Tonsillectomy has been proposed for IgAN patients because of the implication of tonsillar mocosa on the formation of the abnormal IgA and, consequently, the immune complexes and deposits in the glomeruli.

In most of the cases, tonsillectomy was combined with oral or intravenous steroid treatment, so it has been difficult to assess results and distinguish if those are to be accredited to the steroid therapy or the tonsillectomy itself. Another variable to take of note is that tonsillectomy is usually performed in childhood when IgAN is in very early stages and where spontaneous remissions are more common than in adulthood.

RCTs regarding tonsillectomy in IgAN are quite limited and results have been controversial. Many previous studies have indicated reduction of proteinuria and improved renal outcomes in IgAN patients, [57-59] but recent multicentered RCTs of tonsillectomy combined with steroid pulses showed no additional benefit over steroids alone on remission of proteinuria and hematuria. [60]

On the other hand, another metanalysis of 4 studies demonstrated lower rates of progression to ESRD in tonsillectomy/steroid treated patients compared to those receiving only steroid treatment. [61]

A combination of mizoribine with tonsillectomy and steroids seem to be promising. [62] Mizoribine is a purine synthesis inhibitor similar to MMF. It has been used in IgAN Japan patients with good short-term results. In a recent study 18 IgAN patients with wild renal impairment underwent bilateral tonsillectomy and were administered steroids in combination with 100 to 150 mg of mizoribine daily divided in 3 doses. Decrease of hematuria and proteinuria and improvement of eGFR was observed suggesting that this regimen can be used in IgAN patients with impaired renal function who wish to reduce steroid assumption.

However, due to the limited RCTs and data, KDIGO guidelines suggest that tonsillectomy should not be used as a treatment for IgAN, but preserve it for IgAN patients with recurrent tonsillitis and hematuria. [46]

vi. Intravenous Immunoglobulin

High dose intravenous globulin has been used in IgAN patients with heavy proteinuria and renal impairment. [63] Patients received intravenously 1gr/kg per day for 2 consecutive days each month for 3 months, followed by intramuscular 0.35ml/kg twice a month for 6 months.

Decrease of proteinuria, hematuria, and increased GFR was observed. Histologic examination revealed a decrease of IgA and C3 deposits.

Lack of RCTs however limits knowledge on both effectiveness and adverse effects. The potential benefits of this regimen need to be evaluated and confirmed by well-designed trials.

vii. Treatment of Crescentic IgAN

Crescentic IgAN is defined as an IgAN presenting crescents in more than 50% of the glomeruli in a renal biopsy, associated clinically with rapidly progressive renal disease.

This variant of IgAN has a poor prognosis, therefore various therapeutic regimens have been proposed including steroids, cytotoxic agents, and plasmapheresis. Results have been neither uniform nor consistent.

Plasmapheresis seems to be able to stabilize renal function and prevent progression to ESRD but withdrawal of this treatment has been associated with relapse and progression of the disease. [64]

Observational studies regarding treatment of cresentic IgAN concluded that immunosuppressive agents such as cyclophospamide associated with corticosteroids could be helpful. [31, 65, 66] Given the limitation of studies on plasmapheresis, there is only poor-quality evidence to support its use on crescentic IgAN.

2. Post-Infectious glomerulonephritis

Post-infectious glomerulonephritis (PIGN) is a quite common immune complex-mediated primary glomerulonephritis that develops following an infection, affecting mainly children and occasionally young adults and the elderly. Despite the disease is secondary to infections, it is considered as primary glomerulonephritis, since the kidney is the organ targeted from the immunological events triggered from the infection, while extrarenal manifestations are the consequence of impaired renal function.

The most common causative agent is streptococcus. In fact, post-streptococcal glomerulonephritis (PSGN) is the archetype of PIGN- followed by staphylococcus and other Gram-negative bacteria. Other infectious agents with reported association to PIGN are:

- Bacterial: Streptococcus pneumoniae, S. viridans, S.pyogenes, S. equi, S. constellatus, Staphylococcus aureus, S. epidermidis, S. albus Mycobacterium leprae, M. tuberculosis, Neisseria meningitis, N. gonorrhoeae, Listeria monocytogenes,

Treponema pallidum, Coxiella brunettii, Leptospira interrogans, mycoplasma pneumoniae.

- Viral: HIV, Hepatitis A virus, Coxsackie B virus, ECHO virus, mumps virus, rotavirus, infuenza virus, Epstein-Barr Virus, Varicella zoster, Cytomegalovirus, Parvovirus B19, adenovirus, Hepatitis B and C virus
- Protozoal: Plasmodium falciparum, P. Malariae, Toxoplasma gondii, Trypanosoma cruzi, T. Bruci, Leishmania donovani
- Fungal: Candida
- Helminthic: Shistostoma mansoni, S. Haematobium,Trichinella spiralis, Wuchereria bancrofti

Classically, PIGN develops following upper respiratory tract or skin infections, although recently other sites of infection, such as urinary tract, gastrointestinal tract, lungs, and heart, have been correlated to the disease. It manifests with a sudden onset of hematuria and proteinuria, thus nephritic syndrome within a mean time of 1 to 3 weeks from the infectious episode. [67, 68]

There is a tendency for complete remission and spontaneous recovery within a few weeks from the onset in children, while prognosis in young adults and especially in the elderly is less favorable, probably because in the elderly atypical sites of infection and non-common infectious agents such as virus, protozoa and Gram positive bacteria are often the cause of the disease, originating atypical morphologic variants of PIGN including IgA-dominant acute PIGN.

In this context, poststreptococcal, atypical and IgA-dominant PIGN will be treated separately.

2.1. Poststreptococcal Glomerulonephritis

PSGN is the most common form of PIGN, resulting from the upper respiratory tract (pharyngitis) or skin (impetigo) infections caused by group A β-hemolytic streptococci. [69, 70] It mainly affects children, while in adults and elderly it is more rare, showing prevalence in males over females.

Clinical presentation may present asymptomatic forms to nephritic or nephrotic syndrome, manifesting after a latency period of 2 to 6 weeks.

Etiology and Pathogenesis

Seegal and Earl in 1941 were the first to introduce the concept of nephritogenic streptococci after noticing that not all patients with rheumatic fever presented acute PSGN. Since then, different strains have been evaluated as nephritogenic, and in the last decades it has been proved that both M and T proteins of the bacterial wall show nephritogenicity although it mainly concerns certain M protein serotypes.

M protein serotypes 1, 2, 4 and 12, which are involved in upper respiratory infections, and 25, 45, 49, 55, 57 and 60, mostly related to skin infections, have shown strong nephritogenic potential. [71] Also, non-group A streptococci such as group C have been associated to epidemic PSGN suggesting that nephritogenic strains may be present in other streptococci groups. [72]

The overall risk of developing acute PSGN seems to be related to M protein serotypes and the site of infection, with skin infections showing higher risk rates.

Several mechanisms have been proposed for the pathogenesis, including circulating immune complex formation with streptococcal antigens and their glomerular deposition with consequent complement activation, autoimmune response and delayed hypersensitivity.

Immune complex formation and autoimmune processes seemed to be more plausible, given the constant evidence of immune complex deposition and presence of complement components on the glomeruli; therefore, PSGN is largely recognized as an immune complex disease.

The two most widely proposed theories on PSGN include deposition of circulating immune complexes and *in situ* formation of antibody-antigen complexes, resulting from antibody interaction with streptococcal components or components of the glomerulus itself, due to a cross-reaction of antibodies against streptococcal cell membranes. This process is also called molecular mimicry, because antibodies interact with antigenic determinants common in both nephritogenic streptococci and glomerulus. [73] Antibodies against basement membrane collagen type IV, laminin, and heparin sulfate proteoglycan have been proposed as target antigens of molecular mimicry in PSGN. [74]

Nephritogenic streptococci produce and release into the circulation proteins that act as antigens and have a particular affinity for sites of the glomerulus. Some of these antigens bind to circulating immune antistreptococcal antibodies forming circulating immune complexes, while others bind to sites of the glomerulus that serve as fixed antigens, forming in situ immune complexes with the anti-streptococcal antibodies.

Once these nephritogenic antigens bind to these sites of the glomeruli they activate the alternative pathway of the complement by interacting directly with properdin. Complement activation leads to increase permeability of the GBM with consecutive circulating immune complexes deposition, deposition of the C3 component, IgG deposition recruitment of inflammatory cells and mediators such as leukocytes, cytokines and growth factors that promote proliferation of intrinsic cells and induce tissue damage.

Activation of the lectin pathway of complement has also been reported as a possible pathogenic mechanism in PSGN patients, [75] but low complement mannan-binding lectin levels excluded this possibility. [76] Classical pathway can be activated during the first two weeks of the disease, but later is inhibited through C4b-binding protein. [77]

Complement regulatory factors, such as factor H and factor H-like protein 1 (FHL-1), submit proteolysis by streptococcal proteases, abolishing their effect on complement activation that results to be exacerbated.

Several streptococcal proteins have been evaluated for their nephritogenic potential but a definitive nephritogenic antigen has not yet been identified. The most pronounced among all proteins suggested are nepghritis-strain associated protein (NSAP) and nephritis-associated plasmin receptor (NAPlr).

NSAP is a 47kD streptokinase-like protein produced by strains of streptococci isolated in PSGN patients. [78] This protein has antigenic properties and it is able to bind to glomeruli and cause depletion of complement products such as C3a and C4a. [79]

NAPlr is a 43kD plasmin-binding protein with glyceraldeyde-3-phosphate dehydrogenase (GAPDH) activity, present in the glomeruli of all PSGN patients. [80] NAPlr binds to GBM and the mesangial matrix, where it captures and activates plasmin-causing degradation of the GBM, thus glomerular damage. It can also activate the alternative complement pathway, facilitating immune complexes, and complement component deposition in the subepithelium. [81]

Another proposed nephritogenic antigen is streptococcal pyogenic exotoxin B (SPE), a cationic plasmin-binding protease secreted by pyogenic streptococcus. SPEB and its precursor zSPEB increase cytokine production (IL-6, TNFa, IL-8), leukocyte proliferation, and production of adhesion molecules, inducing inflammation, immune complex formation, and consecutively glomerular damage. [82] There is strong evidence that SPEB is the major antigen involved in the pathogenesis of PSGN, but further studies are required to determine the causative antigen.

There is also increasing evidence of an underlying genetic predisposition and susceptibility in the basis of PSGN. Major histocompatibility-complex antigens HLA-DR4, HLA-DR1 and HLA-DRB1*03011 presented higher incidence rates in PSGN patients. [83, 84] Also, polymorphisms of the endothelial nitric oxide synthease gene intron 4a/b (eNOS4a/b), was associated with PSGN in children and represents an important risk factor for nephrotic syndrome and progression of the disease. [85]

However, the correlation of HLA antigens to PSGN development is still under investigation, therefore no definitive conclusions on the genetic predisposition of PSGN can be made to date.

Incidence and Prevalence

PSGN primarily affects children aged between 2 and 12 years with a peak at 5-6 years. It is quite rare in ages below 2 years, [67] probably due to decreased immunogenicity of the children. Young adults and the elderly may also be affected but incidence rates are significantly lower. In adults, there is a peak in the fourth decade of life. The male to female ratio ranges from 2:1 to 3:1.

In the past decades, the overall incidence has decreased more likely due to improvement on socioeconomic, nutritional and health case conditions. [87, 88] Remarkably, in recent years, a slight increase in the incidence of PSGN has been reported, especially in the elderly.

The estimated global incidence of PSGN is 472,000 cases per year, of which 404,000 reported cases refer to children. 456,000 cases occur in less developed countries. [89] Incidence in developed countries account for 0.3 per 100,000 per year, [90] while in developing countries it may reach up to 28.5 cases per 100,000 per year. [67] Epidemics of PSGN are quite rare and are mainly limited to Africa, West India, and the Middle East, and in populations with poor hygienic conditions and malnutrition.

Racial predisposition is hard to define given that PSGN is reported in all races. However, in the developed world, PSGN seems to prevail in Caucasian male adults and in the developing world in black male children.

In the USA, 1.5% of the patients with PSGN reach ESRD. [12] Males prevail over females and mainly affect patients between 20 and 64 years of age. Caucasians seem to be more susceptible than African Americans. 21.5% of these patients die within one year from renal replacement treatment initiation.

Pathology

In PSGN, renal biopsy is not usually required, unless initial presentation of the disease is atypical, with characteristics that raise doubts on the diagnosis.

In the acute phase, light microscopy reveals a global and diffuse involvement of the glomeruli. The glomerular tuft appears enlarged and dilated, often filling the urinary space, and hypercellular due to endogenous cellular proliferation and infiltration of inflammatory cells, such as neutrophylic polymorphonucleare granulocytes, monocytes and rarely eosinophils, macrophages, and lymphocytes. Proliferating cells are mainly endothelial cells but there is also mesangial and epithelial proliferation.

The capillary walls are thickened and in more severe cases, glomeruli appear bloodless as the edema impedes glomerular perfusion.

In biopsies using high power magnification, tiny nodules may be identified on the epithelial site of the glomerular capillary, corresponding to the "humps" observed in electron microscopy.

In severe cases, formation of crescents and adhesions with the Bowman's capsule may be seen. Necrotizing alternations of the glomeruli are rarely observed.

After the acute phase, the histologic picture is less severe, although diffuse mesangial hypercellularity may persist for several months.

Independently from the phase of the disease, tubular involvement is limited, unless there is extensive glomerular damage with proteinuria. In that case, protein cylinders, intraluminal RBCs, and RBC casts may be present. Tubular atrophy may also be observed. Interstitial damage is variable, but usually non-extensive. Interstitial edema and focal inflammation may be found.

On immunofluorescence, diffuse irregular granular deposits of IgG, IgM and predominantly C3 on the glomeruli and in the mesangium may be observed during the first 3 weeks of the disease, a histologic picture characterized by Sorger et al, [91] who described three different immunofluorescence patterns of PSGN, as "starry sky pattern". Deposition of IgA, IgE, and C1q has also been reported but they are usually absent.

In more severe cases with persistent nephrotic range proteinuria, deposits of IgG and C3 may be confluent or linearly packed, corresponding to the subepithelial humps observed in electron microscopy. This pattern is called the "garland pattern" and has the worst long-term prognosis among histological patterns of PSGN.

In resolving or healed phases of the disease, granular deposition of C3 confined in the mesangium is observed, called the "mesangial pattern".

On electron microscopy, the characteristic subepithelial electron-dense deposits called "humps" are observed. Humps are quite numerous during the first weeks from the onset of the disease, decreasing within 6 weeks as the disease resolves, leaving translucent areas that separate humps from the lamina densa. Electro-dense deposits may also be seen in the mesangium, in the lamina densa, and the subendothelium.

Clinical Manifestations

The typical manifestation of PSGN is the abrupt onset of hematuria edema and rarely hypertension 2 to 3 weeks from the upper respiratory infection or 3 to 6 weeks from skin infection. Subclinical forms are more frequent than clinical forms, occurring in more than 50% of PSGN patients, discovered only by urinanalysis where abnormalities are observed. Microscopic hematuria and reduction of serum complement levels are the first appearing features. Full-blown nephritic syndrome may occur with abrupt onset of oliguria, proteinuria, edema, and hypertension.

Edema can frequently be the only symptom and it is present in 85% of the patients. It usually appears periorbitally but it may involve the whole body, giving origin to edema ansarca. The degree of edema depends on the extension of the glomerular damage, degree of hypoalbuminemia and sodium and fluid retention. Pulmonary edema has been reported, even in the absence of other PSGN symptoms. [92]

Macroscopic hematuria is present in 30 to 50% of PSGN patients, especially in childhood. It disappears within a few days while microscopic hematuria usually persists for 1 to 4 years from the onset of nephritis. [89]

Proteinuria is typically present, but nephrotic syndrome rarely occurs. Proteinuria may persist for months.

Hypertension is mainly due to fluid retention, manifesting with headache. Hypertension resolves in 1 to 2 weeks, but in some cases is complicated by hypertensive encephalopathy, with severe hypertension (>200/120 mmHg) and CNS dysfunction symptoms such as confusion, seizures, visual disturbances, and in more severe cases, aphasia, and coma.

Anemia may also be present, but in most cases, it is due to hemodiluition. Rarely, autoimmune hemolytic anemia may occur.

Different immunofluorescence patterns present as different clinical pictures. The "garland pattern" is associated with severe proteinuria or nephrotic syndrome, while the "mesangial pattern" is mostly associated with the resolving phase of the disease where symptoms are less pronounced. The presence of crescents is related to increased serum levels and progression to ESRD.

Prognosis

Clinical course is usually favorable with resolution of edema within 5 to 10 days from the onset and normalization of the blood pressure in 8 to 10 weeks. Microscopic hematuria may persist for more than 1 year. In elderly patients, clinical course may be less favorable due to concomitant pathologies, including cardiovascular disease and diabetes. [67, 71] Acute renal failure with severe proteinuria and hypertension occasionally occur.

Prognosis is generally good, especially in children, with complete recovery and good long-term outcomes. Only less than 1% of the children present progression of the renal disease, usually after 10 to 15 years of follow up. Renal failure is usually associated with the presence of crescents, presenting with persistent proteinuria, hematuria, hypertension, and progressive decrease of GFR.

Mortality rates are quite low, accounting for 5 to 9% in adults and less than 1% in children.

Diagnostic Considerations

Kidney biopsy is generally not recommended in PSGN given that history of recent respiratory and skin infection, along with increased titers of streptococcal antibodies, are considered sufficient to establish diagnosis. Kidney biopsy should be reserved for cases of normocomplementemia, rapid deterioration of renal function, and recurrent episodes of macroscopic hematuria.

Streptococcal antibodies include antistreptolysin (ASO), antihyaluronidase (AHase), antistreptokinase (ASKase), nicotinamide adenine dinucleotidase (ant NADase), and anti-DNAse antibodies. All streptococcal antibodies are commonly present in streptococcal infections; however, ASO titer can be falsely low or negative.

Complement levels are usually low, especially C3 components levels. C4 is commonly within the normal range. Duration of low complement levels period is limited to 6 to 8 weeks. If they persist longer than that, differential diagnosis with other low complement glomerular diseases should be made.

Urinanalysis shows proteinuria that rarely exceeds 3(+). RBCs and RBC casts are observed in 60% of the cases.

Total blood count may show normochromic and normocytic anemia. White blood cell and platelet counts are usually normal. Creatinine and urea levels may be increased. These alternations are typically transient and resolve within weeks or months.

Finally, renal ultrasonography reveals normal to slightly enlarged kidneys with increased echogenicity.

Treatment

Treatment of PSGN is mainly supportive, consisting of salt restriction and blood pressure control. A low sodium and low protein diet is indicated when edema and hypertension are present. If acute renal failure with oliguria is established potassium intake should be limited in order to prevent hyperkaliemia.

If these measures are not sufficient to control hypertension, diuretics and anti-hypertensive agents should be administered. ACEIs and loop diuretics provide good results but β-blockers and calcium channel blockers may also be helpful.

Antibiotics should be administered in order to eliminate the pathogenic antigen or in case of persisting streptococcal infection.

Steroid therapy has also been successfully used in cases of PSGN with nephritic range proteinuria and renal insufficiency, [94, 95] but their efficacy has not been widely proven, [96] therefore their use is not indicated in typical PSGN cases. Favorable results have also been reported in patients treated with plasmapheresis plus steroids. [97]

Cyclophosphamide, azathioprine, dypiridamole, and cyclosporine have also been used in PSGN patients but the results were disappointing. [98]

Vaccination against group A streptococci is indicated, in order to prevent spread of the disease to families and other people in close contact.

2.2. Atypical PIGN

Atypical forms of PIGN are increasingly presenting in both children and adults, particularly in the elderly. The underlying infection is not the typical streptococcal infection but usually includes staphylococcal and Gram negative and more rarely viral or protozoal infection. In the elderly, staphylococcal infections are 3 times more common than streptococcal infections.

Sites of infection are also atypical. Skin infections, pneumonia, urinary tract infections, osteomyelitis, and endocarditis are far more common than upper respiratory infection.

There seems to be prevalence in alcoholics, drug abusers, immunocompromised, and diabetic patients. Malignancy may also be a predisposing condition. The male to female ratio is 3:1.

In these patients, the latent period between infection and onset of the kidney disease is hard to define, given that in most of the cases the underlying infection is unrecognized, as non specific symptoms of the infection and fever are frequently absent.

Clinical presentation is characterized by microscopic hematuria while macroscopic hematuria is present in 20% of the cases. Nephrotic syndrome and impaired renal function occur more frequently than in typical forms. Most of the patients present arterial hypertension.

Prognosis in atypical PIGN patients is worse than in typical cases. Immunocompromised and elderly patients with age-related diseases such as diabetes and cardiovascular disease show higher levels of serum creatinine and proteinuria.

On biopsy, the most common histologic patterns are diffuse endocapillary proliferative and exudative glomerulonepritis, followed by mesangial proliferative and finally crescentic and necrotizing glomerulonephritis. Immunofluorescence reveals "starry sky pattern" in most of the cases, and "mesangial pattern".

The "garland pattern" accounts for less than 8% of the cases. [91] C3 is the dominant deposited complement component. IgG and IgM deposits are present. C1q deposits are often present but in smaller quantity. IgA deposits, in some cases, are the dominant deposits giving origin in a separate entity, the IgA-dominant PIGN.

On electron microscopy, subepithelial and intramembrane dense deposits are seen. Mesangial deposits are present in almost 90% of the cases.

Treatment approach is similar to the typical PSGN. Immunocompromized patients should be treated as soon as possible. Use of steroids in these cases has been reported to be effective. [99]

2.3. IgA-dominant PIGN

Another atypical increasingly recognized morphologic variant of PIGN is the IgA-dominant acute PIGN. The mainly involved pathogenic agent is Staphylococcus aureus, followed by Gram-negative bacteria. The sites of infection are skin, lungs, and heart. The mean time of presentation is 4 weeks from the infection.

IgA-dominant PIGN affects only young adults and elderly. There are no reported cases of IgA PIGN in children. Males prevail over females with a ratio of 3.9:1. [100] Caucasians are more predisposed compared to African Americans. The average age of diagnosis is 60 years.

Diabetes, malignancy, IV drug abuse and immunosuppression are predisposing factors for the disease.

Clinical manifestations include hematuria, proteinuria, hypertension, and in more severe cases, acute renal failure with nephriotic syndrome. Extrarenal symptoms include purpura, arthritis, and abdominal pain.

On biopsy, endocapillary proliferative, mesangial proliferative and rarely crescentic glomerulonephritis may be observed. On immunofluorescence, there is sole or dominant IgA deposition, with IgA_1 kappa to lambda ratio greater in mesangial staining. [101] C3 deposition is also common while positive staining for C1q is rare.

Serum IgA levels are increased, particularly in diabetic patients, while complement components are decreased in circulation.

Acute renal failure at presentation, intercurrent staphylococcal infection, hypocomplementemia, and presence of subepithelial humps on electron microscopy favor IgA-dominant PIGN. [102-104]

Treatment is similar to PIGN, consisting of antibiotics, antihypertensives, diuretics, and steroids administration.

Prognosis is worse than typical PIGN, with up to 40% of the patients progressing to ESRD.

3. Membranoproliferative Glomerulonephritis

Membranoproliferative or mesangiocapillary glomerulonephritis (MPGN) is a term employed to describe a histological pattern of glomerular injury due to a variety of immune-mediated disorders, characterized by subendothelial and mesangial deposition of immune complexes and/or complement factors, diffuse proliferative lesions of the mesangium and thickening of the capillary walls because of reduplication of the GBM, which assumes a "double-contour" appearance.

Major clinical classification includes primary or idiopathic and secondary MPGN. Secondary cases, where the underlying etiology can be identified are far more common than primary cases. Primary or idiopathic MPGN is a diagnosis of exclusion where the exact cause of the disease is not discovered.

A histopathologic classification based on ultrastructural appearance subdivides MPGN into 3 types. Type I is characterized by subendothelial and mesangial deposits, type III is considered a variant of type I with subendothelial and subepithelial deposits, while type II, also called dense deposit disease (DDD), presents characteristic intramembranous electro-dense deposits. Because of its unique histopathologic features, DDD is largely considered a distinct disease entity, conventionally classified as MPGN due to the similarities in light microscopy with the other MPGN variants.

Advances on the pathogenic pathways in MPGN, led nephrologists into proposing a new classification that subdivides it into immune complex mediated and complement mediated. [105] Attention to the composition of the deposits by immunofluorescence allowed distinction of immunoglobulin-negative lesions with isolated C3 complement component deposition from immunoglobulin-mediated MPGN.

Incidence of MPGN is quite limited, approximately 3 to 5 patients per million and is decreasing in developed countries, while in developing countries it remains elevated, probably due to elevated hepatitis C incidence that causes MPGN type I. [106, 107]

It presents with nephrotic syndrome and hypertension and slowly progresses to ESRD. The age of onset varies, but it is more common in late childhood and adolescence.

Etiology and Pathogenesis

In the past, most of the MPGN cases were thought to be idiopathic, probably due to diagnostic difficulties. Over time, as serological and pathological study methods improved making underlying causes easier to identify, cases previously recognized as idiopathic were redefined as secondary.

Causes of secondary MPGN include autoimmune diseases, chronic infections, hereditary diseases, neoplasms, paraproteinemias, and cryoglobulinemias:

- Bacterial infections: visceral abscesses, bacterial endocarditis, infected ventriculoatrial or venticuloperitoneal shunt, infected indwelling catheters
- Viral infections: Hepatitis c, Hepatitis B, HIV
- Other infections: mycoplasma, malaria, leprosy, scistosomiasis, filariasis
- Autoimmune diseases: Systemic lupus erythematosous, scleroderma, Sjögren's syndrome
- Malignancies: chronic lemphocytic leukemia, non-Hodgkin lymphoma, thymoma, renal cell carcinoma, lung carcinomas
- Paraproteinemias and cryoglobulimemias: light chain deposition disease, heavy chain deposition disease, monoclonal IgG deposition, hereditary deficiency of complement componenets (C1q, C2, C3, C4), inherited Factor H deficiency, gene polymorphism of Factor B and Factor H-related proteins
- Other Causes: chronic liver disease-cirrhosis, cystic fibrosis, sarcoidosis, Sickle cell disease, hemolytic uremic syndrome

Although not all pathogenic mechanisms have been clearly understood yet, it has been accepted for some 30 years that complement activation and consecutive hypocomplementemia are the basis of all three types of the disease.

The complement system is an important part of the innate immunity that can induce inflammatory responses, consisting of the classic, the alternative and the mannose-binding lectin pathway, all converging into a common final pathway with the formation of C3 convertase (C3bBb). C3bBb in presence of factor B and D, splits C3 in C3a and C3b. The association of C3b to C3bBb forms the C5b convertase (C42b3b), which activates the cascade of the formation of the membrane attack complex (MAC or C5b-9). MAC induces cell injury and lysis.

The classic pathway is activated by the interaction of C1q to the Fc portion of IgG or IgM of the immune complex form *in situ* or deposited on the glomeruli while the alternative pathway is continually activated through spontaneous generation and activation of C3b. These mechanisms are under control by regulating and inhibiting proteins such as factor H and I.

MPGN type I results from nephritogenic immune complexes formed in situ or deposition of immune complexes formed in circulation by interaction with antibodies, of infectious, neoplastic or other endogenous agents that are recognized as antigens. Immune complexes are deposited in the mesangium and subendothelial space of the capillary walls.

Once deposited, the immune complexes activate the complement cascade through the classical pathway with successive formation of MAC that directly injures the capillary wall, and release of chemotactic factors, cytokines, and growth factors that promote leukocyte accumulation, mesangial proliferation, and matrix expansion.

Leukocytes release oxidants and proteases that injure the capillary walls. Damage of the capillary walls through the complement cascade and leukocytes causes proteinuria and decrease of the GFR. Activation of the complement system through the mannose-binding pathway has also been reported in patients with MPGN type I. [108]

MPGN type II or dense deposit disease (DDD) is associated with multiple complement abnormalities, both inherited or acquired, that lead to uncontrolled and continual systemic activation of the alternative pathway of the complement cascade.

In normal subjects, regulation of the complement activation is exercised by factor H and I, and five factor H-related proteins (CFHR1, CFHR2, CFHR3, CFHR4, CFHR5). Factor H mediates and accelerates the breakdown of C3 convertase, and factor I inactivates C3, inhibiting in this way the activation of the alternative pathway. Factor H-related proteins attach to the cell membrane, preventing formation of active complement products. [109, 110]

In case of DDD this regulating mechanism is lost, mainly because of the presence of an IgG or IgM autoantibody, the C3 nephritic factor (C3Nef) that binds the C3 convertase of the alternative pathway, protecting it from the effects of factor H. C3Nef prolongs the half-life of C3 convertase for up to 60 minutes. It is found in 80% of DDD patients, [111] but is also found in approximately 15% of MPGN type I patients as well as in other glomerular and non-glomerular diseases, suggesting its possible contribution to the pathogenesis of other glomerular diseases. [112, 113] A nephritic factor of the classic pathway (C4Nef) that stabilizes the convertase C4b2a was also found in 20% of MPGN patients. [112, 113]

Genetic polymorphisms and mutations in both activating and regulating proteins of the alternative pathway can lead to hyperactivity of C3 and DDD. A mutation in the gene encoding C3 that produces a C3 resistant to C3 convertase has been recently identified. This mutant C3 becomes the predominant circulating complement component, and its deposition to the glomeruli causes DDD.

Genetic polymorphism in the gene-encoding factor H (CFH) could provoke complete factor H deficiency or impair their regulating effect. Tyrosin-402-hisidine (Tyr402His) allele polymorphism is the most commonly polymorphism found in DDD patients with impairment of the regulation of C3 convertase. [114, 115]

Homozygous mutation of CFH provokes complete CFH deficiency with consecutive excessive C3 deposition in the mesangium and capillary walls. [116] Although it is quite rare, four families with complete CFH deficiency and DDD have been reported. [117]

Mutation of the gene encoding CFHR5 results in a CFHR5 less effective in regulating the C3 and C5 convertases. [118, 119] This mutation presents as an autosomal dominant familial microscopic hematuria, first described in Cypriot families. A 1q32 chromosomal deletion of CFHR gene results in expression of a hybrid CFHR2-CFHR5 protein that stabilizes C3 convertase and reduces factor's H regulating effect. [114, 118]

Finally, polymorphisms of factor B, membrane co-factor protein, and factor I associated to MPGN have been reported. [115, 120]

Pathogenesis of MPGN type III may be related to a slow-acting nephritic factor, called nephritic factor of the terminal pathway (NeFt), present in 60 to 80% of MPGN type III patients. NeFt stabilizes the properdin dependent C3 convertase of the alternative pathway with resulting uncontrolled activation of the common terminal pathway of the complement and formation of the MAC with consecutive glomerular damage. [121]

Genetic mutations related to MPGN type III are rare and not yet widely identified. To date, only a familial form of autosomal dominant MPGN type III has been reported, due to mutation of 1q31-32 gene band that regulates the C3 convertase activity. [123, 124]

Pathology and Classification

The typical histopathologic feature of MPGN on light microscopy consists of diffuse mesangial hypercellularity, endocapillary proliferation with thickening of the capillary walls, assuming "double contour" appearance, all resulting in lobular prominence of the glomerular tufts.

Based on electron microscopy findings MPGN is classified into 3 types: MPGN type I, MPGN type II and MPGN type III.

MPGN type I is the most common variant, characterized by deposits of immune complexes and complement components. In light microscopy, hypercellularity due to influx of circulating leucocytes, mononuclear cells (mesangial interposition) and increased mesangial proliferation, along with diffuse endocapillary proliferation, give this variant the name of "mesangiocapillary glomerulonephritis". The capillary walls are thickened due to the deposits and the infiltration of inflammatory cells, localized between endothelium and GBM, resulting in a double contour basement membrane.

Crescents are rarely seen but if present, are associated to a worse prognosis. Tubulointerstitial fibrosis and vascular sclerosis may be seen in late stages of the disease, indicating worse outcome.

On immunofluorescence, IgG, IgM, and C3 deposits usually present an irregular capillary and mesangial distribution. C3 deposits may be dominant, especially in secondary forms of MPGN type I.

The electron microscopy reveals electron-dense deposits in mesangial areas and within the GBM, under the lamina densa, described as intramembranous.

MPGN type II or DDD is characterized by the presence of intramembranous and mesangial dense deposits. Although this variant is a unique and separated entity, it is conventionally classified as MPGN due to the similarity of its appearance in light microscopy with the other MPGN variants.

On light microscopy, there is a thickening of the basement membranes of glomeruli, tubules, and Bowman's capsule and diffuse endocapillary proliferation. Crescents and segmental necrotizing lesions are rarely seen.

By immunofluorescence, dense deposits in granular or discontinuous distribution are observed. These deposits predominantly consist of C3 component of the complement although rarely IgM, IgG, and IgA have been observed. [124]

By electron microscopy, the lamina densa of the GBM presents dense granular deposits that can also be found in mesangial areas. Hypercellularity due to mesangial proliferation or mesangial interposition may be present but less accentuated than MPGN type I. Podocytes show foot processes effacement or microvillus transformation.

MPGN type III is similar to MPGN type I, presenting other than subendothelial and mesangial, numerous subepithelial deposits. Hypercellularity is less prominent than in type I.

By immunofluorescence, MPGN type III shows capillary and mesangial deposition of C3 and less often IgG and IgM in a granular distribution.

Based on different patterns of electron deposits and the different appearance of the GBM on electron microscopy, MPGN type III is further classified in two subvariants: the Burkholder variant, characterized by subendothelial and subepithelial deposits often forming spikes similar to those in membranous nephropathy, [125, 126] and the Anders and Strife variant, presenting electron lucent deposits that disrupt the lamina densa giving it a multilayering appearance. [127,128] Given the advances made on both biopsy study and understanding of the pathophysiologic mechanisms underlying MPGN, it is believed that the current classification is obsolete, while a more appropriate and practical approach is considered a classification of MPGN based on both histologic findings and pathogenic mechanisms.

Therefore, Sethi et al., proposed a new classification according to the predominant immunofluorescence findings, dividing MPGN cases in immune complex-mediated and complement mediated. [105]

Complement-mediated MPGN can be further classified into C3 glomerulonephritis with subendothelial and mesangial deposits of C3, corresponding more likely to MPGN type I or intramembranous and subepithelial deposits corresponding to MPGN type III, and DDD wth intramembranous and mesangial C3 deposits. These two variants of MPGN, with isolated C3 deposit staining, are included in the term of C3 glomerulopathies. [129]

Epidemiology

MPGN accounts for 7 to 10% of all glomerulonephritis, with overall incidence of 3 to 5 per million. [106] In the USA, MPGN is found in 6 to 12% of renal biopsies, while in Europe the incidence rates are lower, accounting for less than 5% of biopsy-confirmed glomerulonephritis.

There is a decreasing tendency of its incidence in developed countries, probably due to improvement of controlling infections, in socioeconomic conditions, and modification of environmental factors. In developing countries incidence remains high, likely due to the high incidence of hepatitis C. [106]

In the USA, Caucasians seem to be more susceptible to the disease than African Americans. MPGN type I predominantly affects women, while in type II there are no significant differences between genders.

The age of onset is variable, ranging between 6 and 30 years, although cases involving the elderly have also been reported.

Of these patients, 25 to 35% will present ESRD and will need renal replacement therapy. According to USRD 2013, incidence rates of ESRD due to MPGN type I are higher in Caucasians, accounting for 73.6% over 18.4% of African Americans, and in case of MPGN type II, 80% over 12.9%. Death rates within 1 year from renal replacement treatment initiation are 11% for MPGN type I and 9.3% for MPGN type II. [12]

Clinical Presentation

Clinical manifestations of MPGN are similar in all types, presenting mainly with microscopic or macroscopic hematuria and asymptomatic proteinuria, usually in the non-nephrotic range. In 10 to 20% of the cases, hematuria is recurrent, similar to IgA nephropathy. Nephrotic syndrome is observed in approximately 40% of the cases, manifesting with periorbital or peripheral edema and rarely anasarca.

In some patients, acute nephrotic syndrome may develop with concomitant oliguria or anuria and acute renal failure. In rare cases, rapidly progressive disease may be observed. Hypertension is also common and often quite severe.

DDD is often associated with partial lipodystrophy, involving mainly the face, trunk, and upper limbs. Vision impairment along with color defects due to the deposition of "drusen bodies" on the basement membrane of the retinal epithelium, choroidal neovascularization and macular degeneration may accompany DDD.

MPGN due to Hepatitis C infection is associated with cryoglobulinemia and usually presents with weakness, arthralgias, and purpura on the extremities. Raynaud's syndrome and peripheral neuropathy may rarely occur.

Prognosis

Prognosis in both children and adults is poor. Renal survival at 10 years from the onset ranges between 50 and 65%. MPGN type I with non-nephrotic proteinuria presents better outcomes than MPGN type I with nephrotic syndrome, where 50% of the patients progress to ESRD within 10 to 20 years from the onset. DDD presents lower survival rates reaching ESRD within 10 to 12 years.

Prognostic factors affecting the outcome include proteinuria, renal function at presentation of the disease, hypertension, and histopathologic features.

MPGN with nephrotic range proteinuria have a worse prognosis, with renal survival lower than 50%. Patients with higher levels of proteinuria, independently if it is of nephrotic or non-nephrotic range, have worse long term prognosis.

Patients presenting high creatinine levels and low GFR at the time of diagnosis will reach ESRD faster than patients with normal renal function will. Reduced GFR at presentation is considered an independent risk factor for the development of ESRD. [130]

Hypertension is also considered an independent risk factor, and in association with nephrotic range proteinuria induces progression to ESRD in less than 10 years from the onset.

Tubulointerstitial fibrosis, segmental glomerulosclerosis, and presence of crescents on the renal biopsy indicate poor outcome and lower renal survival rates.

Hyperlipidemia and thromboembolic tendency due to proteinuria along with anemia and secondary hyperparathyroidism are complications that negatively affect prognosis.

Diagnosis

Primary MPGN is a diagnosis of exclusion, after no secondary causes provoking the disease have been identified. Identification of underlying conditions is fundamental given that misdiagnosis may lead to incorrect treatment choices and negatively affect prognosis.

However, the definitive diagnosis is reached with biopsy, where mesangial hypercellularity, endocapillary proliferation with double contour appearance of the capillary walls are observed in light microscopy, a histologic picture common for all types of MPGN.

Persistent hypocomplementemia with predominantly decreased C3 serum levels is observed. C1q levels may also be decreased, especially in MPGN type I, suggesting activation of the classical complement pathway. Terminal complement components C5, C8 and C9 serum levels may be low, but they are usually within the normal range.

C3Nef autoantibody is present in more than 70% of MPGN type II cases, suggesting activation of the alternative complement pathway. Factor H serum levels may also be low. NFt is present in 60 to 80% of MPGN type II patients.

Treatment

Given the heterogeneity of underlying causes, histologic findings and clinical manifestations of MPGN, an optimal treatment regimen is not presently available. It is important however to identify and thoroughly evaluate possible underlying diseases and conditions before any specific treatment consideration is made.

The initial therapeutic approach consists of supportive antihypertensive and antiproteinuric treatment. KDIGO guidelines recommend lowering the blood pressure in less than 130mmHg of systolic and less than 80mmHg of diastolic arterial blood pressure, using ACEIs or ARBs alone or in combination, for their double antihypertensive and antiproteinuric activity, keeping in mind limitations in case of advanced renal disease with low GFR. [131]

Calcium channel blockers may also be helpful. Loop diuretics are indicated in case of edema, alone or in combination with albumin infusions. Potassium sparing diuretics could also be used but caution is advised due to elevated risk of hyperkaliemia.

In primary MPGN, specific treatment regimens should be preserved for patients with nephrotic syndrome and progressive decrease of renal function, or in patients with impaired renal function at the time of presentation of the disease.

Costicosteroids

Alternate-day administration of corticosteroids in high doses, seem to benefit children with MPGN types I and II with nephrotic syndrome. It has been demonstrated in various studies that this regimen preserves renal function and increases renal survival. Outcomes seem to be better in MPGN type I. [132] It is believed that initiation of the therapy before irreversible kidney injury is established is fundamental, and provides favorable outcomes.

Initial steroid doses in MPGN nephrotic children are 2 to 2.5mg/kg on alternate days, up to a maximum of 80mg, followed by tapering at 1 to 1.5mg/kg every other day at 2 years and 0.2 to 1mg/kg at 4 years of treatment. Corticosteroid therapy should be administered for a minimum of 2 years and continue with a maintenance dose of 20mg every other day for 3 to 10 years. [133]

If after 1 year of treatment, no improvement is observed in proteinuria and/or renal function, withdrawal of steroids and initiation of a more aggressive treatment should be considered.

In adults, 1mg/kg daily of prednisone for 3 to 6 months is recommended. If patients show no improvement, steroid therapy should be interrupted and immunosuppressive therapy with MMF, tacrolimus, or cyclosporine A should be initiated. [134]

Calcineurin Inhibitors

Cyclosporine A and tacrolimus have both been suggested for the treatment of MPGN, but complete remission of proteinuria has been rarely obtained. [135,136]

Suggested doses were 4 to 6mg/kg daily of Cyclosporine A and 0.1 to 0.15mg/kg per day for tacrolimus, usually accompanied by low doses of steroids.

However, results remain controversial and in association with increased risk for nephrotoxicity, these agents are not recommended for the treatment of MPGN.

Alkylating Agents

Cyclophosphamide administration showed unfavorable results in most MPGN cases. However, in a recent case report, a combination of cyclophosphamide in IV pulses with steroids and plasma exchange therapy provided complete remission of proteinuria and normalization of GFR. Repeated biopsy showed disappearance of crescent formations, but dense deposits persisted. [137]

In contrast, in a RCT carried out by Cattran et al, no benefit was found in treating MPGN types I and II with cyclophosphamide, warfarin and dipiridamole. [138]

Cyclophosphamide may be of help in HCV-mediated glomerulonephritis as it is able to block cryoglobulin production. Suggested doses are 2mg/kg per day for 2 to 4 months. [139]

Inhibitors of Purine Synthesis

Although data on the efficacy of MMF are limited, short-term results seem to be favorable. A combination of MMF with high doses of steroids significantly reduces proteinuria and stabilized renal function. Based on the low quality evidence of efficacy of immunosuppressive agents plus steroids in the treatment of MPGN, KDIGO guidelines suggest oral cyclophosphamide or MMF plus corticosteroids for up to 6 months. [134, 140]

Biological Immunomodulators

Rituximab is a chimeric monoclonal antibody against the CD20 antigen of B cells that has been used with success in the treatment of minimal change disease, membranous nephropathy, and focal segmental glomerulosclerosis. [141] Recent small non-controlled studies and anecdotal reports point out the possibility of application of rituximab in MPGN type I, especially if HCV-related and in the treatment of refractory MPGN. [142]

Suggested doses are 375mg/m^2 given intravenously once a week for 4 consecutive weeks, while others suggest 1000mg intravenously every two weeks. [143]

Obtaining a complete or partial remission in MPGN type I, suggests a role of B cells in its pathogenesis. Eculizumab is a humanized anti-C5 monoclonal antibody that inhibits the formation of C5a and consecutively the terminal membrane attack complex (MAC or C5-9) of the final common complement pathway.

It has been successfully used in the treatment of paroxysmal nocturnal hemoglobinuria (PHN) and in the atypical hemolytic uremic syndrome (aHUS), [144, 145] diseases, both caused by complement activation abnormalities. It is reasonable that inhibition of the formation of C5-9 complex could protect from complement-mediated kidney injury; therefore, eculizumab was considered a good alternative for the treatment of DDD and MPGN type I. [146-148]

It was administered at doses of 900mg per week for 5 consecutive weeks, followed by doses of 1200mg every two weeks in a MPGN type I patient non responding to MMF and steroid treatment. [146] In another case report of recurrent DDD after transplantation, the patient received 900mg of eculizumab once a week for two weeks, followed by 600mg every 14 days. [148]

In both cases, complete remission was obtained, suggesting a role of eculizumab in both refractory and recurrent MPGN. However, further evaluation and large RCTs are required to ensure efficacy and safety of eculizumab in the therapy of MPGN.

Other Therapeutic Measures

High doses of recombinant human interferone-α are suggested in cases of HCV-mediated MPGN, in order to reduce the load of infectious virions. Combination of interferon-α to ribavirin seems quite promising but unfortunately, relapse is very common.

Use of anticoagulants is also indicated in MPGN cases, given the hypercoagulative state of nephrotic syndrome.

4. Rapidly Progressive Glomerulomephritis

Rapidly progressive or crescentic glomerulonephritis (RPGN or CrGN) is a term referring to a group of glomerular disorders having as common characteristic the presence of crescents in more than 50% of the glomeruli and rapid deterioration of renal function. GFR may decline at least 50% within a few days or in best case within 3 months from the onset.

In most of the cases, RPGN is associated with underlying conditions, such as infectious diseases, multisystem diseases, consumption of certain drugs or other glomerular diseases. Regardless the underlying cause, if not timely diagnosed and treated, RPGN leads to severe glomerular injury and ESRD.

Classification

Based on immunopathologic features, RPGN can be classified into 4 types:

Type I, also called anti-GBM antibody disease or anti GBM glomerulonephritis, characterized by linear deposition of antibodies (IgG) along the GBM. These antibodies are directed against type IV collagen, and sometimes cross-react with the basement membrane of the alveoli, producing Goodpasture syndrome. The cases where renal deposition of anticollagen antibodies is present are considered idiopathic. It accounts for 10 to 20% of RPGN cases. 10% of these patients may be ANCAs.

Type II or immune-complex RPGN is characterized by glomerular deposition of immune complexes. It is usually secondary to infectious diseases and connective tissue disorders (Henoch–Schönlein purpura, lupus, cryoglobulinemias) but it can also be idiopathic

Type III or pauci-immune RPGN is distinguished by the presence of a few, or total absence of immune deposits or anti-GBM antibodies. In most of the cases, it is secondary to systemic ANCA-associated diseases such as Wegener's granulomatosis and Churg-Strauss syndrome. In some rare cases, it may be isolated to the glomerulus and these are considered primary or idiopathic. This is most common type of RPGN, accounting for 50 to 55% of all cases.

Type IV, also called "double antibody" positive disease is characterized by the presence of features of both types I and III, thus anti-GBM antibodies and ANCA-antibodies.

Idiopathic forms of RPGN are quite rare, and present with deposition of immune complexes but without any obvious underlying cause, or as the pauci-immune RPGN but without ANCA antibodies.

Epidemiology

Idiopathic RPGN is quite uncommon, accounting for less than 10% of the patients with primary gloemrulonephritis. The overall incidence in the USA is estimated at 7 cases per 1 million persons per year. It occurs mainly between the second and the sixth decade of life with a peak between the fourth and sixth decade. RPGN type I occurs mostly in younger age, while types I and II occur in older adults.

Gender differences are hard to evaluate. Most studies reveal a male-to-female ratio of 1:1, but there seems to be a predilection for males in types I and III. However, according to USRD 2013, of patients with RPGN reaching ESRD, women prevailed slightly with 51.4% over 48.6 of men. [12] There is also a predilection for Caucasians (82.1%) over African Americans (13.1%) in the USA.

More than 50% of the patients present with renal failure at the onset. These patients present increased risk for ESRD and increased mortality rates regardless of any treatment, conventional or immunosuppressive. [149] 18.1% of patients with ESRD due to RPGN die within the first year of renal replacement treatment. [12]

Etiology and Pathogenesis

Etiology of RPGN is variable and not all causes are known. In idiopathic forms, causes are unknown, there is no association to systemic features and no infectious, neoplastic or autoimmune diseases that can be identified. Different types of secondary forms of RPGN are associated to different underlying causes:

- Infectious Diseases: infective endocarditis, Hepatitis B, Hepatitis C, HIV
- Multisystem Diseases: Systemic lupus erythematosus, Henoch–Schönlein purpura, Wegener's granulomatosis, Goodpasture syndrome, malignancies
- Drugs: Allopurinol, propylthiouracil, hydralazine, rifampicin
- Other glomerular diseases: membranoproliferative glomerulonephritis, IgA nephropathy (Berger's Disease), membranous glomerulonephritis

Pathogenesis of each one of the RPGN types has been accurately defined and described.

In type I RPGN, the pathogenic mechanism consists of the deposition of antibodies against the alpha-3 chain in the C-terminal non-collagenous domain (NC1) of type IV collagen of the GBM. Alpha-3 (IV) NC1 domain presents 2 epitopes (EA, EB) located close to each other that are inaccessible to antibody binding. Endogenous oxidants and certain subpopulations of anti-GBM antibodies have the potential of revealing the epitopes and form a bond. This bond activates the complement cascade with consecutive injury of the GBM. Lymphocytes T CD4 and CD8 induce migration of polymorphonuclear neutrophils and macrophages at the site of glomerular injury, which contributes to the crescent formation. [150].

In type II PRGN, formation *in situ* or in circulation of immune complexes and their deposition on the glomerular tufts with subsequent activation of the complement cascade is the mechanism involved. The antigens may be endogenous (nuclear or tumor antigens) or esogenous, including viruses, bacteria or environmental factors.

Type III or pauci-immune RPGN is an anti-neutrophil cytoplasmic antibody (ANCA) mediated disease. ANCAs are directed against myeloperoxidase (MPO) or against proteinase-3 (PR-3). Anti-MPO ANCAs have a perinuclear distribution on immunofluorescensce while anti-PR-3 ANCAs are mostly located in the cytoplasm. ANCAs activate the neutrophils by union of (Fab')2 fragments to antigens on the neutrophils' surfaces. [151] Activated neutrophils cause endothelial necrosis of the glomerular capillaries, [152] and release factors that activate the alternative pathway of the complement cascade aggravating the glomerular injury. [153]

In type IV or "double antibody" positive RPGN, both anti-GBM and ANCA-mediated mechanisms contemporaneously take place.

Regardless of the pathogenic mechanism, all types of RPGN converge in a common pathogenic pathway, the crescents formation. Crescents are defined as the presence of 2 or more layers of proliferating cells in Bowman's space and are a histological marker of severe injury to the capillary wall. [154]

Severe injury of the capillary walls due to any of the mechanisms previously described, lead to the GBM rupture with formation of gaps, also called rents or holes. These gaps may also be seen in Bowman's capsule. [155] Circulating cells such as monocytes, macrophages, fibroblasts, lymphocytes, plasma proteins, inflammatory mediators and coagulation factors enter from the interstitium to the Bowman's space. At this site, intrusive cells are proliferating, while coagulating factors promote conversion of fibrogen to fibrin, the protein mostly contributing to crescent formation. The fibrin along with the proliferating cells, line the Bowman's capsule into layers, which is the final form of the crescents. [154,156]

Crescents may contain mainly cells without collagen and they are called cellular or epithelial crescents, or in more advanced stages, contain both cells and collagen produced by the fibroblasts, referred to as fibroepithelial or fibrocellular crescents. In very advanced stages of the disease, crescents contain only fibrous tissue without any cells and are called fibrous crescents. Presence of fibrous crescents is associated with glomerular sclerosis and worse outcome.

Crescents may fill the Bowman's space partially or totally and they are called respectively circumscribed or circumferential. Presence of circumferential crescents in more than 80% of the glomeruli is characteristic of advanced renal disease and associated with poor prognosis.

Pathology

RPGN or CrGN, based on histological findings, may also be called proliferative extracapillary glomerulonephritis, since the common element characterizing this diseases' collection is the proliferation of epithelial and infiltrating cells, occurring outside the capillary tuft, and fibrous proliferation, both occupying the Bowman's space. However, histological findings may vary according the underlying pathogenic mechanism and stage of the disease.

Type I or anti-GBM antibody-mediated glomerulonephritis is characterized by linear deposition of IgG on the glomerular capillary and it is considered a small-vessel vasculitis. It may manifest as isolated renal disease, or in cases that the antibodies cross-react with pulmonary alveolar capillaries, RPGN is accompanied by pulmonary hemorrhage, referred to as Goodpasture syndrome. In this context, only the renal histological findings will be reported.

By light microscopy, the glomeruli present segmental or global fibrinoid necrosis with rupture of the GBM. In the early stages, there are no crescents, deposits, or proliferating cells and fibrinoid necrosis is the only histological finding. As the disease advances, ruptures on the Bowman's capsule may be seen, with periglomerular fibrosis and infiltration of neutrophils, monocytes, macrophages, and in some cases multinucleated giant cells forming granuloma-like lesions. The non-affected glomeruli may be normal but more often they present moderate mesangial proliferation with mesangial matrix expansion. The interstitium shows periglomerular infiltrates of leukocytes and other inflammatory cells, with fibrosis. Tubules may present epithelial degeneration with cellular desquamation, cytoplasmic vacuolation and tubular dilatation or tubular necrosis in acute renal failure, while in chronic patients tubular atrophy may be seen.

Immunofluorescence reveals strong linear deposition of IgG. C3 staining may also be positive but distribution is granular and discontinuous. Rarely dominant IgA linear deposits may be observed. Occasionally, linear tubular basement membrane deposits of IgG may be seen because of cross-reaction of anti-GBM antibodies with the tubular basement membranes.

By electron microscopy, no immune-complex electron dense deposits are detected. GBM ruptures and electron-dense fibrin tactoids are present in areas of crescent formation.

In type II or immune-complex mediated RPGN there are granular deposits of IgG, IgM or IgA on the capillary walls and the mesangium, with mesangial or/and endocapillary proliferation. Given that any immune-complex mediated disease may progress to RPGN, other pathological features depend on the underlying glomerular or systemic disease. These diseases include SLE, post-infectious glomerulonephritis, Henoch–Schönlein purpura and cryoglobulinemias.

Type III or pauci-immune RPGN is characterized by the absence or paucity of antibody or immune-comlex deposition despite that 80 to 85% of these patients present ANCAs against MPO or PR-3. ANCA positive pauci-immune RPGN may be divided into 4 supgroups according to its association with ANCA-mediated vasculitis:

- Renal-limited vasculitis or pauci-immune necrotizing and crescentic GN
- Renal involvement in microscopic polyangiitis. Microscopic polyangiitis is a necrotizing arteritis that involves small and medium-sized arteries. It often presents with renal and pulmonary involvement.
- Renal involvement in Wegener's granulomatosis, a necrotizing vasculitis affecting small and medium-sized vessels, presenting granulomatous inflammation of the pulmonary tissue. Of note, in Wegener's granulomatosis, granulomas do not occur in the kidney.
- Renal involvement in Churg-Strauss syndrome, also known as eosinophilic granulomatosis with polyangiitis, affects small and medium-sized vessels with abnormally high levels of eosinophils, often presenting with asthma, abdominal pain, and gastrointestinal hemorrhage.

Although clinical manifestations vary, the histopathology is similar in all 4 supgroups of pauci-immune RPGN, with common characteristics the fibrinoid necrosis and crescent formation.

By light microscopy, glomerular necrosis, focal and segmental or diffuse and global is present, often with collapsing glomerular capillaries, accompanied by cellular or fibrous crescents, depending on the stage of the disease. Bowman's capsule is ruptured and may present granulomatous lesions. Of note, in Wegener's granulomatosis, renal granulomas rarely occur.

By immunofluorescence, no immunoglobulins, immune-complexes, or complement components are identified. Rarely, in necrotizing areas, IgM and C3 may be found. In Churg-Strauss syndrome, eosinophils may be present, but not in remarkable numbers.

On electron microscopy, no electron-dense deposits are identified. Bowman's capsule and the GBM present ruptures and urinary space is occupied by crescents, cellular or fibrous. Podocyte processes present focal effacement.

Clinical Manifestations

RPGN presents as nephritic syndrome with hematuria (dysmoprhic red blood cells), erythrocyte casts, and proteinuria lower than 3g/24h. Rarely proteinuria exceeds 3g/24h, thus nephrotic syndrome is quite uncommon. The onset may be abrupt, manifesting with macroscopic hematuria, edema, and hypertension. Severe or malignant hypertension rarely occurs. Occasionally, patients do not present hematuria, but the reason why this happens is not well understood. Non-specific symptoms of renal failure, such as weakness, malaise, anorexia, vomiting and weight loss may be present. If the disease is progressed, oliguria or anuria with fluid retention is common. In case of Wegener's granulomatosis, Goodpasture syndrome and microscopic polyangiitis, hemoptysis and pulmonary hemorrhage may occur. If this is protracted in time, iron deficiency and anemia may arise. Cutaneous manifestations such as leukocytoplastic vasculitis (also called palpable purpura), ulcerations, erythematous and granulomatous nodules may manifest in case of microscopic polyangiitis, Wegener's granulomatosis, or Churg-Strauss syndrome. Nervous system involvement presents mainly with mononeuritis multiplex and seizures in microscopic polyangiitis and Churg-Strauss syndrome. Abdominal pain and occult gastrointestinal hemorrhage due to ischemic ulceration is relatively common in Churg-Strauss syndrome.

Diagnosis

Accurate and urgent diagnosis is crucial and probably the most important factor affecting prognosis in patients with RPGN. Although renal biopsy is the only diagnostic procedure able to establish a definitive diagnosis and determine the severity of the disease, serologic tests are recommended to always accompany renal biopsy, as they are essential for the identification of underlying conditions. Serology should include antinuclear antibodies (ANA), ANCA anti-MPO and anti-PR3, anti-GBM antibodies, complement components, and cryoglobulins.

ANAs titer is usually negative in patients with ANCA-mediated RPGN. If positive, SLE should be suspected.

ANCAs are best measured with ELISA subtyping and indirect immunofluorescence that present 85% sensitivity and 95% specificity in renal-limited ANCA-mediated RPGN. In case of ANCA, positive vasculitis underlying RPGN, the ANCA type (p-ANCA, c-ANCA) is not pathognomonic as they can both be found in different vasculitis. However, high titer of c-ANCA with PR3 specificity suggests Wegener's granulomatosis, while high titer of p-ANCA with MPO specificity suggests diagnosis of microscopic polyangiitis.

Anti-GBM antibodies are best measured by ELISA and in most of the cases are IgG, while rarely IgAs may be dominant. [157] High titer of anti-GBM antibodies suggests RPGN type I. Of note, Routgers et al, in a review of the Limburg renal biopsy registry reported the coexistence of anti-GBM antibodies along with anti-MPO ANCAs in 46 patients with RPGN. Renal survival was similar to patients with Anti MPO ANCAs only. [158]

In some RPGN patients, neither anti-GBM antibodies nor ANCAs are detected. These patients with the progression of the disease develop pulmonary manifestations such as hemoptysis and pulmonary hemorrhage, suggesting that non-0antibody RPGN belongs to the ANCA positive disorders. [159,160]

Complement component C3 and C4 levels are typically normal in patients with RPGN type I, but may be increased in RPGN type II.

Total blood count usually shows leukocytosis and anemia and in case of Churg-Strauss syndrome, eosinophilia may be present.

Erythrocyte sedimentation rate is in general elevated suggesting active disease.

Serum creatinine levels are elevated, often exceeding 2mg/dL, while serum potassium concentration varies according to the degree of renal failure.

Urinanalysis reveals dysmorphic hematuria with red cell casts and proteinuria. In 24h urine collection, proteinuria ranges from 1 to 4 g/24h although nephrotic range proteinuria is rarely seen in RPGN.

Imaging studies should include renal ultrasound in order to exclude obstructive nephropathy and chest x-ray in cases that Goodpasture syndrome or Wegener's granulomatosis is suspected.

Prognosis

RPGN is in general considered a disease of poor outcome, as renal survival in the absence of specific treatment is less than 6 months. If renal function is impaired at the onset of the disease, ESRD may be reached in a few days or in the best-case scenario, within 3 months. If renal damage is quite extensive with circumferential crescents in more than 85% of the glomeruli, especially if fibrocellular or fibrous with glomerular capillary collapse and sclerosis, prognosis is unfavorable even under specific treatment.

If lesions are limited in less than 30% of the glomeruli, prognosis may be positive, but even in this case spontaneous remissions are extremely rare.

The most important factor affecting outcome in RPGN is the timing of treatment initiation. Whatever the underlying cause is, urgent and accurate diagnosis and rapid specific treatment initiation is essential for renal survival as with early treatment there is a possibility to minimize the degree of irreversible renal damage.

Increased serum creatinine levels associated with oligo-anuria are indicators of extensive renal damage and worse prognosis. However, a certain level of serum creatinine corresponding to irreversible renal damage below which no response will be obtained even under specific aggressive treatment that has not been identified yet. Therefore, empiric therapy with high doses of prednisone should be initiated immediately in patients with severe disease even before biopsy results are obtained.

Pathogenic subtypes of RPGN slightly affect prognosis, as outcomes in both ANA-mediated and anti-GBM antibody-mediated diseases are unfavorable. Double-antibody disease has similar prognosis to ANCA and anti-GBM antibody disease, [161,162] although Rutgers et al., suggest that ANCA/anti-GBM disease has a worse outcome compared to ANCA positive or anti-GBM disease alone. [158] It seems though that high titers of anti-GBM antibodies are more associated with poor prognosis than high ANCA titers. [163]

In contrast, persistence of ANCA positivity even after treatment is associated with higher risk of relapses, especially if antibodies are anti-PR-3 ANCA, [164,165] while anti-GBM glomerulonephritis rarely present relapses, as antibodies usually disappear spontaneously after 12 to 18 months. [166]

Treatment

i. Treatment of Anti-GBM Antibody Disease

The aim of the treatment of anti-GBM disease is to remove the already circulating autoantibodies and prevent their further production. Treatment should be initiated as soon as diagnosis is confirmed or in case renal biopsy results are expected but diagnosis is highly suspected. The therapeutic regimen recommended by the KDIGO guidelines 2012 includes corticosteroids, cyclophosphamide, plus plasmapheresis. [46]

Corticosteroids should be administered intravenously for the first 2 weeks, for 3 consecutive days at doses of 500 to 1000mg/day of methylprednisolone followed by oral prednisone of 1mg/kg/day up to a maximum of 80mg/day. Tapering should follow, over 6 to 9 months. Suggested doses of cyclophosphamide are 2mg/kg/day for up to 3 months. Suggested doses of cyclophosphamide are 2mg/kg/day for up to 3 months. [46]

A large retrospective study conducted in Hammersmith hospital, included 85 patients treated with prednisone at doses of 1mg/kg/day, oral cyclophosphamide at doses of 2 to 3 mg/kg/day and daily plasmapheresis for 14 days or until the anti-GBM antibodies disappeared. [167] The one-year survival ranged from 82 to 100% according to the initial serum creatinine levels.

Plasmapheresis results are quite helpful given that anti-GBM antibodies disappear twice as fast as in patients receiving corticosteroids and cyclophosphamide alone. [168] Sessions of plasmapheresis should be withdrawn when anti-GBM antibodies are not detectable. Thus, anti-GBM antibody titers should be monitored closely.

Extensive renal damage with presence of crescent in 85 to 100% of the glomeruli is associated with poor renal survival and need for renal replacement treatment. These patients usually do not respond even under aggressive therapy and require chronic dialysis treatment. [169] In patients with crescents in 100% of the glomeruli, who are dialysis dependent at the time of diagnosis, no treatment should be initiated since it would be futile, unless pulmonary hemorrhage is present. In that case, aggressive therapy should be administrated independently from the kidney damage and prognosis.

Maintenance therapy is not required in anti-GBM disease as relapses are quite rare, accounting for less than 3%. [167] In most of the cases, anti-GBM antibodies disappear within 12 to 18 months. [166] In case of relapse, the initial treatment should be retaken, as it is effective in re-obtaining remission. [166]

If kidney transplantation is considered, anti-GBM antibodies titers should be monitored regularly and the procedure should take place only after antibodies have been undetectable for at least 6 months, although recurrent anti-GBM disease in kidney transplants is very rare. [170]

ii. Treatment of ANCA Positive Pauci-Immune Glomerulonephritis

Treatment of ANCA-associated pauci-immune glomerulonephritis consists primarily in combination of high dose corticosteroids and cyclophosphamide. This combination has dramatically improved prognosis of ANCA positive diseases, therefore its application in ANCA-associated pauci-immune glomerulonephritis is reasonable. If patients present advanced renal disease requiring dialysis, this treatment may be futile, although a clear end-point over which no response will be obtained, has not yet been identified. In any case, patients with pauci-immune glomerulonephritis associated with extrarenal manifestations should receive treatment regardless the degree of renal damage.

Corticosteroids should be administered at doses of 0.75g/m^2 per day for 3 consecutive days for 3-4 weeks, up to a maximum of 1g/day followed by oral prednisone at doses of 1mg/kg/day up to 60mg for 4 weeks. Prednisone should then be tapered by 10mg/day every week and administered on alternate days for 2 to 3 months.

Others suggest pulses of methylprednisolone at doses of 1gr, [149] while others are more hesitant, using 500mg/day. Till now there are no data demonstrating higher efficacy of

1000mg over 500mg, therefore nephrologists conventionally prefer 500mg-dosing due to better patient tolerance.

Use of corticosteroids as monotherapy is not recommended as patients receiving it, present 3 times higher risk of relapse compared to combination therapy with cyclophosphamide, which improved remission rates from 55 to 85% decreased risk of relapses at about 35%. [165]

Cyclophosphamide can be administered orally or intravenously, as both ways show similar remission and relapsing rates, but use of IV cyclophosphamide seems to be correlated to less and lower intense adverse events, given that the cumulative amount of cyclophosphamide in IV administration is halved. [171,172] Cumulative doses higher than 36g have been related to high risk of malignancy, especially melanomas. [173]

In the oral regimen, cyclophosphamide should be administered at doses of 1.5 to 2mg/kg/day. Doses should be reduced in patients older than 60 years and in patients with severe renal impairment, with GFR lower than 20ml/min. If leukocytes drop to less than 3000/mm^3 doses should also be reduced. [46]

When the intravenous administration is chosen, recommended doses are 0.75g/m^2 every 3 to 4 weeks. [46] An alternative to this regimen is the administration of 15mg/kg IV every 3 weeks for 3 months. In the IV route, as in the oral regimen, age of the patient, GFR, and white cell count should be monitored in order to adjust doses when necessary.

Duration of cyclophosphamide administration should be 3 months, but in some cases, a 6-month course is recommended. Longer treatment courses (up to 12 months) have also been considered, but there are no data suggesting significant difference in renal survival or in relapsing rates compared to 6-month courses. [165]

If after 3 months of therapy, no partial or complete remission is achieved, or if patients' condition requires dialysis, cyclophosphamide should be withdrawn. If patients without severe kidney damage show intolerance or have contraindications for the use of cyclophosphamide, rituximab is an effective alternative. [46] In fact, in two recent RCTs, comparison of cyclophosphamide versus rituximab showed no significant differences in remission or relapsing rates and adverse events. [174,175] Suggested doses of rituximab are 375mg/m^2 every week for 4 weeks or 500mg every week for 4 weeks in combination with methylprednisolone pulses. [46] Use of rituximab in cases of severe kidney dysfunction provided disappointing results. [176] Lack of RCTs analyzing its efficacy and safety, in these cases, limits its use.

Plasmapheresis should be added at the initial combination treatment in case of severe renal dysfunction requiring dialysis, in patients who present rapid increase of serum creatinine levels and in patients with diffuse pulmonary hemorrhage. [149] It should be performed 3 times a week, combined with glucocorticoids and cyclophosphamide in severe renal disease or daily if pulmonary hemorrhage occurs, until hemorrhage stops and then every other day until ANCA antibodies are no longer detectable.

Plasmapheresis is related to higher rates of kidney recovery and reduction of mortality due to alveolar hemorrhage, [149,177] but its efficacy on patients without severe renal disease remains controversial and further investigations are required.

If complete remission is achieved after 3 months of cyclophosphamide plus corticosteroids, maintenance therapy with azathioprine for at least 18 months is recommended. [46] Suggested doses are 1 to 2mg/kg/day. An alternative approach could be low dose of prednisone or continuation of cyclophosphamide. However, long courses of cyclophosphamide do not appear to be superior in maintaining remission compared to azathioprine. [178]

If patients show intolerance of azathioprine or have contraindications, mycophenolate mofetil (MMF) appears to be an alternative although a recent RCT showed higher rates of relapse compared to azathioprine. [179] Suggested doses are 1g twice daily.

If patients are intolerant to both azathioprine and MMF, methotrexate at doses of 0.3mg/kg per week, up to a maximum dose of 25mg/week could also be used. Efficacy is similar to azathioprine but severity of adverse events is greater when methotrexate is used. [180] Methotrexate is contraindicated in patients with severe renal dysfunction (GFR < 30ml/min) and caution at dosing in patients with GFR lower than 60ml/min is advised, due to high risk of adverse events. [46]

If relapses occur, it is recommended to repeat the course of the initial therapy. If patients are resistant to cyclophosphamide plus corticosteroids, rituximab should be added at the initial therapy at doses of $375mg/m^2$ weekly for 4 weeks or 500mg IV for 4 weeks.

In alternative to rituximab, IV immunoglobulin could be used, at doses of 0.5g/kg/day. [181, 182] Although this treatment seems to decrease serum ANCA titers and to be well tolerated by the patients, efficacy and safety remain controversial. Therefore, it is recommended as a rescue therapy in patients resistant to other treatments. [182]

ANCA negative patients are treated with the same regimen as ANCA positive patients, while in double antibody disease; addition of plasmapheresis to immunomodulating treatment is indicated. [46]

Finally, if transplantation is considered, it is wise to delay it until complete remission for at least 12 months is maintained. [183] Titers of ANCAs should be monitored before transplantation is performed, although it doesn't appear to be an association between ANCA titers and recurrence in transplantation. [183] The overall recurrence of ANCA positive pauci-immune glomerulonephritis in kidney transplant recipients is around 5%.

References

[1] D'Amico G. The commonest glomerulonephritis in the world: IgA nephropathy. *Q. J. Med.* 1987 Sep;64(245):709-27.

[2] Huang HD, Lin FJ, Li XJ, Wang LR, Jiang GR. Genetic polymorphisms of the renin-angiotensin-aldosterone system in Chinese patients with end-stage renal disease secondary to IgA nephropathy. *Chin. Med. J.* (Engl). 2010 Nov;123(22):3238-42.

[3] Berger J, Hinglais N. [Intercapillary deposits of IgA-IgG*]. J. Urol. Nephrol.* (Paris). 1968 Sep;74(9):694-5. [Article in French]

[4] Donadio JV, Grande JP. IgA nephropathy. N Engl J Med. 2002 Sep 5;347(10):738-48.

[5] Alexopoulos E. Treatment of primary IgA nephropathy. *Kidney Int.* 2004 Jan;65(1):341-55.

[6] Geddes CC, Rauta V, Gronhagen-Riska C, Bartosik LP, Jardine AG, Ibels LS, et al. A tricontinental view of IgA nephropathy. *Nephrol. Dial Transplant.* 2003 Aug;18(8):1541-8.

[7] Mubarak M. The Oxford classification of IgA nephropathy: a role model for classifying other renal diseases. *Saudi J. Kidney Dis Transpl.* 2011 Sep;22(5):897-900.

[8] Mubarak M. Oxford classification of IgA nephropathy: Broadening the scope of the classification. *J. Nephropathol.* 2012 Apr;1(1):13-6.

[9] Working Group of the International IgA Nephropathy Network and the Renal Pathology Society, Cattran DC, Coppo R, Cook HT, Feehally J, Roberts IS, Troyanov S, et al. The Oxford classification of IgA nephropathy: rationale, clinicopathological correlations, and classification. *Kidney Int.* 2009 Sep;76(5):534-45.

[10] Berthoux F, Mohey H, Laurent B, Mariat C, Afiani A, Thibaudin L. Predicting the risk for dialysis or death in IgA nephropathy. *J. Am. Soc. Nephrol.* 2011 Apr;22(4):752-61.

[11] Nair R, Walker PD. Is IgA nephropathy the commonest primary glomerulopathy among young adults in the USA? *Kidney Int.* 2006 Apr;69(8):1455-8.

[12] US Renal Data System: Annual Data Report 2013, Reference Tables: ESRD, Vol. 2 : 335-358.

[13] Barratt J, Feehally J, Smith AC. Pathogenesis of IgA nephropathy. *Semin. Nephrol.* 2004 May;24(3):197-217.

[14] Barratt J, Eitner F, Feehally J, Floege J. Immune complex formation in IgA nephropathy: a case of the 'right' antibodies in the 'wrong' place at the 'wrong' time? *Nephrol. Dial Transplant.* 2009 Dec;24(12):3620-3.

[15] Gharavi AG, Moldoveanu Z, Wyatt RJ, Barker CV, Woodford SY, Lifton RP, et al. Aberrant IgA1 glycosylation is inherited in familial and sporadic IgA nephropathy. *J Am. Soc. Nephrol.* 2008 May;19(5):1008-14.

[16] Brezzi B, Del Prete D, Lupo A, Magistroni R, Gomez-Lira M, Bernich P, et al. Primary IgA nephropathy is more severe in TGF-beta1 high secretor patients. *J. Nephrol.* 2009 Nov-Dec;22(6):747-59.

[17] Lai KN, Leung JC, Chan LY, Saleem MA, Mathieson PW, Tam KY, et al. Podocyte injury induced by mesangial-derived cytokines in IgA nephropathy. N*ephrol. Dial Transplant.* 2009 Jan;24(1):62-72.

[18] Xue C, Nie W, Xu J, Dai B, Mei CL. C509T and T869C polymorphisms of transforming growth factor β1 and the risk of IgA nephropathy: a meta-analysis. *Chin. Med. J.* (Engl). 2013 Dec;126(23):4562-7.

[19] Beerman I, Novak J, Wyatt RJ, Julian BA, Gharavi AG. The genetics of IgA nephropathy. *Nat. Clin. Pract. Nephrol.* 2007 Jun;3(6):325-38.

[20] Harden PN, Geddes C, Rowe PA, McIlroy JH, Boulton-Jones M, Rodger RS, et al. Polymorphisms in angiotensin-converting-enzyme gene and progression of IgA nephropathy. *Lancet.* 1995 Jun 17;345(8964):1540-2.

[21] Suzuki S, Suzuki Y, Kobayashi Y, Harada T, Kawamura T, Yoshida H, et al. Insertion/deletion polymorphism in ACE gene is not associated with renal progression in Japanese patients with IgA nephropathy. *Am. J. Kidney Dis.* 2000 May;35(5):896-903.

[22] Frimat L, Philippe C, Maghakian MN, Jonveaux P, Hurault de Ligny B, Guillemin F, et al. Polymorphism of angiotensin converting enzyme, angiotensinogen, and angiotensin II type 1 receptor genes and end-stage renal failure in IgA nephropathy: IGARAS--a study of 274 Men. J. Am. Soc. Nephrol. 2000 Nov;11(11):2062-7.

[23] Xia YF, Huang S, Li X, Yang N, Huang J, Xue C, et al. A family-based association study of megsin A23167G polymorphism with susceptibility and progression of IgA nephropathy in a Chinese population. Clin. Nephrol. 2006 Mar;65(3):153-9.

[24] Goto M, Wakai K, Kawamura T, Ando M, Endoh M, Tomino Y. A scoring system to predict renal outcome in IgA nephropathy: a nationwide 10-year prospective cohort study. *Nephrol. Dial. Transplant.* 2009 Oct;24(10):3068-74.

[25] D'Amico G, Napodano P, Ferrario F, Rastaldi MP, Arrigo G. Idiopathic IgA nephropathy with segmental necrotizing lesions of the capillary wall. *Kidney Int.* 2001 Feb;59(2):682-92.

[26] Tomino Y, Sakai H; Special Study Group (IgA Nephropathy) on Progressive Glomerular Disease. Clinical guidelines for immunoglobulin A (IgA) nephropathy in Japan, second version. *Clin. Exp. Nephrol.* 2003 Jun;7(2):93-7.

[27] Herzenberg AM, Fogo AB, Reich HN, Troyanov S, Bavbek N, Massat AE, et al. Validation of the Oxford classification of IgA nephropathy. *Kidney Int.* 2011 Aug;80(3):310-7.

[28] Shi SF, Wang SX, Jiang L, Lv JC, Liu LJ, Chen YQ, et al. Pathologic predictors of renal outcome and therapeutic efficacy in IgA nephropathy: validation of the Oxford classification. *Clin. J. Am. Soc. Nephrol.* 2011 Sep;6(9):2175-84.

[29] Nasri H, Sajjadieh S, Mardani S, Momeni A, Merikhi A, Madihi Y, et al. Correlation of immunostaining findings with demographic data and variables of Oxford classification in IgA nephropathy. *J. Nephropathol.* 2013 Jul;2(3):190-5.

[30] Ohsawa I, Kusaba G, Ishii M, Sato N, Inoshita H, Onda K, et al. Extraglomerular C3 deposition and metabolic impacts in patients with IgA nephropathy. *Nephrol. Dial Transplant.* 2013 Jul;28(7):1856-64.

[31] Tang Z, Wu Y, Wang QW, Yu YS, Hu WX, Yao XD, et al. Idiopathic IgA nephropathy with diffuse crescent formation. *Am. J. Nephrol.* 2002 Sep-Dec;22(5-6):480-6.

[32] Reich HN, Troyanov S, Scholey JW, Cattran DC; Toronto Glomerulonephritis Registry. Remission of proteinuria improves prognosis in IgA nephropathy. *J. Am. Soc. Nephrol.* 2007 Dec;18(12):3177-83.

[33] Zhou J, Chen Y, Liu Y, Shi S, Li X, Wang S, et al. Plasma uric acid level indicates tubular interstitial leisions at early stage of IgA nephropathy. *BMC Nephrol.* 2014 Jan 14;15(1):11.

[34] Kalantari S, Rutishauser D, Samavat S, Nafar M, Mahmudieh L, Rezaei-Tavirani M, et al. Urinary prognostic biomarkers and classification of IgA nephropathy by high resolution mass spectrometry coupled with liquid chromatography. *PLoS One.* 2013 Dec 5;8(12):e80830.

[35] Zhou J, Chen Y, Liu Y, Shi S, Wang S, Li X, et al. Urinary uromodulin excretion predicts progression of chronic kidney disease resulting from IgA nephropathy. *PLoS One.* 2013 Aug 22;8(8):e71023.

[36] Maiguma M, Suzuki Y, Suzuki H, Okazaki K, Aizawa M, Muto M, et al. Dietary zinc is a key environmental modifier in the progression of IgA nephropathy. *PLoS One.* 2014 Feb 28;9(2):e90558.

[37] Tanaka S, Ninomiya T, Katafuchi R, Masutani K, Tsuchimoto A, Noguchi H, et al. Development and validation of a prediction rule using the Oxford classification in IgA nephropathy. *Clin. J. Am. Soc. Nephrol.* 2013 Dec;8(12):2082-90.

[38] Harmankaya O, Oztürk Y, Baştürk T, Obek A, Kiliçarslan I. Efficacy of immunosuppressive therapy in IgA nephropathy presenting with isolated hematuria. *Int. Urol. Nephrol.* 2002;33(1):167-71.

[39] Sarafidis PA, Khosla N, Bakris GL. Antihypertensive therapy in the presence of proteinuria. Am. J. Kidney Dis. 2007 Jan;49(1):12-26.

[40] Gharavi AG, Yan Y, Scolari F, Schena FP, Frasca GM, Ghiggeri GM, et al. IgA nephropathy, the most common cause of glomerulonephritis, is linked to 6q22-23. *Nat Genet.* 2000 Nov;26(3):354-7.

[41] Li PK, Kwan BC, Chow KM, Leung CB, Szeto CC. Treatment of early immunoglobulin A nephropathy by angiotensin-converting enzyme inhibitor. *Am. J. Med.* 2013 Feb;126(2):162-8.

[42] Yang Y, Ohta K, Shimizu M, Nakai A, Kasahara Y, Yachie A, et al. Treatment with low-dose angiotensin-converting enzyme inhibitor (ACEI) plus angiotensin II receptor blocker (ARB) in pediatric patients with IgA nephropathy. *Clin. Nephrol.* 2005 Jul;64(1):35-40.

[43] Donadio JV, Grande JP. The role of fish oil/omega-3 fatty acids in the treatment of IgA nephropathy. *Semin. Nephrol.* 2004 May;24(3):225-43.

[44] Hogg RJ, Lee J, Nardelli N, Julian BA, Cattran D, Waldo B, et al; Southwest Pediatric Nephrology Study Group. Clinical trial to evaluate omega-3 fatty acids and alternate day prednisone in patients with IgA nephropathy: report from the Southwest Pediatric Nephrology Study Group. *Clin J Am Soc Nephrol.* 2006 May;1(3):467-74.

[45] Hogg RJ, Fitzgibbons L, Atkins C, Nardelli N, Bay RC; North American IgA Nephropathy Study Group. Efficacy of omega-3 fatty acids in children and adults with IgA nephropathy is dosage- and size-dependent. *Clin. J. Am. Soc. Nephrol.* 2006 Nov;1(6):1167-72.

[46] Kidney Disease: Improving Global Outcomes (KDIGO) Glomerulonephritis Work Group. KDIGO Clinical Practice Guideline for Glomerulonephritis. *Kidney inter.,* Suppl. 2012; 2: 139–274.

[47] Lv J, Xu D, Perkovic V, Ma X, Johnson DW, Woodward M, et al; TESTING Study Group. Corticosteroid therapy in IgA nephropathy. *J. Am. Soc. Nephrol.* 2012 Jun;23(6):1108-16.

[48] Pozzi C, Bolasco PG, Fogazzi GB, Andrulli S, Altieri P, Ponticelli C, et al. Corticosteroids in IgA nephropathy: a randomised controlled trial. *Lancet.* 1999 Mar 13;353(9156):883-7.

[49] Pozzi C, Andrulli S, Del Vecchio L, Melis P, Fogazzi GB, Altieri P, Ponticelli C, Locatelli F. Corticosteroid effectiveness in IgA nephropathy: long-term results of a randomized, controlled trial. *J. Am. Soc. Nephrol.* 2004 Jan;15(1):157-63.

[50] Manno C, Torres DD, Rossini M, Pesce F, Schena FP. Randomized controlled clinical trial of corticosteroids plus ACE-inhibitors with long-term follow-up in proteinuric IgA nephropathy. *Nephrol. Dial Transplant.* 2009 Dec;24(12):3694-701.

[51] Ballardie FW, Roberts IS. Controlled prospective trial of prednisolone and cytotoxics in progressive IgA nephropathy. *J. Am. Soc. Nephrol.* 2002 Jan;13(1):142-8.

[52] Pozzi C, Andrulli S, Pani A, Scaini P, Del Vecchio L, Fogazzi G, et al. Addition of azathioprine to corticosteroids does not benefit patients with IgA nephropathy. *J. Am. Soc. Nephrol.* 2010 Oct;21(10):1783-90.

[53] Kim YC, Chin HJ, Koo HS, Kim S. Tacrolimus decreases albuminuria in patients with IgA nephropathy and normal blood pressure: a double-blind randomized controlled trial of efficacy of tacrolimus on IgA nephropathy. *PLoS One.* 2013 Aug 19;8(8):e71545.

[54] Chen X, Chen P, Cai G, Wu J, Cui Y, Zhang Y, et al. [A randomized control trial of mycophenolate mofeil treatment in severe IgA nephropathy]. Zhonghua Yi Xue Za Zhi. 2002 Jun 25;82(12):796-801. [Article in Chinese]

[55] Tang SC, Tang AW, Wong SS, Leung JC, Ho YW, Lai KN. Long-term study of mycophenolate mofetil treatment in IgA nephropathy. *Kidney Int.* 2010 Mar;77(6): 543-9.

[56] Onishi A, Sugiyama D, Tsuji G, Nakazawa T, Kogata Y, Tsuda K, et al. Mycophenolate mofetil versus intravenous cyclophosphamide for induction treatment of proliferative lupus nephritis in a Japanese population: a retrospective study. *Mod. Rheumatol.* 2013 Jan;23(1):89-96.

[57] Xie Y, Chen X, Nishi S, Narita I, Gejyo F. Relationship between tonsils and IgA nephropathy as well as indications of tonsillectomy. *Kidney Int.* 2004 Apr;65(4):1135-44.

[58] Akagi H, Kosaka M, Hattori K, Doi A, Fukushima K, Okano M, et al. Long-term results of tonsillectomy as a treatment for IgA nephropathy. *Acta. Otolaryngol. Suppl.* 2004 Dec;(555):38-42.

[59] Komatsu H, Fujimoto S, Hara S, Sato Y, Yamada K, Kitamura K. Effect of tonsillectomy plus steroid pulse therapy on clinical remission of IgA nephropathy: a controlled study. *Clin. J. Am. Soc. Nephrol.* 2008 Sep;3(5):1301-7.

[60] Kawamura T, Yoshimura M, Miyazaki Y, Okamoto H, Kimura K, Hirano K, et al; The Special IgA Nephropathy Study Group. A multicenter randomized controlled trial of tonsillectomy combined with steroid pulse therapy in patients with immunoglobulin A nephropathy. *Nephrol. Dial Transplant.* 2014 Mar 3. [Epub ahead of print]

[61] Wang Y, Chen J, Wang Y, Chen Y, Wang L, Lv Y. A meta-analysis of the clinical remission rate and long-term efficacy of tonsillectomy in patients with IgA nephropathy. *Nephrol. Dial Transplant.* 2011 Jun;26(6):1923-31.

[62] Kaneko T, Shimizu A, Tsuruoka S, Iino Y, Katayama Y. Efficacy of steroid pulse therapy in combination with mizoribine following tonsillectomy for immunoglobulin A nephropathy in renally impaired patients. *J. Nippon. Med. Sch.* 2013;80(4):279-86.

[63] Rostoker G, Desvaux-Belghiti D, Pilatte Y, Petit-Phar M, Philippon C, Deforges L, et al. High-dose immunoglobulin therapy for severe IgA nephropathy and Henoch-Schönlein purpura. *Ann. Intern. Med.* 1994 Mar 15;120(6):476-84.

[64] Coppo R, Basolo B, Giachino O, Roccatello D, Lajolo D, Mazzucco G, et al. Plasmapheresis in a patient with rapidly progressive idiopathic IgA nephropathy: removal of IgA-containing circulating immune complexes and clinical recovery. *Nephron.* 1985;40(4):488-90.

[65] Tumlin JA, Lohavichan V, Hennigar R. Crescentic, proliferative IgA nephropathy: clinical and histological response to methylprednisolone and intravenous cyclophosphamide. *Nephrol. Dial Transplant.* 2003 Jul;18(7):1321-9.

[66] Pankhurst T, Lepenies J, Nightingale P, Howie AJ, Adu D, Harper L. Vasculitic IgA nephropathy: prognosis and outcome. *Nephron. Clin. Pract.* 2009;112(1):c16-24.

[67] Rodriguez-Iturbe B, Musser JM. The current state of poststreptococcal glomerulonephritis. *J. Am. Soc. Nephrol.* 2008 Oct;19(10):1855-64.

[68] Nadasdy T, Hebert LA. Infection-related glomerulonephritis: understanding mechanisms. *Semin.Nephrol.* 2011 Jul;31(4):369-75.

[69] Blyth CC, Robertson PW, Rosenberg AR. Post-streptococcal glomerulonephritis in Sydney: a 16-year retrospective review. *J. Paediatr. Child Health.* 2007 Jun;43(6): 446-50.

[70] Sanjad S, Tolaymat A, Whitworth J, Levin S. Acute glomerulonephritis in children: a review of 153 cases. *South Med. J.* 1977 Oct;70(10):1202-6.

[71] Nordstrand A, Norgren M, Holm SE. Pathogenic mechanism of acute post-streptococcal glomerulonephritis. *Scand. J. Infect Dis.* 1999;31(6):523-37.

[72] Rodríguez-Iturbe B, Batsford S. Pathogenesis of poststreptococcal glomerulonephritis a century after Clemens von Pirquet. *Kidney Int.* 2007 Jun;71(11):1094-104.

[73] Kraus W, Dale JB, Beachey EH. Identification of an epitope of type 1 streptococcal M protein that is shared with a 43-kDa protein of human myocardium and renal glomeruli. *J. Immunol.* 1990 Dec 15;145(12):4089-93.

[74] Kefalides NA, Pegg MT, Ohno N, Poon-King T, Zabriskie J, Fillit H. Antibodies to basement membrane collagen and to laminin are present in sera from patients with poststreptococcal glomerulonephritis. *J. Exp. Med.* 1986 Mar 1;163(3):588-602.

[75] Ohsawa I, Ohi H, Endo M, Fujita T, Matsushita M, Fujita T. Evidence of lectin complement pathway activation in poststreptococcal glomerulonephritis. *Kidney Int.* 1999 Sep;56(3):1158-9.

[76] Skattum L, Akesson P, Truedsson L, Sjöholm AG. Antibodies against four proteins from a Streptococcus pyogenes serotype M1 strain and levels of circulating mannan-binding lectin in acute poststreptococcal glomerulonephritis. *Int. Arch. Allergy Immunol.* 2006;140(1):9-19.

[77] Levy M, Sich M, Pirotzky E, Habib R. Complement activation in acute glomerulonephritis in children. *Int. J. Pediatr. Nephrol.* 1985 Jan-Mar;6(1):17-24.

[78] García R, Rubio L, Rodríguez-Iturbe B. Long-term prognosis of epidemic poststreptococcal glomerulonephritis in Maracaibo: follow-up studies 11-12 years after the acute episode. *Clin. Nephrol.* 1981 Jun;15(6):291-8.

[79] Peake PW, Pussell BA, Karplus TE, Riley EH, Charlesworth JA. Post-streptococcal glomerulonephritis: studies on the interaction between nephritis strain-associated protein (NSAP), complement, and the glomerulus. *APMIS.* 1991 May;99(5):460-6.

[80] Winram SB, Lottenberg R. The plasmin-binding protein Plr of group A streptococci is identified as glyceraldehyde-3-phosphate dehydrogenase. *Microbiology.* 1996 Aug;142 (Pt 8):2311-20.

[81] Yoshizawa N, Yamakami K, Fujino M, Oda T, Tamura K, Matsumoto K, et al. Nephritis-associated plasmin receptor and acute poststreptococcal glomerulonephritis: characterization of the antigen and associated immune response. *J. Am. Soc. Nephrol.* 2004 Jul;15(7):1785-93.

[82] Mosquera J, Romero M, Viera N, Rincon J, Pedreáñez A. Could streptococcal erythrogenic toxin B induce inflammation prior to the development of immune complex deposits in poststreptococcal glomerulonephritis? *Nephron. Exp. Nephrol.* 2007;105(2):e41-4.

[83] Bakr A, Mahmoud LA, Al-Chenawi F, Salah A. HLA-DRB1* alleles in Egyptian children with post-streptococcal acute glomerulonephritis. *Pediatr. Nephrol.* 2007 Mar;22(3):376-9.

[84] Ahn SY, Ingulli E. Acute poststreptococcal glomerulonephritis: an update. *Curr. Opin. Pediatr.* 2008 Apr;20(2):157-62.

[85] Dursun H, Noyan A, Matyar S, Buyukcelik M, Soran M, Cengiz N, et al. Endothelial nitric oxide synthase gene intron 4 a/b VNTR polymorphism in children with APSGN. *Pediatr. Nephrol.* 2006 Nov;21(11):1661-5.

[86] Shet A, Kaplan EL, Johnson DR, Cleary PP. Immune response to group A streptococcal C5a peptidase in children: implications for vaccine development. *J. Infect. Dis.* 2003 Sep 15;188(6):809-17.

[87] Markowitz M. Changing epidemiology of group A streptococcal infections. *Pediatr. Infect. Dis. J.* 1994 Jun;13(6):557-60.

[88] Ilyas M, Tolaymat A. Changing epidemiology of acute post-streptococcal glomerulonephritis in Northeast Florida: a comparative study. *Pediatr. Nephrol.* 2008 Jul;23(7):1101-6.

[89] Yoshizawa N. Acute glomerulonephritis. *Intern. Med.* 2000 Sep;39(9):687-94.

[90] Carapetis JR, Steer AC, Mulholland EK, Weber M. The global burden of group A streptococcal diseases. *Lancet Infect. Dis.* 2005 Nov;5(11):685-94.

[91] Sorger K, Gessler U, Hübner FK, Köhler H, Schulz W, Stühlinger W, et al. Subtypes of acute post-infectious glomerulonephritis. Synopsis of clinical and pathological features. *Clin Nephrol.* 1982 Mar;17(3):114-28.

[92] Yap HK, Chia KS, Murugasu B, Saw AH, Tay JS, Ikshuvanam M, et al. Acute glomerulonephritis--changing patterns in Singapore children. *Pediatr. Nephrol.* 1990 Sep;4(5):482-4.

[93] Bergholm AM, Holm SE. Effect of early penicillin treatment on the development of experimental poststreptococcal glomerulonephritis. *Acta. Pathol. Microbiol. Immunol.* Scand C. 1983 Aug;91(4):271-81.

[94] Zeledon JI, McKelvey RL, Servilla KS, Hofinger D, Konstantinov KN, Kellie S, et al. Glomerulonephritis causing acute renal failure during the course of bacterial infections. Histological varieties, potential pathogenetic pathways, and treatment. *Int. Urol. Nephrol.* 2008;40(2):461-70.

[95] Okuyama S, Wakui H, Maki N, Kuroki J, Nishinari T, Asakura K, et al. Successful treatment of post-MRSA infection glomerulonephritis with steroid therapy. *Clin. Nephrol.* 2008 Oct;70(4):344-7.

[96] Raff A, Hebert T, Pullman J, Coco M. Crescentic post-streptococcal glomerulonephritis with nephrotic syndrome in the adult: is aggressive therapy warranted? *Clin. Nephrol.* 2005 May;63(5):375-80.

[97] Suyama K, Kawasaki Y, Suzuki H. Girl with garland-pattern poststreptococcal acute glomerulonephritis presenting with renal failure and nephrotic syndrome. *Pediatr. Int.* 2007 Feb;49(1):115-7.

[98] Roy S 3rd, Murphy WM, Arant BS Jr. Poststreptococcal crescenteric glomerulonephritis in children: comparison of quintuple therapy versus supportive care. *J. Pediatr.* 1981 Mar;98(3):403-10.

[99] Moroni G, Pozzi C, Quaglini S, Segagni S, Banfi G, Baroli A, et al. Long-term prognosis of diffuse proliferative glomerulonephritis associated with infection in adults. *Nephrol. Dial Transplant.* 2002 Jul;17(7):1204-11.

[100] Baldwin DS, Gluck MC, Schacht RG, Gallo G. The long-term course of poststreptococcal glomerulonephritis. *Ann. Intern. Med.* 1974 Mar;80(3):342-58.

[101] Chui SH, Lam CW, Lewis WH, Lai KN. Light-chain ratio of serum IgA1 in IgA nephropathy. *J. Clin. Immunol.* 1991 Jul;11(4):219-23.

[102] Nasr SH, Markowitz GS, Whelan JD, Albanese JJ, Rosen RM, Fein DA, et al. IgA-dominant acute poststaphylococcal glomerulonephritis complicating diabetic nephropathy. *Hum. Pathol.* 2003 Dec;34(12):1235-41.

[103] Haas M, Racusen LC, Bagnasco SM. IgA-dominant postinfectious glomerulonephritis: a report of 13 cases with common ultrastructural features. *Hum. Pathol.* 2008 Sep;39(9):1309-16.

[104] Wen YK, Chen ML. Discrimination between postinfectious IgA-dominant glomerulonephritis and idiopathic IgA nephropathy. Ren. Fail. 2010 Jun;32(5):572-7.

[105] Sethi S, Fervenza FC. Membranoproliferative glomerulonephritis: pathogenetic heterogeneity and proposal for a new classification. *Semin. Nephrol.* 2011 Jul;31(4):341-8.

[106] Smith RJ, Alexander J, Barlow PN, Botto M, Cassavant TL, Cook HT, et al; Dense Deposit Disease Focus Group. New approaches to the treatment of dense deposit disease. *J Am Soc Nephrol.* 2007 Sep;18(9):2447-56.

[107] Fabrizi F. Hepatitis C virus, cryoglobulinemia, and kidney: novel evidence. *Scientifica* (Cairo). 2012;2012:128382.

[108] Lhotta K, Würzner R, König P. Glomerular deposition of mannose-binding lectin in human glomerulonephritis. *Nephrol. Dial Transplant.* 1999 Apr;14(4):881-6.

[109] Zipfel PF, Skerka C. Complement regulators and inhibitory proteins. *Nat. Rev. Immunol.* 2009 Oct;9(10):729-40.

[110] Ferreira VP, Pangburn MK, Cortés C. Complement control protein factor H: the good, the bad, and the inadequate. *Mol. Immunol.* 2010 Aug;47(13):2187-97.

[111] West CD, Witte DP, McAdams AJ. Composition of nephritic factor-generated glomerular deposits in membranoproliferative glomerulonephritis type 2. *Am. J. Kidney Dis.* 2001 Jun;37(6):1120-30.

[112] Frémeaux-Bacchi V, Weiss L, Demouchy C, May A, Palomera S, Kazatchkine MD. Hypocomplementaemia of poststreptococcal acute glomerulonephritis is associated with C3 nephritic factor (C3NeF) IgG autoantibody activity. *Nephrol. Dial Transplant.* 1994;9(12):1747-50.

[113] Gewurz AT, Imherr SM, Strauss S, Gewurz H, Mold C. C3 nephritic factor and hypocomplementaemia in a clinically healthy individual. *Clin. Exp. Immunol.* 1983 Oct;54(1):253-8.

[114] Abrera-Abeleda MA, Nishimura C, Smith JL, Sethi S, McRae JL, Murphy BF, et al. Variations in the complement regulatory genes factor H (CFH) and factor H related 5 (CFHR5) are associated with membranoproliferative glomerulonephritis type II (dense deposit disease*). J. Med. Genet.* 2006 Jul;43(7):582-9.

[115] Abrera-Abeleda MA, Nishimura C, Frees K, Jones M, Maga T, Katz LM, et al. Allelic variants of complement genes associated with dense deposit disease. *J. Am. Soc. Nephrol.* 2011 Aug;22(8):1551-9.

[116] Levy M, Halbwachs-Mecarelli L, Gubler MC, Kohout G, Bensenouci A, Niaudet P, et al. H deficiency in two brothers with atypical dense intramembranous deposit disease. *Kidney Int.* 1986 Dec;30(6):949-56.

[117] Pickering MC, Cook HT. Translational mini-review series on complement factor H: renal diseases associated with complement factor H: novel insights from humans and animals. *Clin. Exp. Immunol.* 2008 Feb;151(2):210-30.

[118] Gale DP, de Jorge EG, Cook HT, Martinez-Barricarte R, Hadjisavvas A, McLean AG, et al. Identification of a mutation in complement factor H-related protein 5 in patients of Cypriot origin with glomerulonephritis. *Lancet*. 2010 Sep 4;376(9743):794-801.

[119] Athanasiou Y, Voskarides K, Gale DP, Damianou L, Patsias C, Zavros M, et al. Familial C3 glomerulopathy associated with CFHR5 mutations: clinical characteristics of 91 patients in 16 pedigrees. *Clin. J. Am. Soc. Nephrol*. 2011 Jun;6(6):1436-46.

[120] Heurich M, Martínez-Barricarte R, Francis NJ, Roberts DL, Rodríguez de Córdoba S, Morgan BP, et al. Common polymorphisms in C3, factor B, and factor H collaborate to determine systemic complement activity and disease risk. *Proc. Natl. Acad. Sci. U S A*. 2011 May 24;108(21):8761-6.

[121] West CD, McAdams AJ. Membranoproliferative glomerulonephritis type III: association of glomerular deposits with circulating nephritic factor-stabilized convertase. *Am. J. Kidney Dis*. 1998 Jul;32(1):56-63.

[122] Neary JJ, Conlon PJ, Croke D, Dorman A, Keogan M, Zhang FY, et al. Linkage of a gene causing familial membranoproliferative glomerulonephritis type III to chromosome 1. *J. Am. Soc. Nephrol*. 2002 Aug;13(8):2052-7.

[123] Licht C, Schlötzer-Schrehardt U, Kirschfink M, Zipfel PF, Hoppe B. MPGN II-genetically determined by defective complement regulation? *Pediatr. Nephrol*. 2007 Jan;22(1):2-9.

[124] Nakopoulou L. Membranoproliferative glomerulonephritis. *Nephrol. Dial Transplant*. 2001;16 Suppl 6:71-3.

[125] Burkholder PM, Marchand A, Krueger RP. Mixed membranous and proliferative glomerulonephritis. A correlative light, immunofluorescence, and electron microscopic study. *Lab. Invest*. 1970 Nov;23(5):459-79.

[126] Fervenza FC, Sethi S, Glassock RJ. Idiopathic membranoproliferative glomerulonephritis: does it exist? *Nephrol. Dial Transplant*. 2012 Dec;27(12):4288-94.

[127] Strife CF, McEnery PT, McAdams AJ, West CD. Membranoproliferative glomerulonephritis with disruption of the glomerular basement membrane. *Clin. Nephrol*. 1977 Feb;7(2):65-72.

[128] Anders D. [Membranoproliferative glomerulonephritis]. *Dtsch Med. Wochenschr*. 1977 Sep 9;102(36):1295-6. [Article in German]

[129] Royer P, Habib R, Vermeil G, Mathieu H, Alizon M. [Prolonged glomerulonephritis in children. Apropos of 4 anatomical aspects revealed by renal biopsy]. Ann Pediatr (Paris). 1962 Mar 2;9:173-87. [Article in French]

[130] Glassock, R. J. (2009) Membranoproliferative Glomerulonephritis, in Evidence-Based Nephrology (eds D. A. Molony and J. C. Craig), Wiley-Blackwell, Oxford, UK.

[131] Kidney Disease: Improving Global Outcomes (KDIGO) CKD Work Group. KDIGO 2012 Clinical Practice Guideline for the Evaluation and Management of Chronic Kidney Disease. *Kidney inter*., Suppl.2013;3:1–150.

[132] Braun MC, West CD, Strife CF. Differences between membranoproliferative glomerulonephritis types I and III in long-term response to an alternate-day prednisone regimen. *Am. J. Kidney Dis*. 1999 Dec;34(6):1022-32.

[133] Levin A. Management of membranoproliferative glomerulonephritis: evidence-based recommendations. *Kidney Int Suppl*. 1999 Jun;70:S41-6.

[134] Jones G, Juszczak M, Kingdon E, Harber M, Sweny P, Burns A. Treatment of idiopathic membranoproliferative glomerulonephritis with mycophenolate mofetil and steroids. *Nephrol. Dial Transplant.* 2004 Dec;19(12):3160-4.

[135] Kiyomasu T, Shibata M, Kurosu H, Shiraishi K, Hashimoto H, Hayashidera T, et al. Cyclosporin A treatment for membranoproliferative glomerulonephritis type II. Nephron. 2002 Jul;91(3):509-11.

[136] Haddad M, Lau K, Butani L. Remission of membranoproliferative glomerulonephritis type I with the use of tacrolimus. *Pediatr. Nephrol.* 2007 Oct;22(10):1787-91.

[137] Krmar RT, Holtbäck U, Linné T, Berg UB, Celsi G, Söderberg MP, et al. Acute renal failure in dense deposit disease: complete recovery after combination therapy with immunosuppressant and plasma exchange. *Clin. Nephrol.* 2011 Feb;75 Suppl 1:4-10.

[138] Cattran DC, Cardella CJ, Roscoe JM, Charron RC, Rance PC, Ritchie SM, et al. Results of a controlled drug trial in membranoproliferative glomerulonephritis. *Kidney Int.* 1985 Feb;27(2):436-41.

[139] Kamar N, Rostaing L, Alric L. Treatment of hepatitis C-virus-related glomerulonephritis. *Kidney Int.* 2006 Feb;69(3):436-9.

[140] Bayazit AK, Noyan A, Cengiz N, Anarat A. Mycophenolate mofetil in children with multidrug-resistant nephrotic syndrome. *Clin. Nephrol.* 2004 Jan;61(1):25-9.

[141] Jayne D. Role of rituximab therapy in glomerulonephritis. *J. Am. Soc. Nephrol.* 2010 Jan;21(1):14-7.

[142] Bestard O, Cruzado JM, Ercilla G, Gomà M, Torras J, Serón D, et al. Rituximab induces regression of hepatitis C virus-related membranoproliferative glomerulonephritis in a renal allograft. *Nephrol. Dial Transplant.* 2006 Aug;21(8):2320-4.

[143] Dillon JJ, Hladunewich M, Haley WE, Reich HN, Cattran DC, Fervenza FC. Rituximab therapy for Type I membranoproliferative glomerulonephritis. *Clin. Nephrol.* 2012 Apr;77(4):290-5.

[144] Hillmen P, Young NS, Schubert J, Brodsky RA, Socié G, Muus P, et al. The complement inhibitor eculizumab in paroxysmal nocturnal hemoglobinuria. *N. Engl. J. Med.* 2006 Sep 21;355(12):1233-43.

[145] Legendre CM, Licht C, Muus P, Greenbaum LA, Babu S, Bedrosian C, et al. Terminal complement inhibitor eculizumab in atypical hemolytic-uremic syndrome. *N. Engl. J. Med.* 2013 Jun 6;368(23):2169-81.

[146] Radhakrishnan S, Lunn A, Kirschfink M, Thorner P, Hebert D, Langlois V, et al. Eculizumab and refractory membranoproliferative glomerulonephritis. *N. Engl. J. Med.* 2012 Mar 22;366(12):1165-6.

[147] Bomback AS, Smith RJ, Barile GR, Zhang Y, Heher EC, Herlitz L, et al. Eculizumab for dense deposit disease and C3 glomerulonephritis. *Clin. J. Am. Soc. Nephrol.* 2012 May;7(5):748-56.

[148] McCaughan JA, O'Rourke DM, Courtney AE. Recurrent dense deposit disease after renal transplantation: an emerging role for complementary therapies. *Am. J. Transplant.* 2012 Apr;12(4):1046-51.

[149] Jayne DR, Gaskin G, Rasmussen N, Abramowicz D, Ferrario F, Guillevin L, et al; European Vasculitis Study Group. Randomized trial of plasma exchange or high-dosage methylprednisolone as adjunctive therapy for severe renal vasculitis. *J. Am. Soc Nephrol.* 2007 Jul;18(7):2180-8.

[150] Hudson BG, Tryggvason K, Sundaramoorthy M, Neilson EG. Alport's syndrome, Goodpasture's syndrome, and type IV collagen. *N. Engl. J. Med.* 2003 Jun 19;348(25):2543-56.
[151] Kettritz R, Jennette JC, Falk RJ. Crosslinking of ANCA-antigens stimulates superoxide release by human neutrophils. *J. Am. Soc. Nephrol.* 1997 Mar;8(3):386-94.
[152] Jennette JC, Falk RJ. New insight into the pathogenesis of vasculitis associated with antineutrophil cytoplasmic autoantibodies. *Curr. Opin. Rheumatol.* 2008 Jan;20(1):55-60.
[153] Xiao H, Schreiber A, Heeringa P, Falk RJ, Jennette JC. Alternative complement pathway in the pathogenesis of disease mediated by anti-neutrophil cytoplasmic autoantibodies. *Am. J. Pathol.* 2007 Jan;170(1):52-64.
[154] Jennette JC. Rapidly progressive crescentic glomerulonephritis. *Kidney Int.* 2003 Mar;63(3):1164-77.
[155] Lan HY, Nikolic-Paterson DJ, Atkins RC. Involvement of activated periglomerular leukocytes in the rupture of Bowman's capsule and glomerular crescent progression in experimental glomerulonephritis. *Lab. Invest.* 1992 Dec;67(6):743-51.
[156] Bonsib SM. Glomerular basement membrane discontinuities. Scanning electron microscopic study of acellular glomeruli. *Am. J. Pathol.* 1985 Jun;119(3):357-60.
[157] Border WA, Baehler RW, Bhathena D, Glassock RJ. IgA antibasement membrane nephritis with pulmonary hemorrhage. *Ann. Intern. Med.* 1979 Jul;91(1):21-5.
[158] Rutgers A, Slot M, van Paassen P, van Breda Vriesman P, Heeringa P, Tervaert JW. Coexistence of anti-glomerular basement membrane antibodies and myeloperoxidase-ANCAs in crescentic glomerulonephritis. *Am. J. Kidney Dis.* 2005 Aug;46(2):253-62.
[159] Woodworth TG, Abuelo JG, Austin HA 3rd, Esparza A. Severe glomerulonephritis with late emergence of classic Wegener's granulomatosis. Report of 4 cases and review of the literature. Medicine (Baltimore). 1987 May;66(3):181-91.
[160] Falk RJ, Hogan S, Carey TS, Jennette JC. Clinical course of anti-neutrophil cytoplasmic autoantibody-associated glomerulonephritis and systemic vasculitis. The Glomerular Disease Collaborative Network. *Ann. Intern. Med.* 1990 Nov 1;113(9): 656-63.
[161] Cui Z, Zhao MH, Xin G, Wang HY. Characteristics and prognosis of Chinese patients with anti-glomerular basement membrane disease. *Nephron. Clin. Pract.* 2005;99(2):c49-55.
[162] Lindic J, Vizjak A, Ferluga D, Kovac D, Ales A, Kveder R, et al. Clinical outcome of patients with coexistent antineutrophil cytoplasmic antibodies and antibodies against glomerular basement membrane. *Ther. Apher. Dial.* 2009 Aug;13(4):278-81.
[163] Lionaki S, Jennette JC, Falk RJ. Anti-neutrophil cytoplasmic (ANCA) and anti-glomerular basement membrane (GBM) autoantibodies in necrotizing and crescentic glomerulonephritis. *Semin. Immunopathol.* 2007 Nov;29(4):459-74.
[164] Sanders JS, Huitma MG, Kallenberg CG, Stegeman CA. Prediction of relapses in PR3-ANCA-associated vasculitis by assessing responses of ANCA titres to treatment. *Rheumatology* (Oxford). 2006 Jun;45(6):724-9.
[165] Hogan SL, Falk RJ, Chin H, Cai J, Jennette CE, Jennette JC, et al. Predictors of relapse and treatment resistance in antineutrophil cytoplasmic antibody-associated small-vessel vasculitis. *Ann. Intern. Med.* 2005 Nov 1;143(9):621-31.

[166] Levy JB, Lachmann RH, Pusey CD. Recurrent Goodpasture's disease. *Am. J. Kidney Dis.* 1996 Apr;27(4):573-8.

[167] Levy JB, Turner AN, Rees AJ, Pusey CD. Long-term outcome of anti-glomerular basement membrane antibody disease treated with plasma exchange and immunosuppression. *Ann. Intern. Med.* 2001 Jun 5;134(11):1033-42.

[168] Johnson JP, Moore J Jr, Austin HA 3rd, Balow JE, Antonovych TT, Wilson CB. Therapy of anti-glomerular basement membrane antibody disease: analysis of prognostic significance of clinical, pathologic and treatment factors. Medicine (Baltimore). 1985 Jul;64(4):219-27.

[169] Levy JB, Hammad T, Coulthart A, Dougan T, Pusey CD. Clinical features and outcome of patients with both ANCA and anti-GBM antibodies. *Kidney Int.* 2004 Oct;66(4):1535-40.

[170] Joshi K, Nada R, Minz M, Sakhuja V. Recurrent glomerulopathy in the renal allograft. *Transplant. Proc.* 2007 Apr;39(3):734-6.

[171] de Groot K, Harper L, Jayne DR, Flores Suarez LF, Gregorini G, Gross WL, et al; EUVAS (European Vasculitis Study Group). Pulse versus daily oral cyclophosphamide for induction of remission in antineutrophil cytoplasmic antibody-associated vasculitis: a randomized trial. *Ann. Intern. Med.* 2009 May 19;150(10):670-80.

[172] Walters GD, Willis NS, Craig JC. Interventions for renal vasculitis in adults. A systematic review. *BMC Nephrol.* 2010 Jun 24;11:12.

[173] Faurschou M, Sorensen IJ, Mellemkjaer L, Loft AG, Thomsen BS, Tvede N, et al. Malignancies in Wegener's granulomatosis: incidence and relation to cyclophosphamide therapy in a cohort of 293 patients. *J. Rheumatol.* 2008 Jan;35(1):100-5.

[174] Jones RB, Tervaert JW, Hauser T, Luqmani R, Morgan MD, Peh CA, et al; European Vasculitis Study Group. Rituximab versus cyclophosphamide in ANCA-associated renal vasculitis. *N. Engl. J. Med.* 2010 Jul 15;363(3):211-20.

[175] Stone JH, Merkel PA, Spiera R, Seo P, Langford CA, Hoffman GS, et al; RAVE-ITN Research Group. Rituximab versus cyclophosphamide for ANCA-associated vasculitis. *N. Engl. J. Med.* 2010 Jul 15;363(3):221-32.

[176] Aries PM, Hellmich B, Voswinkel J, Both M, Nölle B, Holl-Ulrich K, et al. Lack of efficacy of rituximab in Wegener's granulomatosis with refractory granulomatous manifestations. *Ann. Rheum. Dis.* 2006 Jul;65(7):853-8.

[177] Holguin F, Ramadan B, Gal AA, Roman J. Prognostic factors for hospital mortality and ICU admission in patients with ANCA-related pulmonary vasculitis. *Am. J. Med. Sci.* 2008 Oct;336(4):321-6.

[178] Jayne D, Rasmussen N, Andrassy K, Bacon P, Tervaert JW, Dadoniené J, et al; European Vasculitis Study Group. A randomized trial of maintenance therapy for vasculitis associated with antineutrophil cytoplasmic autoantibodies. *N. Engl. J. Med.* 2003 Jul 3;349(1):36-44.

[179] Hiemstra TF, Walsh M, Mahr A, Savage CO, de Groot K, Harper L, et al; European Vasculitis Study Group (EUVAS). Mycophenolate mofetil vs azathioprine for remission maintenance in antineutrophil cytoplasmic antibody-associated vasculitis: a randomized controlled trial. *JAMA.* 2010 Dec 1;304(21):2381-8.

[180] Pagnoux C, Mahr A, Hamidou MA, Boffa JJ, Ruivard M, Ducroix JP, et al; French Vasculitis Study Group. Azathioprine or methotrexate maintenance for ANCA-associated vasculitis. *N. Engl. J. Med.* 2008 Dec 25;359(26):2790-803.

[181] Jayne DR, Chapel H, Adu D, Misbah S, O'Donoghue D, Scott D, et al. Intravenous immunoglobulin for ANCA-associated systemic vasculitis with persistent disease activity. *QJM*. 2000 Jul;93(7):433-9.

[182] Basok A, Shnaider A, Tovbin D, Rogachev B. Successful use of high dose intravenous immunoglobulin in rapidly progressive crescentic glomerulonephritis with vasculitis. *Isr. Med. Assoc. J.* 2001 Jun;3(6):453-4.

[183] Little MA, Hassan B, Jacques S, Game D, Salisbury E, Courtney AE, et al. Renal transplantation in systemic vasculitis: when is it safe? *Nephrol. Dial Transplant.* 2009 Oct;24(10):3219-25.

Section C. Secondary Glomerulonephritis

Chapter IV

Secondary Non-Proliferative Glomerulonephritis

Abstract

Diabetic nephropathy is the most common glomerular disease among primary and secondary glomerulonephritis, caused by longstanding diabetes of both type I and type II and it is considered as a non proliferative glomerular disease as mesangial cell proliferation, which occurs in its course, is less pronounced and less significant than mesangial matrix expansion. Renal amyloidosis is more rare than diabetic nephropathy and results from the deposition of fibrous protein aggregates called amyloid in the glomeruli, capillaries, mesangium, and interstitium. Histopathologic patterns in renal biopsy may vary according to the site of amyloid deposition. In most of the cases, glomerular deposition predominates and can be accompanied by vascular and interstitial deposits. This chapter focuses on renal histological patterns, classification, diagnosis, and treatment of the above mentioned diseases.

1. Diabetic Nephropathy

Diabetic nephropathy (DN) is a long-term complication of both types I and II diabetes mellitus (DM), and the leading cause of ESRD worldwide, [1] affecting 25 to 40% of patients with long standing diabetes. [2] In the USA, DN is the most common cause of ESRD requiring renal replacement treatment, [3] accounting for more than 30% of patients enrolled in long-term dialysis. [4]

DN is a clinical syndrome first described by Clifford Wilson and Paul Kimmelstiel in 1936, [5] defined by persistent proteinuria (>300mg/24h) and progressive decline of renal function as recognized by increased plasma creatinine levels and decreased GFR, often accompanied by diabetic vasculopathies and other end-organ complications such as retinopathy. [6]

Common risk factors for DN development are long-term duration of diabetes, poor control of glycemia and hypertension and presence of albuminuria. Genetic predisposition may also play a role.

Currently, strict glycemic control and blood pressure treatment are the most effective therapeutic interventions; unfortunately, they offer partial protection as they can only slow down, but fail to prevent progression of DN.

Typically, LN presents with proteinuria, hypertension, active urine sediment, and in some cases renal insufficiency. Moreover, cases of asymptomatic lupus nephritis are not lacking. [5]

Presence of LN in SLE patients is a strong predictor of poor outcome [6] therefore early diagnosis and determination of reliable biomarkers for LN, are crucial for evaluating the disease and improving prognosis. [7]

Epidemiology

DN, as aforementioned, is the most common cause of ESRD in the USA. [3] Prevalence of DN has practically doubled in this country over the last 20 years, probably in proportion to the increase of diabetes prevalence. [7, 8]

It has been estimated that approximately 7 million people are affected from diabetic kidney disease in the USA. [8] Disparities in prevalence among different racial and ethnic groups exist, despite the common therapeutic approaches and recommendations for glycemic and blood pressure control applied to all these patients.

In the USA, DN is more frequent in Africans Americans, Asian Americans, and Native Americans, probably due to genetic susceptibility to nephropathy as a complication of diabetes. [9]

Interestingly, in two successive generations of Pima Indians, a group of indigenous Americans living in central and southern Arizona, presenting type II DM before 20 years of age, nephropathy occurred in almost 50% of them. Approximately 15% of these patients progressed to ESRD, [10] suggesting that susceptibility to renal disease is inherited, independently of diabetes. [10]

Caucasians with type I DM are more likely to develop DN, although DN shows a higher overall prevalence in type II diabetic patients, as type II DM is more prevalent compared to DM type I. [11]

Worldwide, the majority of ESRD patients due to DN suffer from type II DM, although if untreated, patients with type I DM are more likely to develop DN and ESRD.

This is attributed to the increasing prevalence of DM type II in both developed and developing countries and to the currently available treatments for DM and hypertension that provide longer survival, thus more time of exposure to the risk for development of DN and ESRD.

Finally, higher incidence of ESRD due to DN in developed countries may be associated with genetic predisposition, socioeconomic status, accessibility to screening programs, and other factors. [12]

Natural History

Natural history of DN varies according to the type of diabetes underlying the disease, and the presence or absence of microalbuminuria (>30 and < 300mg/34h). Patients with type I

DM for more than 5 years and microalbuminuria are more likely to develop DN. [13] Almost 80% of type I diabetic patients will present overt nephropathy, defined as more than 300mg of albumin excreted daily (macroalbuminuria). [14] 20% of microalbuminuric and 80% of macroalbuminuric patients will reach ESRD requiring dialysis within 10 years from the onset. [15] Concomitant presence of elevated blood pressure is an early predictor of progression of the disease. [16].

In type II diabetic patients, it is hard to evaluate the exact duration of diabetes before the onset of nephropathy as in most of the cases they remain undiagnosed for 5 to 10 years, until a complication or an event stimulates patients to request medical attention. However, 20% of type II diabetic patients will progress to ESRD within 10 years from diagnosis. [14] Although the percentage is lower than DM type I, total numbers of DM type II and type I patients with DN are similar, due to prevalence of DM type II, presenting rates 5 to 10 times higher than DM type I. Hypertension is usually present at the time of DN diagnosis, in contrast to type I DM, where it develops after microalbuminuria [17]

Development of DN is a long lasting process, including five stages. Stage I is characterized by glomerular hyperfiltration and hyperperfusion, with GFR being normal or more often increased. Kidneys are hypertrophic, increased by 20% of the original sized. Albuminuria and hypertension are usually absent.

Stage II is considered as the "quiet stage", as there is no clinical symptom, and takes place two years after the onset of the disease. This stage is characterized by basement membrane thickening and mesangial expansion. GFR returns to normal values.

Stage III is the stage of manifestation of nephropathy. At this point, albuminuria ranges between 30 and 300mg/24h and blood pressure may be normal or increased.

At Stage IV proteinuria exceeds 300mg/24h and GFR decreases below 60ml/min/1.73m^2. Blood pressure is normally elevated. This stage is considered irreversible.

Stage V corresponds to ESRD, as GFR is below 15ml/min/1.73m^2 and requires renal replacement treatment.

These steps however do not always take place. During this process, microalbuminuria may present variable course, making its progression to macroalbuminuria unpredictable. [18] Therefore, microalbuminuria may not always lead to nephropathy. [18] Indeed, more than 40% of diabetic patients may reach stage II and II of the process without proceeding further, and stay at this point till the end of their lives.

On the other hand, microalbuminuria is not the only pathogenetic factor determining the development of DN. Metabolic, hemodynamic and genetic factors also contribute, thus predicting progression to DN is practically impossible.

Presence of albuminuria and DN increases mortality in both type I and type II DM. Microalbuminuria is considered an independent predictor of cardiovascular morbidity, as it reflects a generalized endothelial dysfunction and it has been associated with increased coronary and peripheral vascular disease in the non-diabetic population.[19] Patients with type I and albuminuria present a mortality up to 200 times higher, compared to the general population. [20]

In type II diabetics with albuminuria, mortality may be even higher, as its prevalence peaks in patients older than 65 years. Age is associated with comorbidities that may worsen the clinical course.

Early diagnosis of DM, intense glycemic and blood pressure control, early referral to a nephrologist and initiation of renoprotective treatment may delay progression to ESRD and reduce mortality. [21, 22]

Pathogenesis

Pathogenesis

Pathogenesis of DN is very complex and not completely elucidated. Interaction of hemodynamic and metabolic factors, along with genetic predisposition, contributes to the development, clinical course, and outcomes of diabetic nephropathy. Inflammation and oxidative stress also seem to play an important role in the establishment of kidney injury.

i. Hemodynamic Pathways

Glomerular hyperfiltration and hyperperfusion occur early in the course of DN development. Longstanding exposure to even mildly elevated serum glucose has been associated with increased blood pressure and kidney volume expansion. [23] The mechanism linking hyperglycemia to hyperfiltration and consecutive renal damage is not completely understood, but it is thought that glucose-dependent processes lead to an increase of different vasoactive mediators, such as insulin-like growth factor I (IGF-I), transforming growth factor β1 (TGF-β1), vascular endothelial growth factor (VEGF), nitric oxide and activation of renin-angiotensin system (RAS). [24, 25] These factors are involved in a defective autoregulation that results in decreased resistance of both afferent and efferent arterioles of the glomeruli and consecutive hyperfiltration. As demonstrated by an experimental model, IGF-I upregulation may be the key to kidney volume expansion, afferent arteriolar dilatation, and GFR increase. [26]

RAS plays a double role in development of DN. Besides regulation of systemic and renal hemodynamics; RAS seem to have profibrotic effects and promotes mesangial expansion and glomerulosclerosis. Mesangial angiotensin II stimulates production of TGF-β1 in mesangial cells, podocytes, and tubular epithelial cells, which in its turn stimulates synthesis of mesangial matrix proteins and collagen, contributing to cellular hypertrophy. [27, 28] It may also inhibit mesangial matrix degradation as it decreases collagenase levels. [27] TGF-β1 may induce genes to encode connective tissue growth factor and heat shock proteins that have fibrogenic effects. Profibrogenic effects of TGF-β1 can be inhibited by the bone morphogenetic protein 7 (BMP7), [28, 29], but its expression in diabetes is decreased. [28, 30]

Angiotensin II and TGF-β1 stimulate expression of vascular endothelial growth factor (VEGF), a cytokine implicated in neovascularization and probably in GBM thickening. VEGF stimulates production of the α3 chain of collagen IV, an important component of GBM. Its role in the pathogenesis of DN is considered controversial as levels of VEGF mRNA were decreased in DN patients, [31, 32] although some authors believe that this is attributable to podocyte loss and progression of renal disease. [31] VEGF expression stimulates production of endothelial nitric oxide (NO) that leads to vasodilatation and hyperfiltration. With the progression of DN and renal damage, VEGF levels decrease, leading to local NO deficiency that contributes to Kimmelstiel-Wilson lesion, a pathologic hallmark of DN. Administration of ACEIs reduces stimulation and serum levels of TGF-β1 and angiotensin II, thereby improves renal fibrosis, delays progression of DN and improves renal function. [28, 33]

Endothelin-I, a potent vasoconstrictor may also contribute to DN. Binding of endothelin-I to mesandial cell endothelin-I receptor stimulates mesangial cell proliferation and hypertrophy. [34]

ii. Hyperlycemia

Hyperglycemia is considered a significant factor for the development of DN, as increased serum and mesangial glucose concentrations induce mesangial cell proliferation and hypertrophy, increased mesangial matrix production, and basement membrane thickening, directly damaging the glomeruli. [35, 36]

Production of different vasoactive cytokines under stimulation of hyperglycemia, also increase mesangial cell proliferation and mesangial matrix expansion. Furthermore, upregulation of growth factors due to hyperglycemia, as VEGF, increases permeability of the filtration barrier to proteins, promoting albuminuria. [37]

Although not all mechanisms by which hyperglycemia incite kidney damage have been clarified yet, four different pathways have been proposed: glycation and generation of advanced glycation end products (AGEs), activation of protein kinase C, the aldose reductase pathway, and the hexosamine pathway. [38, 39]

iia. Glycation and Advanced Glycation End Products

In chronic hyperglycemia, a part of the excess glucose reversibly binds through a nonenzymatic process, the Maillard reaction, or glycation, to free amino acids from circulating tissue proteins, forming early glycation end products. These products submit rearrangement generating irreversible advanced glycation end products (AGES).

AGEs bind to specific receptors, the RAGE, present in tubular cells and podocytes, where it is upregulated under the stimulus of angiotensin II. [40] This bond mediates inflammatory processes, modulates cells activation, alternates signaling pathways, and increases expression of cytokines, growth factors, and hormones. Effects of AGEs on podocytes are reduced migration, cell hypertrophy, and apoptosis. [41, 42] Similarly, on mesangial cells, AGEs induce cell hypertrophy, fibronectin synthesis, and apoptosis. [43] Thus, formation and accumulation of AGEs induce glomerulosclerosis and albuminuria. [44]

AGEs are normally excreted in the urine. In patients with kidney disease and diabetes, circulating concentrations of AGEs were increased. [45] In animal models, infusion of glycation products increased intraglomerular pressure and induced hyperfiltration with consecutive increases of GFR, [46] albuminuria, and glomerulosclerosis. [44]

iib. Protein Kinase C

Protein kinase C (PKC) is a family of serine/threonine kinases consisting of 12 isoforms, activated when bonding with calcium and/or dialcylglycerol (DAG). DAG was increased in renal glomeruli of diabetic animal models. [47-49] Activation of PKC promotes development of DN. [50] PKC activation reinforces actions of angiotensin II, increases production of vasodilatatory prostaglandins, and modulates NO production thereby regulating renal hemodynamics. [51-55] Also PKC activation mediates actions of VEGF, increasing capillary permeability. [56]

Additionally, PKC increases capillary permeability directly by phosphorylation of cytoskeletal proteins of endothelial cells or indirectly by increasing expression of VEGF. [56- 59]

Furthermore, PKC increases expression of TGF-β1 in mesangial cells, promoting mesangial matrix expansion. [60]

iic. Aldose-Reductase Pathway or Polyol Patway

Aldose reductase is a NADPH-dependent enzyme that catalyzes the reduction of glucose to sorbitol, which is the initial event in the aldose-reductase, also called the polyol pathway. [61] Then, sorbitol submits NAD-linked oxidation, catalyzed by sorbitol dehydrogenase, generating fructose with concomitant production production of NADH. [61] Aldose reductase is located in the cornea, retina, lenses, and in the kidney tissues often insulted in diabetes. [62] Under hyperglycemic conditions, the excess glucose activates aldose reductase, triggering the polyol pathway. Activation of the polyol pathway leads to PKC activity, with resulting loss of mesangial cell contractility. [63]

Increased concentrations of glucose induce overexpression of aldose reductase in mesangial cells, which increases the fibronectin expression of the mesangial matrix. [64]

Moreover, production and accumulation of excess sorbitol in the cells provokes osmotic damage. [65] In animal models, increased concentrations of sorbitol and fructose were associated with metabolic changes of renal medulla including oxygen tension, oxygen consumption, pH, and lactate/piruvate ratio, suggesting a role of the polyol pathway in acute kidney injury. [66]

Aldose reductase inhibitors may reduce PKC activity, [67] decrease fibronectin expression [64, 68] and ameliorate metabolic profile of renal cells, [66] but they seem to have no effect on mesangial expansion, [69] suggesting that they might prevent but not reverse kidney damage.

iid. Hexosamine Pathway

Hexosamine pathway, an important process guaranteeing the synthesis of glycoproteins, proteoglycans and lipids, has been reported to be involved in the development of DN. [70]

Hexokinase is an enzyme that phosphorylates six-carbon sugars into hexose-phosphate. In the hexosamine pathway, glucose transported in the cells is phosphorylated by hexokinase into glucose phosphate and subsequently transformed into fructose-6-phosphate by isomerization. Fructose-6-phosphate is then converted to glucosamine-6-phosphate (GluN-6-P), a reaction catalyzed by the rate-limiting enzyme Glutamine/fructose-6-phosphate amidotransferase (GFAT), using glutamine as an amino donor. [71, 72] GluN-6-P is further converted to uridine-5-diphosphate-N-acetylglucosamine (UDP-GluNAc), a common precursor of glycoproteins, proteoglycans, glycosaminoglycans, and glycolipids.

Glucosamine (Glu-N) may use the glucose-transporters to enter the cells, skipping the GFAT effect, and then be phosphorilated into GluN-6-P by hexokinase. Thus, glucosamine provides the same hexosamine pathway mediated effects as glucose. Hyperglycemia increases production of glucosamine and its metabolites, and promotes their accumulation in the cells.

In addition, Glu-N induces translocation of PKC isoenzymes in mesangial cells, enhancing its activity.

In diabetic conditions, high glucose and angiotensin II concentrations activate the GFAT promoter in mesangial cells. [73] Glucosamine was found to significantly increase production and activation of TGF-β1, with subsequent mesangial matrix expansion, more than glucose did. [74] In vitro, doubling UDP-GluNAc concentration increased TGF-β1 mRNA levels approximately two-fold. [75] [76] In addition, glucosamine induces translocation of PKC isoenzymes in mesangial cells, enhancing its activity. [76] Furthermore, overexpression of GFAT leads to increased expression of fibronectin in mesangial cells promoting fibrosis. [77] These data indicate the involvement of the hexosamine pathway in the development of DN.

iii. Inflammation and Cytokines

Inflammation is a crucial component in the development and progression mechanisms of DN, as it appears to be the final pathway of metabolic, hemodynamic and biochemical derangements. Renal inflammation is characterized by glomerular and tubulointerstitial infiltration of neutrophils, macrophages, lymphocytes and other cells. [78] Once kidney tissue is damaged, neutrophils infiltrate the site of injury in order to phagocyte apoptotic cells, following the pathway indicated by interleukins produced by macrophages. Macrophages derive from differentiation of circulating monocytes. Monocytes and macrophages produce the monocyte chemotactic protein-1 (MCP-1) a chemokine that recruits other monocytes and dendritic cells to the site of injury. MCP-1 plays an important role in the inflammation process of DN, as its depletion in diabetic animal models reduced macrophage accumulation in renal tissue and attenuated inflammation and renal damage. [79] Type II diabetic patients with DN excrete high levels of MCP-1 in the urine; therefore, MCP-1 is considered a marker of tubular injury. [80]

Activated macrophages produce different proinflammatory and profibrotic factors including TNF-α, IL-1, IL-6, IL-18, and TGF-β.

TNF-α is an adipokine mainly produced by activated macrophages but it can also be produced by monocytes and CD4+ T lymphocytes as well as by mesangial, endothelial, glomerular, and tubular cells. [81-84] This factor has a wide variety of biological effects that promote diabetic nephropathy. Other than recruitment of monocytes and macrophages, TNF-α alters endothelial permeability, [85] contributes to glomerular hemodynamic changes increasing GFR, [86-89] and to sodium retention and renal hypertrophy. [90] This factor is excreted with the urine and it can be considered a biomarker of DN. [91]

IL-1 alters glomerular hemodynamics by affecting prostaglandin synthesis, [92] increases vascular endothelial cell permeability, [93] stimulates mesangial and fibroblast proliferation, [94] and increases hyaluron generation in renal proximal tubular epithelial cells. [95]

IL-6 is produced by macrophages and T cells but is also expressed in adipocytes, endothelial, and mesangial cells. Overexpression of IL-6 has been associated to GBM thickening and mesangial proliferation and expansion. [96-99]

IL-18 is produced by macrophages that stimulate natural killer (NK) cells and T cells to release interferon γ, IL-1 and TNF-α and increases expression of intercellular adhesion molecule-1 (ICAM-1) on endothelial cells, macrophages, and lymphocytes facilitating their adhesion. [101] IL-18 is also produced by monocytes, macrophages, T cells, and tubular epithelial cells. [102]

Other cytokines and factors implicated in inflammatory processes of DN are TGF-β1, VCAM-1, adiponectine, leptin, and resistin.

iv. Prorenin

Prorenin is a component of the RAS and for many years was considered as an inactive form of rennin (or angiotensinogenase), the enzyme that hydrolyzes angiotensinogen to angiotensin I. The discovery of (pro)renin receptor (PRR) by Nguyen in 2002 abrogated this concept. [103] PRR is expressed in mesangial cells, podocytes, renal vessels and distal renal tubules and although it can bind both rennin and prorenin, it has a higher affinity for prorenin.

In diabetic patients, activity and components of RAS are increased due to its chronic stimulation by different factors including prorenin that increases in a disproportional manner compared to rennin, [103-105] even before the occurrence of microalbuminuria, [106] probably due to increased production. [107] The main site of prorenin production is the kidney but it may also originate from other tissues, such as eyes and ovaries. [108, 109]

Prorenin is converted to renin under the proteolytic effect of proconvertase-1 and cathepsin B, [110,111] but it is activated in a non-proteolytic way through its bond to the PRR. PRR is expressed in mesangial cells, podocytes, renal vessels and distal renal tubules and although it can bind both rennin and prorenin it has a higher affinity for prorenin. [112] The overexpression of PRR, and its bond to prorenin, increases angiotensin II production, bypassing the enzymatic process of prorenin transformation. [107] This bond also mediates activation of mitogen-activated protein kinase (MAPK) and increases production of TGF-β1, which increases plasminogen activator inhibitor-1 (PAI-1) and fibronectin, promoting mesangial matrix expansion in diabetics. [103, 114]

Moreover, PRR-prorenin bond increases production of VEGF, ICAM-1, TNF-α, and IL-β in diabetic subjects. [115, 116] The effects of PRR-prorenin bond are independent of changes in angiotensin II and RAS. Thus, PRR and protrenin involvement in the development and progression of DN is mainly explained by inflammatory processes.

v. Nephrin

Nephrin is a transmembrane protein of the podocyte that along with other proteins, such as actin, podocin, and CD2AP, contributes to the structure of slit diaphragm and the maintenance of the glomerular filtration barrier. In DN, expression of nephrin is dysregulated. [117, 118]

Reduction of nephrin expression in the glomeruli of both type I and type II diabetes and microalbuminuria, even in absence of histological glomerular lesions, [119] are associated with foot processes effacement and increased width of filtration slits with consecutive loss of selectivity and albuminuria. [119, 120] The mechanism involved in the reduced expression of nephrin may be explained by interaction of glycated proteins to the cell surface receptor RAGE, which expression is upregulated in DN. [119, 121] Indeed; blockade of RAGE prevents reduction of nephrin expression induced by glycated proteins. [119]

Excretion of nephrin in the urine is increased even in early disease (microalbuminuria) but it has also been described in 30% of normoalbuminuric patients, suggesting a role of nephrin in the progression of the disease. [122]

Moreover, decrease of nephrin expression impairs insulin responsiveness of podocytes. Nephrin plays an important role in the insulin-stimulated fusion of glucose-transporters

(GLUT-1 and GLUT-2) to the plasma cell membrane in order to facilitate transport of glucose. In the absence of nephrin, this fusion is interrupted. [123]

vi. Genetic Predisposition

Increasing evidence supports the role of genetic susceptibility and heritability in the development of DN. Given the variety of pathogenic factors cytokines and other molecules underlying the disease and the poorly understood genetic mechanisms, several candidate genes have been studied considering variations on gene expression and epigenetic mechanisms. Polimorphisms in the ACE gene located on chromosome 17q23 were associated with circulating ACE levels, [124] while the ACE DD allele was associated with DNB and persistent microalbuminuria in type I and type II diabetic patients. [125, 126]

Also, polymorphisms in the aldose reductase gene have been associated with increased susceptibility to DN in both type I and type II patients. [127, 128]

Other candidate genes associated with susceptibility, development and progression of DN are TGF-β1 gene, GLUT-1, VEGF, and connective tissue growth factor (CTGF).

Epigenetic mechanisms also have a say in the development of DN. Epigenetic mechanisms could explain the "metabolic memory" phenomenon, thus, patients previously exposed to hyperglycemia develop DN despite strict glycemic control. Indeed studies in endothelial cells showed that glucose-induced histone modifications induce modifications on gene expression, which persist even after glycemia is normalized, leading to DN. [129]

However, knowledge on genetic mechanisms is limited, given the heterogeneity of studied population and the variety and number of genes interlinked between them. Hopefully advances on DN genetic and pharmacogenomics will provide new screening techniques and new therapeutic approaches.

Pathology and Classification

Renal pathological changes occur early in the course of both types I and II DM, before the appearance of microalbuminuria. The main histopathological findings in DN are thickening of the GBM - the earliest morphologic change, mesangial matrix expansion, and glomerular sclerosis, nodular or diffuse.

Abnormalities in the tubulointerstitium as fibrosis and in renal vessels as arteriosclerosis and hyalinosis may also be found in more advanced stages of the disease. The most pathognomonic lesion of DN is the Kimmelstiel-Wilson nodule, a nodular acellular glomerular intercapillary lesion, first described by Kimmelstiel and Wilson in 1936, [5] located in central regions of peripheral glomerular lobules.

Different attempts were made in recent years to classify histologic lesions of DN but their use in clinical practice was limited as only type II DM-induced pathologic alternations were considered. [130, 131] In 2010, Tervaert et al, [132] developed a consensus classification of DN, common to both types I and type II DM-induced nephropathy on behalf of the Renal Pathology Society, considering the structural and functional similarities between them.

This classification consists of 4 different classes, according to the severity of the lesions. Interstitial and vascular lesions are evaluated by a different scoring system created by the same research group. [132]

In Class I, light microscopy shows mild and/or non-specific histologic changes, as glomerular hypertrophy, mesangial expansion and hyperplasia, Kimmelstiel-Wlison lesion, or global sclerosis. Inclusion criteria of other classes should be absent. On electron microscopy, thickening of the GBM without spikes or splitting is observed. Males and females older than 9 years old with GBM width measured directly on electron microscopy larger than 430nm and 395nm, respectively, are considered as class I DN patients.

Class II is divided in 2 subclasses. Class IIa includes patients with mild mesangial expansion in more than 25% of the total mesangium. Patients with severe mesangial expansion in more than 25% of the total mesangium are classified as class IIb DN patients. If mesangial expansion is smaller than the mean area of a capillary lumen, it is considered mild, whereas, a larger one is considered as severe. To be classified as class II, biopsies should not meet the criteria for class III and IV.

Class III is characterized by the presence of at least one convincing Kimmelstiel-Wilson lesion, and the absence of inclusion criteria for class IV, thus glomerulosclerosis. Kimmelstiel-Wilson is a focal nodular acellular lesion with a hyaline core surrounded by mesangial nuclei that seem like crescents. It has been suggested that Kimmelstiel-Wilson nodules formation results from microaneurismatic dilatation of capillaries with dissociation of endothelial cells that disrupt the GBM and mesangium connections, followed by mesangiolysis and accumulation of mesangial matrix, cellular debris. [133]

Class IV corresponds to global glomerular in more than 50% of the glomeruli, which indicates advanced DN, and presence of lesions belonging to all other classes.

Tubular atrophy, interstitial fibrosis, and inflammatory vascular lesions, often accompany glomerular lesions of class II, III and IV. Authors scored interstitial fibrosis according to its extension. A score of 0 was assigned to absence of interstitial fibrosis or tubular atrophy, while involvement of 25% and 50% of the total interstitium and tubule area were respectively scored 1 and 2. If more than 50% of the total interstitium and tubule area was involved a score of 3 was assigned.

Absence of interstitial inflammatory infiltrates around atrophic tubules was scored 0. If infiltrates were limited around the atrophic tubules the score assigned was 1 and in case of their extension to other areas they were scored 2.

Vascular lesions observed in DN are hyalinosis of the efferent arteriole. If afferent arteriole hyalinosis is present, is probably due to concomitant hypertensive nephropathy. Absence of arteriole hyalinosis is scored 0. Presence of 1 or more arterioles with hyalinosis is scored respectively 1 and 2.

Arteriosclerosis in large vessels may also be present in bioptic specimens of DN patients. Therefore, authors scored the extension of intimal thickening in these vessels comparing width of the tunica intima to the width of the media. No intimal thickening was assigned a score of 0, thickening of the intima presenting smaller width that the media was scored 1 and intimal thickening with width bigger than the intima was scored 2.

Other glomerular lesions often observed are capsular drop lesion, consisting of plasma proteins and lipids accumulated in Bowman's capsule, and fibrin cap or hyaline cap lesion, if intramural accumulation of lipids and plasma proteins occurs in glomerular capillaries.

The validity and reproducibility of the DN classification was investigated in a recent Chinese retrospective study. [134] Although authors consider this classification as a promising diagnostic instrument, they suggest that more attention should be paid to tubular and interstitial lesions.

In the course of DN, the earliest histologic findings are associated with hyperfiltration and hypertrophy. On light microscopy, glomeruli are hypertrophic, presenting cellular hyperplasia.

GBM is thickened without spikes or spitting. As the disease progresses, mesangial cellularity and mesangial matrix expansion is detected, but it can also be observed even earlier on electron microscopy.

Although mesangial cell proliferation occurs in the course of diabetic nephropathy, it is less pronounced compared to mesangial matrix expansion, which is the main histological alternation, resulting in renal damage; therefore, DN is not considered a proliferative glomerular disease.

In more advanced stages, Kimmelstiel–Wilson nodules may be observed in central regions of peripheral glomerular lobules, often associated with hyaline caps and capsular drops. Artetriosclerosis of arterioles may also be present. Tubular atrophy, thickening of the tubular basement membrane and tubular vacuolization, along with interstitial fibrosis, often accompany arteriosclerotic lesions.

Immunofluorescence reveals immunoglobulins; albumin and plasma proteins deposited in a linear pattern along the GBM, the Bowman's capsule, and tubular basement membranes.

Electron microscopy shows podocyte processes effacement and mesangial matrix expansion. Sclerotic and hyaline lesions appear electron-dense and GBM thickening is confirmed. Also, electron microscopy provides detailed information of GBM's width.

Diagnosis

Diagnosis of DN is based on the finding of proteinuria in diabetic patients. Type I diabetic patients, usually present albuminuria five years from the onset, while in type II diabetic patients development of proteinuria occurs at least 4 to 7 years from the onset of the disease.

Screening of proteinuria in type II DM patients should be performed at the time of diagnosis, given that in most of these cases diagnosis is delayed. In type I DM patients it is cautious to perform screening 1 year from the onset. Screening should be avoided if conditions that increase urinary albumin excretion (UAE) occur, such as urinary infections, hematuria, fever, uncontrolled hypertension, and cardiac failure, because results will be inaccurate. [135]

Screening methods of albuminuria include:

- Urine dipstic in a morning or random urine spot sample. This test has 100% sensitivity and 93% specificity for diagnosis of proteinuria. However, "trace-positive" results may often be observed in healthy people and they shouldn't be taken into consideration unless it is repeatedly detected.
- 24-hour urine collection: although it is considered an accurate screening test for albuminuria, frequently errors occur, mostly due to incorrect collection of the sample.
- Timed urinary collection: is the collection of urine sample over a specified length of time, usually 4 to 8 hours.

Increase of blood pressure usually accompanies microalbuminuria, therefore monitoring of blood pressure is essential. The target for both type I and type II diabetic adults is to reduce blood pressure to 130/80mmHg. Reduction of blood pressure should take place under strict control, as decrease below 130/80 has been associated with increased mortality. [136]

Measurement of serum creatinine levels and estimation of GFR are the screening tests most frequently used to evaluate renal function. However, both tests could underestimate the severity of the disease. In patients with low muscle mass, low creatinine levels may correspond to important reduction of renal function, and the currently available prediction equations used to estimate GFR, such as the Modification of Diet in Renal Disease Study equation (MDRD) and the Cockcroft-Gault equation, often overestimate clearance. Of note, MDRD is considered more accurate than the Cockcroft-Gault equation and KDIGO guidelines recommend its use for the estimation of GFR. [137]

Biopsy is usually not required, unless there is evidence suggesting other cause of CKD in diabetic patients. Diabetic retinopathy usually precedes diabetic nephropathy. If retinopathy is absent, suspicion of other renal disease should raise and renal biopsy is required. Also, rapidly progressive glomerulonephritis with increasing proteinuria or nephrotic syndrome and rapid reduction of GFR, and presence of active urine sediment suggest other underlying causes of CKD. In these cases, renal biopsy is recommended. [138]

In the early stages of DN, kidney size may be enlarged due to hyperfiltration and hypertrophy. As the disease progresses, kidneys return to normal and then decrease in size due to glomerular sclerosis. If in the ultrasound, the kidneys are hyperechogenic and small, performing biopsy will be of no benefit, as renal tissues will be sclerosing, providing no useful information on the disease.

Treatment

Given that pathogenesis of DN is multifactorial, currently available therapeutic options are directed against the up to date known mechanisms underlying the disease, including glycemia, systemic and glomerular hypertension, activity of RAS and other metabolic, inflammatory and hemodynamic processes.

The goal of all treatment approaches is to decelerate renal impairment processes and delay loss of renal function as well as to prevent cardiovascular events and metabolic complications related to renal failure.

Current therapeutic strategies include lifestyle modification, glycemic control, and blood pressure control.

i. Lifestyle Modification

Nutritional modifications, smoking cessation, decrease of alcohol consumption, and exercise can add benefit to pharmacologic treatments of DN, but unfortunately are frequently neglected.

Reduction of dietary protein intake below 0.8g/kg daily has been associated with reduction of proteinuria in type II diabetic patients with microalbuminuria. [139] Contrarily, another study showed that low protein intake was correlated to low serum albumin concentrations and provided no significant benefit in both type I and type II diabetic patients.

[140] However, dietary protein intake should be personalized for these patients, according to their nutritional status.

High dietary intake of AGEs may also contribute to the development of DN. In animal models, low AGEs diet reduced TGF-β1 expression and creatinine/albumin ratio and improved glomerular lesions. [141] The same benefit of low AGEs diet was also observed in obese non-diabetic subjects. [142] In contrast, high AGEs intake induces insulin resistance contributing to DN. [143]

Pyridoxamine, a vitamer of vitamin B6 that inhibits the Maillard reaction and blocks the formation of AGEs, was successfully used in type I and type II diabetic patients. [144] In this study, pyridoxamine reduced AGEs production and TGF-β1 urinary excretion, but failed to improve serum creatine levels and proteinuria. Other agents with AGEs-reducing properties such as aminoguanidine and benfotiamine have been suggested, but trials were stopped due to toxicity.

Smoking is considered a promoting factor of development and progression of DN in both type I and II patients as it alters renal hemodynamics by increasing endothelin production and impairing endothelial function and affects urinary protein excretion. [145] Cessation of smoking reduced microalbuminuria in 193 patients with newly diagnosed type II DM. [146]

Sodium intake should also be limited as many of the diabetic patients with kidney disease are salt sensitive. Sodium status significantly affects response to ACEIs and AT1 receptor blockers. In a comparison of the effects of adding dietary sodium restriction to ACEIs and AT1 receptor blockers, sodium restriction was found to be more effective, ion lowering proteinuria and blood pressure. [147]

According to KDIGO guidelines, dietary sodium intake should be less than 2.4g/day or less than 100mmol/day in patients with CKD and hypertension. [137]

ii. Glycemic Control

Strict and longstanding control of hyperglycemia halts the development of microalbuminuria in both types I and type II diabetic patients. [148] According to KDIGO guidelines, the target of glucose lowering treatment is the achievement of HbA1c values of around 7% in order to prevent or delay DN and other complications of diabetes such as cardiovascular events and reduced mortality. [137]. However, in elderly type II diabetic patients, intense glycemic control failed to reduce incidence of cardiovascular events and was associated with increased mortality. [149] Patients with already advanced kidney disease (GFR 15- 30 ml/min) had HbA1c levels above 9% but also levels of HbA1c below 6.5% were associated with increased mortality. In these patients, dosing of hypoglycemic agents should be individualized considering risk for hypoglycemia and major comorbidities.

Renoprotective effects of strict glycemic control persist even after glucose control is less intensive, due to metabolic memory. [148] In two clinical trials, patients under intensive glycemic control showed lower medial HbA1c levels compared to patients receiving conservative treatment, even after 4 years from the end of the trials.

Currently available agents are:

- Glitazones: glitazones act by activating the nuclear peroxisome proliferator activated receptor (PPARs), which decreases insulin resistance. These agents are widely used but they have been associated with increased cardiovascular events, including acute myocardial infarction and congestive heart failure. [151]

- Biguanides: these agents reduce hepatic gluconeogenesis and increase insulin sensitivity. Metformin, the most frequently used agent among all biguanides, has been associated with increased risk of lactic acidosis. In patients with chronic kidney disease, dosing of these agents should be reduced as the risk of lactic acidosis is higher and its consequences more severe.
- Sulfonylureas: these agents increase pancreatic insulin production. They are usually well tolerated in patients with GFR>60ml/min but the risk for hypoglycemia is very high in patients with more severe kidney impairment. Use of sulfolylureas in patients with GFR<30ml/min should be avoided.
- Gliptins or dipeptidyl-peptidase inhibitors: these agents block breakdown of incretins, inhibiting glucagone release with following increase of insulin secretion. These agents are handy as they are less likely to induce hypoglycemia but their use in kidney disease with GFR lower than 30ml/min is not recommended given that the kidney eliminates them. Also, their use in type II diabetic patients was associated with increased proliferation, dysplasia, and hyperplasia of α-pancreatic cells that could potentially evolve to tumors. [152]
- α-glucosidase inhibitors are competitive inhibitors of α-glucosidase enzyme that hydrolyzes oligosaccharides to monosaccharides, inhibiting their absorption from the intestine with consecutive reduction of postprandial glycemia. Side effects of these agents are flatulence and diarrhea. These drugs haven't been studied in patients with GFR<25ml/min, therefore their use in these patients should be avoided. [153]
- Sodium-glucose cotransporter inhibitors inhibit renal glucose absorption in the proximal tubule inducing glycosuria and natriuresis. These agents can only be used in patients with GFR>45ml/min. These agents have been associated with increased risk of urinary tract infections due to increased glycosuria. [154]
- Glucagon-like peptid-1 receptor agonists or incretin mimetics are new injectable hypoglycemic agents that induce insulin release and delay of glucagon release and gastric emptying. These agents do not cause hypoglycemias but they haven't been studied in patients with GFR below 30ml/min or ESRD, thus in these populations their use should be avoided.
- Amylin analogs: amylin is a peptid co-secreted with insulin by β-cells of the pancreas that shows a synergic action to insulin in regulating glycemia. Amylin analogs slow gastric emptying and reduce postprandial glycemia. These agents can be administrated in patients with mild to moderate renal disease, but should be avoided in ESRD patients as data on their safety and efficacy in this population are lacking. [155]

iii. Blood Pressure Control

It is well established that arterial hypertension is a major risk factor for the progression of DN. In patients with type II DM, arterial hypertension usually precedes renal disease and probably occurs as part of a metabolic syndrome characterized by obesity, dyslipidemia, insulin resistance, and hypertension. In type I diabetic patients, hypertension develops long after microalbuminuria appears.

Intensive and strict control of hypertension delays progression of DN and improves survival. Indeed, the UK Prospective Diabetes Study showed a 13% reduction of microvascular complications for every 10mmHg decrease in systolic blood pressure. [156]

The target blood pressure levels for patients with DN are continually under discussion. In the past, systolic blood pressure lower than 120-130mmHg were considered the target in these patients, but different trials showed no benefit in renal function, but rather increased risk for hyperkaliemia and renal dysfunction, while there was no improvement in cardiovascular events or mortality rates. [157]

Given that this observation put blood pressure goals below 130/80mmHg in discussion, the recently published KDIGO guidelines recommend to consistently maintain blood pressure at or below 130/90mmHgin in both diabetic and non diabetic patients with proteinuria. [137]

In elderly, the American Diabetes and Aging Guidelines suggest as a target a blood pressure of 140/80-90mmHg, as the risk for hypotension is increased in these patients and associated with cardiovascular events. [158, 159]

However, the target blood pressure goals are difficult to reach, especially in type II diabetic patients, and in most of the cases, as shown from different RCTs, more than 3 antihypertensive agents are required.

Blockade of RAS with ACEIs, ARBs or their combination appears to be beneficial in reducing blood pressure and albuminuria, delaying progression of DN in both type I and type II diabetic patients.

Treatment with these agents should be started as soon as possible, as timely initiation of treatment could provide the greatest benefit in prevention of kidney disease.

Maximizing dosage of RAS blockade is recommended, given that benefits are dose related. Unfortunately, maximal dosing of these agents has been associated with different adverse events, such as hyperkaliemia, hypotension, and increase of serum creatinine levels, limiting their use. If ACEIs are used and serum creatinine levels increase, it doesn't necessarily require withdrawal of the treatment. Rise of creatinine levels in this case is due to long-term renoprotection. A rise of more than 30% of initial serum creatinine levels suggests renal artery stenosis.

Diuretics are used as second line agents and usually in association with RAS blocking agents, helping the achievement of blood pressure goals. Loop diuretics are the most commonly used agents, administered twice a day in order to prevent sodium retention. Thiazide diuretics are also well tolerated. Aldosterone receptor antagonists could also be used, but with caution as their combination to ACEIs or ARBs increases risk for hyperkaliemia.

The direct rennin inhibitor aliskiren, associated with irbesartan or losartan, provided a greater antiproteinuric effect than placebo in type II diabetic patients. [160] However, its use may be limited due to adverse effects such as hypotension, hyperkaliemia, and reduction of GFR.

Dihydropyridine calcium channel blockers can also be used to treat hypertension and they appear to be safe even in elderly diabetic patients, but they are inferior in reducing proteinuria compared to ACEIs. [161] Non-dihydropyridine calcium channel blockers, other than their antihypertensive effects, were found to be comparable to ACEIs in reducing proteinuria. [162]

2. Renal Amyloidosis

Amyloidosis is defined as a group of chronic infiltrative disorders characterized by extracellular deposition of protein aggregates forming insoluble fibrils. These fibrous protein aggregates called amyloid, have a characteristic β-plated sheet configuration with 7.5 to 10nm width and indefinite length, and are resistant to proteolysis [163]. On electron microscopy, they look like fine, rigid, and linear nonbranching fibrils.

To date, 25 different proteins, not related to each other, referred to as amyloidogenic precursor proteins, are known to cause amyloidosis. [164] Classification of amyloidosis is based on the amyloidogenic precursor proteins causing the disease. [164-167]

Renal amyloidosis mostly occurs in the course of AL or AH amyloidosis, and rarely in hereditary or familial forms (ATTR, AFib, AApoAI, AApoAII and ALys).

Pathogenesis

AL or primary amyloidosis is the most common type of amyloidosis, and results from amyloid formation from immunoglobulin light chains, mainly lamda (λ) but also kappa (κ), or from light chain fragments, secreted by monoclonal B cells or plasma cells. This form occurs more frequently in patients with multiple myeloma, Waldenström's macroglobulinemia, or monoclonal gammopathy of undetermined significance (MGUS). [168]

AA amyloidosis, also called secondary or reactive amyloidosis, occurs in the course of longstanding inflammation, such as rheumatoid arthritis, familial Mediterranean fever, psoriatic arthritis, ankylosing spondylitis, granulomatous colitis, and symphilis. Occasionally, patients with SLE, Gaucher's disease, and cystic fibrosis may present AA amyloidosis. AA amylodosis associated with chronic tuberculosis or osteomyelitis is rarely seen, accounting for less than 15% of the cases. [169] Rheumatoid arthritis remains the main cause of AA amyloidosis and its prevalence has increased significantly, accounting for almost 60% of the cases. [169]

AA amyloidosis is the result of overproduction and partial catabolism of serum amyloid A protein (SAA), an apolipoprotein synthesized in the liver that circulates united to HDL lipoproteins. SAA proteins are produced as acute phase proteins, under inflammatory conditions, and exist in two different forms, SAA1 and SAA2. These two proteins are catabolized, generating N-terminal fragments, which are the amyloidogenic precursor proteins.

Progressive accumulation of amyloid fibril protein in the kidney, disrupt its normal architecture with consecutive kidney injury and renal failure, especially if the deposition is extensive. Amyloid deposits are mainly glomerular but they can also be seen in the mesangium, capillary loops, tubuli, and the interstitium.

However, pathogenic mechanisms are quite complicated and it is difficult to say why amyloid deposits to one tissue and not to another. The heterogeneity in tissue distribution suggests a different tissue tropism of amyloidogenic proteins and local tissue characteristics that can promote or prevent amyloid deposition. It has been suggested that mutations, and more interestingly, the position of the mutations, may alter tissue tropism and distribution of amyloidogenic proteins. [170, 171] Indeed, mutation in the amino-terminal portion of Apo AI protein determined kidney, liver, and heart involvement, while mutations in the carboxyl terminal portion was correlated to heart and skin involvement of amyloidosis. [171]

Also, the mesangial cell tropism for λVI light chain proteins suggests that tissue characteristics play an important role. [172, 173] A factor that may explain this phenomenon is the presence of glycosaminoglycans (GAGs) on the GBM. GAGs are polysaccharide chains of hyaluronic acid hexosamine linked to a protein core. GAGs promote and stabilize the β-plated conformation of the fibrils and protect them from proteolysis, facilitating their deposition. [174] Moreover acid PH may also promote fibrillogenesis and deposition of AApoAI amyloid to the medulla. [175] Amyloid P protein (SAP), a protein resistant to proteolysis that coats amyloid fibrils protecting them from digestion, may also contribute to renal amyloidosis.

Amyloidogenic precursors may also have toxic properties that contribute to renal amyloidosis, independently of the extent of amyloid deposits. [165] Direct toxicity of amyloidogenic precursor proteins, presence of amyloidogenic precursors in damaged tissue in absence of amyloid and improvement of organ dysfunction after reduction of precursor protein production supports this mechanism. [164, 172, 176-178] These observations have been made in both renal AA and AL amyloidosis. [179-181]

In patients with renal amyloidosis, biopsies were performed after treatment-induced resolution of proteinuria. Extent of amyloid deposition remained unchanged despite proteinuria remission. [179-181]

Finally, exposure to amyloidogenic light chains induced a macrophage-like phenotype in cultured mesangial cells, changes that weren't observed in mesangial cells exposed to nonamyloidogenic light chains. [172, 173]

Epidemiology

AL amyloidosis is the most common type of systemic amyloidosis in the USA and Western world. Incidence in developed countries is estimated at 9 cases per million inhabitants per year. [182] In the USA incidence ranges between 5.1 and 12.8 million inhabitants per year. [183] AA amyloidosis on the other hand, shows a decreased incidence in Western countries, accounting for 0.5 to 0.86% of all biopsies. [184] In Europe, AA amyloidosis represents approximately 45% of systemic amyloidosis with rheumatoid arthritis as the main cause. [185] Almost 60% of the cases present AL amyloidosis over the age range from 50 to 70 years, while only 10% of the patients are younger. [186] Males are affected twice as often as women.

Incidence of renal amyloidosis is variable. Although incidence in Europe has been estimated at approximately 1%, [187] in some countries of Northern Europe such as Finland, Norway, and Sweden, the incidence is significantly higher. In the UK renal amyloidosis accounts for 2.8% of all kidney biopsies performed, while in Italy a frequency of 2.5% has been reported. [188]

Similarly in India, the incidence of renal amyloidosis is 2% of total renal biopsies. Although, in contrast to European countries where rheumatoid arthritis is the most common cause of renal amyloidosis, there is an increased incidence of AL amyloidosis. In this country, AA amyloidosis is the most frequent type of amyloidosis, and tuberculosis the most common cause.

Prognosis of AL amyloidosis is poor with median survival of less than 2 years. Five-year survival is approximately 20%. Mortality rates are particularly high in case of renal and cardiac involvement. [189, 190]

Pathology

Histopathologic patterns in renal biopsy may vary according to the site of amyloid deposition. In most of the cases, glomerular deposition predominates and can be accompanied by vascular and interstitial deposits. In some cases, predominant vascular or interstitial deposits may also be seen. Intratubular deposition may rarely occur, causing cast nephropathy. Deposits are extracellular eosinophilic and metachromatic.

On light microscopy, mesangial amyloid deposits, which represent the earliest lesion, appear like amorphous acelullar nodules, similar to those in diabetic nephropathy, initially confined in segmental areas to gradually replace the whole mesangial matrix. GBM may also be infiltrated by amyloid deposits, with consecutive thickening and formation of spikes similar to membranous nephropathy.

Tubular and interstitial amyloid deposits induce tubular atrophy, interstitial fibrosis, and inflammation. Capillaries may also be infiltrated by acellular amyloid deposits. Extent amyloid deposition disrupts the normal glomerular architecture and with the progression of the disease, glomeruli become sclerotic. At this point, Cong red staining may not be able to demonstrate the presence of amyloid deposits.

Immunofluorescence reveals Ig light chains in Al amyloidosis but shows negativity for intact Ig, complement components, and fibrin.

On electron microscopy, amyloid appears as 8 to 12nm diameter nonbranching fibrils randomly arrayed in the mesangium, along the GBM, I vessels and tubulointerstitium, in contrast to immunotactoid glomerulopathy where fibrils have a specific parallel orientation and fibrillary glomerulonephritis, with fibrils of 15 to 20nm of diameter. Extent of amyloid deposits may vary from localized and segmental to diffuse, according to the stage of the disease.

In an attempt to associate clinical manifestations and renal outcomes to histologic findings in renal biopsy, different pathologists tried to standardize renal amyloid biopsy by grading histologic patterns and scoring renal amyloid deposition, [191-193] but to date, a detailed histopathologic classification of renal amyloidosis has not yet been established.

Recently, Sen et al., proposed a novel classification, [194] based exclusively on glomerular amyloid deposition similarly to SLE classification. This classification consists of 6 histologic patterns or renal amyloidosis, similar to SLE classification.

Class I or minimal renal amyloidosis is characterized by amyloid deposition in less than 10% of the glomeruli. If amyloid is found on vessels of renal allograft patients without glomerular involvement it should also be classified as class I.

Class II is defined as mesangial minimal deposition and characterized by focal and segmental mesangial deposition in 10 to 25% of the glomeruli. In case of recurrence of amyloidosis in renal transplants, tubulointerstitial lesions may also be observed.

Class III or focal mesangiocapillary amyloid deposition presents focal and segmental deposition in 26 to 50% of the flomeruli accompanied by cortical tubulointerstitial lesions and vascular amyloid deposition.

In class IV or diffuse mesangiocapillary amyloid deposition, amyloid deposits are extended in 50 to 75% of the glomeruli. Interstitial deposits, interstitial fibrosis, tubular atrophy, and sclerotic glomeruli are usually observed.

Class V, or membranous amyloid deposition, is characterized by amyloid deposits along the GBM forming spikes similar to membranous nephropathy. In this class, mesangial amyloid deposition is insignificant.

Class VI or advanced amyloidosis is characterized by diffuse glomerular deposition in more than 76% of the glomeruli, with glomerular amyloid nodules and presence or absence of global glomerular sclerosis. Interstitial fibrosis and tubular atrophy are usually observed in this class.

Authors also developed a scoring system of renal amyloidosis, inspired from the Banff classification of renal allograft pathology and SLE classification. In this scoring system, vascular amyloid deposition, interstitial amyloid deposition, interstitial fibrosis, and tubular atrophy, presence of interstitial inflammatory infiltration and glomerular sclerosis were scored 0 to 4 according to the severity of these lesions. Class of glomerular amyloid deposition was scored 0 to 6 while percentage of glomerular deposition was scored 0 to 5.

However, this classification has limitations. The most important limitation is that only the glomerular form is taken into consideration, whereas vascular and interstitial forms are excluded. [195] Second, the scoring system is quite complicated and this could limit its intraobserver and interobserver reproducibility. [195] Therefore, although this classification seems promising, improvement of scoring system and validations studies are required.

Clinical Manifestations

Amyloidosis can involve almost any organ but mainly affects the kidneys, heart, and liver. Cardiac manifestations include restrictive cardiopathy, arrhythmias, sick sinus syndrome, and myocardial infarction due to coronary arteries infiltration. Cardiac disturbances are common in AL amyloidosis but rarely occur in AA amyloidosis.

Gatrointestinal involvement manifests with macroglosia, hepato-splenomegaly, hepatic dysfunction, bowel motility disturbances (constipation, diarrhea), and hemorrhage.

Peripheral neuropathy is also common, presenting initially with sensory and later with motor deficits.

Gastrointestinal and neurologic involvements are common in both AA and AL amyloidosis.

Skin lesions are more frequent in AA amyloidosis, consisting mainly in purpura located in periorbital areas, or ecchymoses, papules and plaques on the face and trunk.

Another rare but important extrarenal manifestation of Al amyloidosis is the acquired bleeding diathesis due to factor X deficiency, increased fibrinolysis, and platelet dysfunction. [196, 197]

Renal involvement presents with proteinuria, mainly albuminuria, ranging from subnephrotic to massive urinary excretion. Kidney size is usually increased in ultrasound but it can be preserved in initial stages of the disease.

When amyloid is predominantly deposited in the tubulointerstitium and the vasculature, proteinuria is less pronounced but there is significant reduction of GFR.

Proteinuria is usually accompanied by hypoalbuminemia, inducing severe edema, often non responsive to diuretic therapy. Hypotension is usually absent, but it may occur in case of concomitant cardiovascular involvement.

Hematuria is typically absent. Amyloid deposition in the collecting ducts interferes with the concentrating mechanism, inducing nephrogenic diabetes insipidus, [198, 199] whereas deposition in proximal tubules causes tubular acidosis and Fanconi's syndrome. [200]

Diagnosis

Diagnosis of amyloidosis requires demonstration of amyloid deposits in bioptic speciments obtained by renal or other tissues such as rectum, salivary glands, subcutaneous abdominal fat, liver, and skin.

Congo red staining is the gold standard in the diagnosis of amyloidosis as it gives a characteristic orange-red appearance to the amyloid fibrils on light microscopy and an apple-green birefringence under polarized light, due to intercalation of Congo-red color into amyloid fibrils.

All above-mentioned tissues could be stained with Congo red to evaluate the presence of amyloid. As renal and liver biopsy are invasive procedures, less invasive methods such as salivary gland and rectal biopsies could be used, given that they present more than 80% sensitivity.

Subcutaneous abdominal fat biopsy can also confirm amyloidosis, as Congo red staining on these tissues presents 80 to 90% sensitivity for AL amyloidosis and 65 to 75% for AA amyloidosis. [201] However, absence of Congo red positivity in this tissue does not necessarily exclude amyloidosis, and in that case, if the disease is suspected, a more invasive procedure should be considered.

Indeed, misdiagnosis is less likely to occur with renal biopsy especially under electron microscopy, although in cases of minimal amyloid deposition, the disease could be misdiagnosed as minimal change disease. [202]

Congo red fluorescence and thioflavin T assay could also be used to increase sensitivity of detecting amyloid deposits. [204] Immunohistochemistry, immunoelectron microscopy, and Western blot technique could also be performed after diagnosis of amyloidosis to determine the type of the deposited amyloid. [204-206]

Treatment

i. AL Amyloidosis

Therapy of AL amyloidosis aims at the elimination of clonal plasma and B cells that produce amyloidognic precursor proteins.

In the past, the most frequently used therapeutic regimen has been melphalan (an alckylating agent) associated to prednisolone, administrated orally in 4 to 7 day cycles every 6 weeks for 2 years. This treatment was rarely successful in obtaining hematologic response, [207, 208] thus negativity of serum and urine for a monoclone protein less than 5% plasma cells in the bone marrow, and absence of signs of monoclonal light chain production. [209]

Oral melphalan (M) at doses of $10mg/m^2$/day with high doses of dexamethasone (Dex) (40mg/day) administrated in 4 day cycles showed better results in eradicating light chain production. [210]

Highs doses of intravenously administrated melphalan (HDM) (140 to $200mg/m^2$) followed by autologous stem cell transplantation (SCT), presented higher hematologic response rates, reaching up to 50% of treated patients. [211, 212] Effects of HDM/SCT regimen have also been evaluated in AL with renal involvement. [178] In this study, 65 patients with AL amyloidosis and urinary protein excretion higher than 1g/24h received HDM/SCT treatment and were followed for at least 12 months. Of the 65 patients, only 50 survived for more than 12 months. Among the patients with complete hematologic response, 71% also showed renal response with reduction of proteinuria and improvement of hypoalbuminemia and hypercholesterolemia. This finding suggested an association between hematologic and renal response, but this remains controversial as another study failed to prove such connection. [213]

There is also concern on the safety of this regimen as severe complications due to toxicity have been frequently reported. Splenic rapture, bleeding diathesis due to thrombocytopenia, and acute renal failure may limit its use. Acute renal failure is more likely to occur in patients with already impaired renal function and AL patients with cardiac involvement. [214]

Dialysis can be required in AL amyloidosis with renal and/or cardiac involvement, but this treatment is often cumbersome due to hemodynamic instability, bleeding diathesis and difficulties in vascular access. Peritoneal dialysis could be a valid alternative for these patients. However, survival rates are similar for both procedures.

Renal transplantation may be considered after complete hematologic response but is often limited by cardiac involvement.

ii. AA Amyloidosis

Treatment of AA amyloidosis aims at the underlying inflammatory predisposing disease. Suppression of inflammation whatever the underlying cause is reduces SAA production and clinical manifestations and improves survival.

To date different cytotoxic agents and antinflammatories have been used. Chlorambucil was successfully used in patients with juvenile inflammatory arthritis, and azathioprine showed delay of the disease progression in patients with rheumatoid arthritis. Use of colchicine was also beneficial in AA amyloidosis due to familial Mediterranean fever. Antimicrobial therapy for tuberculosis and osteomyelitis and surgical excision of abscesses, have also been helpful.

TNF antagonists may reduce interaction of AA fibrils to advanced glycation end products, preventing AA-mediated cell toxicity. [215, 216]

Eprodisate, a new compound with structure similar to heparin sulfate, competitively binds to glycosaminoglycans-binding sites of SAA-inhibiting fibril polymerization and amyloid deposition. [217] In a multicentered randomized double blind trial, 124 patients with AA amyloidosis and renal involvement were treated with 800 to 2400 mg of oral eprodisate daily, in two divided doses. [218] Treatment delayed decline of renal function but failed to improve renal protein excretion. A limit on its use in AA amyloidosis-induced renal disease is that eprodisate is primarily excreted by the kidneys and requires dosage adjustment in order to avoid side effects, such as gastrointestinal disorders, infections, arthralgias, headache, dizziness, and renal failure. [219, 220]

References

[1] Remuzzi G, Schieppati A, Ruggenenti P. Clinical practice. Nephropathy in patients with type 2 diabetes. *N. Engl. J. Med.* 2002 Apr 11;346(15):1145-51.

[2] Collins AJ, Foley RN, Chavers B, Gilbertson D, Herzog C, Johansen K, et al. 'United States Renal Data System 2011 Annual Data Report: Atlas of chronic kidney disease & end-stage renal disease in the United States.' *Am. J. Kidney Dis.* 2012 Jan;59(1 Suppl 1):A7, e1-420.

[3] Held PJ, Port FK, Webb RL, Wolfe RA, Garcia JR, Blagg CR, e al. The United States Renal Data System's 1991 annual data report: an introduction. *Am. J. Kidney Dis.* 1991 Nov;18(5 Suppl 2):1-16.

[4] Raparia K, Usman I, Kanwar YS. Renal morphologic lesions reminiscent of diabetic nephropathy. *Arch. Pathol. Lab. Med.* 2013 Mar;137(3):351-9.

[5] Kimmelstiel P, Wilson C. Benign and Malignant Hypertension and Nephrosclerosis: A Clinical and Pathological Study. *Am. J. Pathol.* 1936 Jan;12(1):45-82.3.

[6] Eknoyan G, Hostetter T, Bakris GL, Hebert L, Levey AS, Parving HH, et al. Proteinuria and other markers of chronic kidney disease: a position statement of the national kidney foundation (NKF) and the national institute of diabetes and digestive and kidney diseases (NIDDK). *Am. J. Kidney Dis.* 2003 Oct;42(4):617-22.

[7] Deshpande SD, Putta S, Wang M, Lai JY, Bitzer M, Nelson RG, et al. Transforming growth factor-β-induced cross talk between p53 and a microRNA in the pathogenesis of diabetic nephropathy. *Diabetes.* 2013 Sep;62(9):3151-62.

[8] de Boer IH, Rue TC, Hall YN, Heagerty PJ, Weiss NS, Himmelfarb J. Temporal trends in the prevalence of diabetic kidney disease in the United States. *JAMA.* 2011 Jun 22;305(24):2532-9.

[9] Young BA, Maynard C, Boyko EJ. Racial differences in diabetic nephropathy, cardiovascular disease, and mortality in a national population of veterans. *Diabetes Care.* 2003 Aug;26(8):2392-9.

[10] Pettitt DJ, Saad MF, Bennett PH, Nelson RG, Knowler WC. Familial predisposition to renal disease in two generations of Pima Indians with type 2 (non-insulin-dependent) diabetes mellitus. *Diabetologia.* 1990 Jul;33(7):438-43.

[11] Cowie CC, Port FK, Wolfe RA, Savage PJ, Moll PP, Hawthorne VM. Disparities in incidence of diabetic end-stage renal disease according to race and type of diabetes. *N Engl. J. Med. 1989* Oct 19;321(16):1074-9.

[12] Nguyen NT, Magno CP, Lane KT, Hinojosa MW, Lane JS. Association of hypertension, diabetes, dyslipidemia, and metabolic syndrome with obesity: findings from the National Health and Nutrition Examination Survey, 1999 to 2004. *J. Am. Coll Surg.* 2008 Dec;207(6):928-34.

[13] Groop PH, Thomas MC, Moran JL, Wadèn J, Thorn LM, Mäkinen VPet al; FinnDiane Study Group. The presence and severity of chronic kidney disease predicts all-cause mortality in type 1 diabetes. *Diabetes.* 2009 Jul;58(7):1651-8.

[14] Mogensen CE. Microalbuminuria predicts clinical proteinuria and early mortality in maturity-onset diabetes. *N. Engl. J. Med.* 1984 Feb 9;310(6):356-60.

[15] Hovind P, Rossing P, Tarnow L, Smidt UM, Parving HH. Progression of diabetic nephropathy. *Kidney Int.* 2001 Feb;59(2):702-9.

[16] Nielsen S, Schmitz A, Rehling M, Mogensen CE. The clinical course of renal function in NIDDM patients with normo- and microalbuminuria. *J. Intern. Med.* 1997 Feb;241(2):133-41.

[17] Adler S. Diabetic nephropathy: Linking histology, cell biology, and genetics. *Kidney Int.* 2004 Nov;66(5):2095-106.

[18] Steinke JM, Sinaiko AR, Kramer MS, Suissa S, Chavers BM, Mauer M; International Diabetic Nephopathy Study Group. The early natural history of nephropathy in Type 1 Diabetes: III. Predictors of 5-year urinary albumin excretion rate patterns in initially normoalbuminuric patients. *Diabetes.* 2005 Jul;54(7):2164-71.

[19] Ziyadeh FN. Mediators of diabetic renal disease: the case for TGF-β as the major mediator. *J. Am. Soc. Nephrol.* 2004 Jan;15 Suppl 1:S55-7.

[20] Gall MA, Borch-Johnsen K, Hougaard P, Nielsen FS, Parving HH. Albuminuria and poor glycemic control predict mortality in NIDDM. *Diabetes.* 1995 Nov;44(11):1303-9.

[21] Jones C, Roderick P, Harris S, Rogerson M. Decline in kidney function before and after nephrology referral and the effect on survival in moderate to advanced chronic kidney disease. *Nephrol. Dial. Transplant.* 2006 Aug;21(8):2133-43.

[22] Chan MR, Dall AT, Fletcher KE, Lu N, Trivedi H. Outcomes in patients with chronic kidney disease referred late to nephrologists: a meta-analysis. *Am. J. Med.* 2007 Dec;120(12):1063-70.

[23] Jacobsen P, Rossing K, Hansen BV, Bie P, Vaag A, Parving HH. Effect of short-term hyperglycaemia on haemodynamics in type 1 diabetic patients. *J. Intern. Med.* 2003 Nov;254(5):464-71.

[24] Wolf G, Ziyadeh FN. Molecular mechanisms of diabetic renal hypertrophy. *Kidney Int.* 1999 Aug;56(2):393-405.

[25] Bak M, Thomsen K, Christiansen T, Flyvbjerg A. Renal enlargement precedes renal hyperfiltration in early experimental diabetes in rats. *J. Am. Soc. Nephrol.* 2000 Jul;11(7):1287-92.

[26] Hirschberg R, Kopple JD. The growth hormone-insulin-like growth factor I axis and renal glomerular function. *J. Am. Soc. Nephrol.* 1992 Mar;2(9):1417-22.

[27] Singh R, Alavi N, Singh AK, Leehey DJ. Role of angiotensin II in glucose-induced inhibition of mesangial matrix degradation. *Diabetes.* 1999 Oct;48(10):2066-73.

[28] Sharma K, Eltayeb BO, McGowan TA, Dunn SR, Alzahabi B, Rohde R, et al. Captopril-induced reduction of serum levels of transforming growth factor-beta1 correlates with long-term renoprotection in insulin-dependent diabetic patients. *Am. J. Kidney Dis.* 1999 Nov;34(5):818-23.

[29] Morrissey J, Hruska K, Guo G, Wang S, Chen Q, Klahr S. Bone morphogenetic protein-7 improves renal fibrosis and accelerates the return of renal function. *J. Am. Soc. Nephrol.* 2002 Jan;13 Suppl 1:S14-21.

[30] Turk T, Leeuwis JW, Gray J, Torti SV, Lyons KM, Nguyen TQ, et al. BMP signaling and podocyte markers are decreased in human diabetic nephropathy in association with CTGF overexpression. *J. Histochem. Cytochem.* 2009 Jul;57(7):623-31.

[31] Baelde HJ, Eikmans M, Lappin DW, Doran PP, Hohenadel D, Brinkkoetter PT, et al. Reduction of VEGF-A and CTGF expression in diabetic nephropathy is associated with podocyte loss. *Kidney Int.* 2007 Apr;71(7):637-45.

[32] Bortoloso E, Del Prete D, Dalla Vestra M, Gambaro G, Saller A, Antonucci F, et al. Quantitave and qualitative changes in vascular endothelial growth factor gene

expression in glomeruli of patients with type 2 diabetes. *Eur. J. Endocrinol.* 2004 Jun;150(6):799-807.

[33] Hilgers KF, Veelken R. Type 2 diabetic nephropathy: never too early to treat? *J. Am. Soc. Nephrol.* 2005 Mar;16(3):574-5.

[34] Sorokin A, Kohan DE. Physiology and pathology of endothelin-1 in renal mesangium. *Am. J. Physiol. Renal. Physiol.* 2003 Oct;285(4):F579-89.

[35] Harris RD, Steffes MW, Bilous RW, Sutherland DE, Mauer SM. Global glomerular sclerosis and glomerular arteriolar hyalinosis in insulin dependent diabetes. *Kidney Int.* 1991 Jul;40(1):107-14.

[36] Heilig CW, Concepcion LA, Riser BL, Freytag SO, Zhu M, Cortes P. Overexpression of glucose transporters in rat mesangial cells cultured in a normal glucose milieu mimics the diabetic phenotype. *J. Clin. Invest.* 1995 Oct;96(4):1802-14.

[37] Chen ZJ, Yang YB, Huang SM. [Expression of VEGF in kidney of diabetic rats]. Sichuan Da Xue Xue Bao Yi Xue Ban. 2007 Jul;38(4):633-6. [Article in Chinese]

[38] Friedman EA. Advanced glycation end-products in diabetic nephropathy. *Nephrol. Dial. Transplant.* 1999;14 Suppl 3:1-9.

[39] Porte D Jr, Schwartz MW. Diabetes complications: why is glucose potentially toxic? *Science.* 1996 May 3;272(5262):699-700.

[40] Rüster C, Bondeva T, Franke S, Tanaka N, Yamamoto H, Wolf G. Angiotensin II upregulates RAGE expression on podocytes: role of AT2 receptors. *Am. J. Nephrol.* 2009;29(6):538-50.

[41] Loeffler I, Rüster C, Franke S, Liebisch M, Wolf G. Erythropoietin ameliorates podocyte injury in advanced diabetic nephropathy in the db/db mouse. *Am. J. Physiol Renal. Physiol.* 2013 Sep 15;305(6):F911-8.

[42] Bondeva T, Rüster C, Franke S, Hammerschmid E, Klagsbrun M, Cohen CD, et al. Advanced glycation end-products suppress neuropilin-1 expression in podocytes. *Kidney Int.* 2009 Mar;75(6):605-16.

[43] Fukami K, Ueda S, Yamagishi S, Kato S, Inagaki Y, Takeuchi M, et al. AGEs activate mesangial TGF-beta-Smad signaling via an angiotensin II type I receptor interaction. *Kidney Int.* 2004 Dec;66(6):2137-47.

[44] Brownlee M. Biochemistry and molecular cell biology of diabetic complications. *Nature.* 2001 Dec 13;414(6865):813-20.

[45] Makita Z, Radoff S, Rayfield EJ, Yang Z, Skolnik E, Delaney V, et al. Advanced glycosylation end products in patients with diabetic nephropathy. *N. Engl. J. Med.* 1991 Sep 19;325(12):836-42.

[46] Sabbatini M, Sansone G, Uccello F, Giliberti A, Conte G, Andreucci VE. Early glycosylation products induce glomerular hyperfiltration in normal rats. *Kidney Int.* 1992 Oct;42(4):875-81.

[47] Craven PA, Davidson CM, DeRubertis FR. Increase in diacylglycerol mass in isolated glomeruli by glucose from de novo synthesis of glycerolipids. *Diabetes.* 1990 Jun;39(6):667-74.

[48] Derubertis FR, Craven PA. Activation of protein kinase C in glomerular cells in diabetes. Mechanisms and potential links to the pathogenesis of diabetic glomerulopathy. *Diabetes.* 1994 Jan;43(1):1-8.

[49] Ishii H, Jirousek MR, Koya D, Takagi C, Xia P, Clermont A, et al. Amelioration of vascular dysfunctions in diabetic rats by an oral PKC beta inhibitor. *Science*. 1996 May 3;272(5262):728-31.
[50] Cherney DZ, Sochett EB, Miller JA. Gender differences in renal responses to hyperglycemia and angiotensin-converting enzyme inhibition in diabetes. *Kidney Int*. 2005 Oct;68(4):1722-8.
[51] Craven PA, Caines MA, DeRubertis FR. Sequential alterations in glomerular prostaglandin and thromboxane synthesis in diabetic rats: relationship to the hyperfiltration of early diabetes. *Metabolism*. 1987 Jan;36(1):95-103.
[52] Perico N, Benigni A, Gabanelli M, Piccinelli A, Ròg M, De Riva C, et al. Atrial natriuretic peptide and prostacyclin synergistically mediate hyperfiltration and hyperperfusion of diabetic rats. *Diabetes*. 1992 Apr;41(4):533-8.
[53] Ruan X, Arendshorst WJ. Role of protein kinase C in angiotensin II-induced renal vasoconstriction in genetically hypertensive rats. *Am. J. Physiol*. 1996 Jun;270(6 Pt 2):F945-52.
[54] Sharma K, Danoff TM, DePiero A, Ziyadeh FN. Enhanced expression of inducible nitric oxide synthase in murine macrophages and glomerular mesangial cells by elevated glucose levels: possible mediation via protein kinase C. *Biochem. Biophys. Res. Commun.* 1995 Feb 6;207(1):80-8.
[55] Craven PA, Studer RK, DeRubertis FR. Impaired nitric oxide-dependent cyclic guanosine monophosphate generation in glomeruli from diabetic rats. Evidence for protein kinase C-mediated suppression of the cholinergic response. *J. Clin. Invest*. 1994 Jan;93(1):311-20.
[56] Aiello LP, Bursell SE, Clermont A, Duh E, Ishii H, Takagi C, et al. Vascular endothelial growth factor-induced retinal permeability is mediated by protein kinase C in vivo and suppressed by an orally effective beta-isoform-selective inhibitor. *Diabetes*. 1997 Sep;46(9):1473-80.
[57] Oliver JA. Adenylate cyclase and protein kinase C mediate opposite actions on endothelial junctions. *J. Cell Physiol.* 1990 Dec;145(3):536-42.
[58] Lynch JJ, Ferro TJ, Blumenstock FA, Brockenauer AM, Malik AB. Increased endothelial albumin permeability mediated by protein kinase C activation. *J. Clin. Invest.* 1990 Jun;85(6):1991-8.
[59] Xia P, Aiello LP, Ishii H, Jiang ZY, Park DJ, Robinson GS, et al. Characterization of vascular endothelial growth factor's effect on the activation of protein kinase C, its isoforms, and endothelial cell growth. *J. Clin. Invest*. 1996 Nov 1;98(9):2018-26.
[60] Koya D, Jirousek MR, Lin YW, Ishii H, Kuboki K, King GL. Characterization of protein kinase C beta isoform activation on the gene expression of transforming growth factor-beta, extracellular matrix components, and prostanoids in the glomeruli of diabetic rats. *J. Clin. Invest.* 1997 Jul 1;100(1):115-26.
[61] Petrash JM. All in the family: aldose reductase and closely related aldo-keto reductases. *Cell. Mol. Life Sci.* 2004 Apr;61(7-8):737-49.
[62] Schrijvers BF, De Vriese AS, Flyvbjerg A. From hyperglycemia to diabetic kidney disease: the role of metabolic, hemodynamic, intracellular factors and growth factors/cytokines. *Endocr. Rev.* 2004 Dec;25(6):971-1010.
[63] Gabbay KH, Merola LO, Field RA. Sorbitol pathway: presence in nerve and cord with substrate accumulation in diabetes. *Science*. 1966 Jan 14;151(3707):209-10.

[64] Huang P, Zhang Y, Jiang T, Zeng W, Zhang N. Role of aldose reductase in the high glucose induced expression of fibronectin in human mesangial cells. *Mol. Biol. Rep.* 2010 Jul;37(6):3017-21.

[65] Kinoshita JH. Mechanisms initiating cataract formation. Proctor Lecture. *Invest Ophthalmol.* 1974 Oct;13(10):713-24.

[66] Palm F, Hansell P, Ronquist G, Waldenström A, Liss P, Carlsson PO. Polyol-pathway-dependent disturbances in renal medullary metabolism in experimental insulin-deficient diabetes mellitus in rats. *Diabetologia.* 2004 Jul;47(7):1223-31.

[67] Derylo B, Babazono T, Glogowski E, Kapor-Drezgic J, Hohman T, Whiteside C. High glucose-induced mesangial cell altered contractility: role of the polyol pathway. *Diabetologia.* 1998 May;41(5):507-15.

[68] Morrisey K, Steadman R, Williams JD, Phillips AO. Renal proximal tubular cell fibronectin accumulation in response to glucose is polyol pathway dependent. *Kidney Int.* 1999 Jun;55(6):2548-72.

[69] Donnelly SM, Zhou XP, Huang JT, Whiteside CI. Prevention of early glomerulopathy with tolrestat in the streptozotocin-induced diabetic rat. *Biochem Cell. Biol.* 1996;74(3):355-62.

[70] Riedl E, Pfister F, Braunagel M, Brinkkötter P, Sternik P, Deinzer M, et al. Carnosine prevents apoptosis of glomerular cells and podocyte loss in STZ diabetic rats. *Cell. Physiol Biochem.* 2011;28(2):279-88.

[71] Marshall S, Bacote V, Traxinger RR. Discovery of a metabolic pathway mediating glucose-induced desensitization of the glucose transport system. Role of hexosamine biosynthesis in the induction of insulin resistance. *J. Biol. Chem.* 1991 Mar 15;266(8):4706-12.

[72] Marshall S, Garvey WT, Traxinger RR. New insights into the metabolic regulation of insulin action and insulin resistance: role of glucose and amino acids. *FASEB J.* 1991 Dec;5(15):3031-6.

[73] James LR, Ingram A, Ly H, Thai K, Cai L, Scholey JW. Angiotensin II activates the GFAT promoter in mesangial cells. *Am. J. Physiol. Renal. Physiol.* 2001 Jul;281(1):F151-62.

[74] Kolm-Litty V, Sauer U, Nerlich A, Lehmann R, Schleicher ED. High glucose-induced transforming growth factor beta1 production is mediated by the hexosamine pathway in porcine glomerular mesangial cells. *J. Clin. Invest.* 1998 Jan 1;101(1):160-9.

[75] Xu G, Lehmann R, Schleicher E, Häring HU, Liebich H. Advantages in the analysis of UDP-sugars by capillary electrophoresis-comparison of the conventional HPLC method with two new capillary electrophoretic micro-procedures. *Biomed. Chromatogr.* 1998 May-Jun;12(3):113-5.

[76] Kolm-Litty V, Tippmer S, Häring HU, Schleicher E. Glucosamine induces translocation of protein kinase C isoenzymes in mesangial cells. *Exp. Clin. Endocrinol. Diabetes.* 1998;106(5):377-83.

[77] Zheng JM, Zhu JM, Li LS, Liu ZH. Rhein reverses the diabetic phenotype of mesangial cells over-expressing the glucose transporter (GLUT1) by inhibiting the hexosamine pathway. *Br. J. Pharmacol.* 2008 Apr;153(7):1456-64.

[78] Ferenbach D, Kluth DC, Hughes J. Inflammatory cells in renal injury and repair. *Semin. Nephrol.* 2007 May;27(3):250-9.

[79] Chow FY, Nikolic-Paterson DJ, Ma FY, Ozols E, Rollins BJ, Tesch GH. Monocyte chemoattractant protein-1-induced tissue inflammation is critical for the development of renal injury but not type 2 diabetes in obese db/db mice. *Diabetologia.* 2007 Feb;50(2):471-80.

[80] Morii T, Fujita H, Narita T, Shimotomai T, Fujishima H, Yoshioka N, et al. Association of monocyte chemoattractant protein-1 with renal tubular damage in diabetic nephropathy. *J. Diabetes Complications*. 2003 Jan-Feb;17(1):11-5.

[81] Jevnikar AM, Brennan DC, Singer GG, Heng JE, Maslinski W, Wuthrich RP, et al. Stimulated kidney tubular epithelial cells express membrane associated and secreted TNF alpha. *Kidney Int*. 1991 Aug;40(2):203-11.

[82] Nakamura T, Fukui M, Ebihara I, Osada S, Nagaoka I, Tomino Y, et al. mRNA expression of growth factors in glomeruli from diabetic rats. *Diabetes.* 1993 Mar;42(3):450-6.

[83] Sugimoto H, Shikata K, Wada J, Horiuchi S, Makino H. Advanced glycation end products-cytokine-nitric oxide sequence pathway in the development of diabetic nephropathy: aminoguanidine ameliorates the overexpression of tumour necrosis factor-alpha and inducible nitric oxide synthase in diabetic rat glomeruli. *Diabetologia*. 1999 Jul;42(7):878-86.

[84] Dong X, Swaminathan S, Bachman LA, Croatt AJ, Nath KA, Griffin MD. Resident dendritic cells are the predominant TNF-secreting cell in early renal ischemia-reperfusion injury. *Kidney Int.* 2007 Apr;71(7):619-28.

[85] Wójciak-Stothard B, Entwistle A, Garg R, Ridley AJ. Regulation of TNF-alpha-induced reorganization of the actin cytoskeleton and cell-cell junctions by Rho, Rac, and Cdc42 in human endothelial cells. *J. Cell. Physiol*. 1998 Jul;176(1):150-65.

[86] Baud L, Ardaillou R. Tumor necrosis factor in renal injury. *Miner Electrolyte Metab.* 1995;21(4-5):336-41.

[87] Gómez-Chiarri M, Ortíz A, Lerma JL, López-Armada MJ, Mampaso F, González E, et al. Involvement of tumor necrosis factor and platelet-activating factor in the pathogenesis of experimental nephrosis in rats. *Lab. Invest.* 1994 Apr;70(4):449-59.

[88] Marsden PA, Brenner BM. Transcriptional regulation of the endothelin-1 gene by TNF-alpha. *Am. J. Physiol*. 1992 Apr;262(4 Pt 1):C854-61.

[89] Marsden PA, Ballermann BJ. Tumor necrosis factor alpha activates soluble guanylate cyclase in bovine glomerular mesangial cells via an L-arginine-dependent mechanism. *J Exp. Med*. 1990 Dec 1;172(6):1843-52.

[90] DiPetrillo K, Coutermarsh B, Gesek FA. Urinary tumor necrosis factor contributes to sodium retention and renal hypertrophy during diabetes. *Am. J. Physiol. Renal. Physiol.* 2003 Jan;284(1):F113-21.

[91] Navarro JF, Mora C, Muros M, García J. Urinary tumour necrosis factor-alpha excretion independently correlates with clinical markers of glomerular and tubulointerstitial injury in type 2 diabetic patients. *Nephrol. Dial Transplant*. 2006 Dec;21(12):3428-34. Epub 2006 Aug 25.

[92] Pfeilschifter J, Pignat W, Vosbeck K, Märki F. Interleukin 1 and tumor necrosis factor synergistically stimulate prostaglandin synthesis and phospholipase A2 release from rat renal mesangial cells. *Biochem. Biophys. Res. Commun*. 1989 Mar 15;159(2):385-94.

[93] Royall JA, Berkow RL, Beckman JS, Cunningham MK, Matalon S, Freeman BA. Tumor necrosis factor and interleukin 1 alpha increase vascular endothelial permeability. *Am. J. Physiol.* 1989 Dec;257(6 Pt 1):L399-410.

[94] Vesey DA, Cheung C, Cuttle L, Endre Z, Gobe G, Johnson DW. Interleukin-1beta stimulates human renal fibroblast proliferation and matrix protein production by means of a transforming growth factor-beta-dependent mechanism. *J. Lab. Clin. Med.* 2002 Nov;140(5):342-50.

[95] Jones S, Jones S, Phillips AO. Regulation of renal proximal tubular epithelial cell hyaluronan generation: implications for diabetic nephropathy. *Kidney Int.* 2001 May;59(5):1739-49.

[96] Coleman DL, Ruef C. Interleukin-6: an autocrine regulator of mesangial cell growth. *Kidney Int.* 1992 Mar;41(3):604-6.

[97] Suzuki D, Miyazaki M, Naka R, Koji T, Yagame M, Jinde K, et al. In situ hybridization of interleukin 6 in diabetic nephropathy. *Diabetes.* 1995 Oct;44(10):1233-8.

[98] Ruef C, Budde K, Lacy J, Northemann W, Baumann M, Sterzel RB, et al. Interleukin 6 is an autocrine growth factor for mesangial cells. *Kidney Int.* 1990 Aug;38(2):249-57.

[99] Dalla Vestra M, Mussap M, Gallina P, Bruseghin M, Cernigoi AM, Saller A, et al. Acute-phase markers of inflammation and glomerular structure in patients with type 2 diabetes. *J. Am. Soc. Nephrol.* 2005 Mar;16 Suppl 1:S78-82.

[100] Sugimoto H, Shikata K, Hirata K, Akiyama K, Matsuda M, Kushiro M, et al. Increased expression of intercellular adhesion molecule-1 (ICAM-1) in diabetic rat glomeruli: glomerular hyperfiltration is a potential mechanism of ICAM-1 upregulation. *Diabetes.* 1997 Dec;46(12):2075-81.

[101] Matsui H, Suzuki M, Tsukuda R, Iida K, Miyasaka M, Ikeda H. Expression of ICAM-1 on glomeruli is associated with progression of diabetic nephropathy in a genetically obese diabetic rat, Wistar fatty. *Diabetes Res. Clin. Pract.* 1996 Apr;32(1-2):1-9.

[102] Melnikov VY, Faubel S, Siegmund B, Lucia MS, Ljubanovic D, Edelstein CL. Neutrophil-independent mechanisms of caspase-1- and IL-18-mediated ischemic acute tubular necrosis in mice. *J. Clin. Invest.* 2002 Oct;110(8):1083-91.

[103] Nguyen G, Delarue F, Burcklé C, Bouzhir L, Giller T, Sraer JD. Pivotal role of the renin/prorenin receptor in angiotensin II production and cellular responses to renin. *J. Clin Invest.* 2002 Jun;109(11):1417-27.

[104] Danser AH, Derkx FH, Schalekamp MA, Hense HW, Riegger GA, Schunkert H. Determinants of interindividual variation of renin and prorenin concentrations: evidence for a sexual dimorphism of (pro)renin levels in humans. *J Hypertens.* 1998 Jun;16(6):853-62.

[105] Sealey JE, Moon C, Laragh JH, Atlas SA. Plasma prorenin in normal, hypertensive, and anephric subjects and its effect on renin measurements. *Circ. Res.* 1977 May;40(5 Suppl 1):I41-5.

[106] Deinum J, Rønn B, Mathiesen E, Derkx FH, Hop WC, Schalekamp MA. Increase in serum prorenin precedes onset of microalbuminuria in patients with insulin-dependent diabetes mellitus. *Diabetologia.* 1999 Aug;42(8):1006-10.

[107] Nguyen G, Danser AH. Prorenin and (pro)renin receptor: a review of available data from in vitro studies and experimental models in rodents. *Exp. Physiol.* 2008 May;93(5):557-63.

[108] Itskovitz J, Sealey JE, Glorioso N, Rosenwaks Z. Plasma prorenin response to human chorionic gonadotropin in ovarian-hyperstimulated women: correlation with the number of ovarian follicles and steroid hormone concentrations. *Proc. Natl. Acad. Sci. U S A*. 1987 Oct;84(20):7285-9.

[109] Berka JL, Stubbs AJ, Wang DZ, DiNicolantonio R, Alcorn D, Campbell DJ, et al. Renin-containing Müller cells of the retina display endocrine features. *Invest Ophthalmol. Vis. Sci*. 1995 Jun;36(7):1450-8.

[110] Reudelhuber TL, Ramla D, Chiu L, Mercure C, Seidah NG. Proteolytic processing of human prorenin in renal and non-renal tissues. *Kidney Int*. 1994 Dec;46(6):1522-4.

[111] Neves FA, Duncan KG, Baxter JD. Cathepsin B is a prorenin processing enzyme. *Hypertension*. 1996 Mar;27(3 Pt 2):514-7.

[112] Nabi AH, Kageshima A, Uddin MN, Nakagawa T, Park EY, Suzuki F. Binding properties of rat prorenin and renin to the recombinant rat renin/prorenin receptor prepared by a baculovirus expression system. *Int. J. Mol. Med*. 2006 Sep;18(3):483-8.

[113] Sakoda M, Ichihara A, Kaneshiro Y, Takemitsu T, Nakazato Y, Nabi AH, et al. (Pro)renin receptor-mediated activation of mitogen-activated protein kinases in human vascular smooth muscle cells. *Hypertens Res*. 2007 Nov;30(11):1139-46.

[114] Huang Y, Wongamorntham S, Kasting J, McQuillan D, Owens RT, Yu L, et al. Renin increases mesangial cell transforming growth factor-beta1 and matrix proteins through receptor-mediated, angiotensin II-independent mechanisms. *Kidney Int*. 2006 Jan;69(1):105-13.

[115] Satofuka S, Ichihara A, Nagai N, Noda K, Ozawa Y, Fukamizu A, et al. (Pro)renin receptor-mediated signal transduction and tissue renin-angiotensin system contribute to diabetes-induced retinal inflammation. *Diabetes*. 2009 Jul;58(7):1625-33.

[116] Matavelli LC, Huang J, Siragy HM. (Pro)renin receptor contributes to diabetic nephropathy by enhancing renal inflammation. *Clin. Exp. Pharmacol. Physiol*. 2010 Mar;37(3):277-82.

[117] Langham RG, Kelly DJ, Cox AJ, Thomson NM, Holthöfer H, Zaoui P, et al. Proteinuria and the expression of the podocyte slit diaphragm protein, nephrin, in diabetic nephropathy: effects of angiotensin converting enzyme inhibition. *Diabetologia*. 2002 Nov;45(11):1572-6.

[118] Kelly DJ, Aaltonen P, Cox AJ, Rumble JR, Langham R, Panagiotopoulos S, et al. Expression of the slit-diaphragm protein, nephrin, in experimental diabetic nephropathy: differing effects of anti-proteinuric therapies. Nephrol. Dial. Transplant. 2002 Jul;17(7):1327-32.

[119] Doublier S, Salvidio G, Lupia E, Ruotsalainen V, Verzola D, Deferrari G, et al. Nephrin expression is reduced in human diabetic nephropathy: evidence for a distinct role for glycated albumin and angiotensin II. *Diabetes*. 2003 Apr;52(4):1023-30.

[120] Bjørn SF, Bangstad HJ, Hanssen KF, Nyberg G, Walker JD, Viberti GC, et al. Glomerular epithelial foot processes, and filtration slits in IDDM patients. *Diabetologia*. 1995 Oct;38(10):1197-204.

[121] Tanji N, Markowitz GS, Fu C, Kislinger T, Taguchi A, Pischetsrieder M, et al. Expression of advanced glycation end products and their cellular receptor RAGE in diabetic nephropathy and nondiabetic renal disease. *J. Am. Soc. Nephrol*. 2000 Sep;11(9):1656-66.

[122] Pätäri A, Forsblom C, Havana M, Taipale H, Groop PH, Holthöfer H. Nephrinuria in diabetic nephropathy of type 1 diabetes. *Diabetes*. 2003 Dec;52(12):2969-74.
[123] Coward RJ, Welsh GI, Koziell A, Hussain S, Lennon R, Ni L, et al. Nephrin is critical for the action of insulin on human glomerular podocytes. *Diabetes*. 2007 Apr;56(4):1127-35.
[124] Rigat B, Hubert C, Alhenc-Gelas F, Cambien F, Corvol P, Soubrier F. An insertion/deletion polymorphism in the angiotensin I-converting enzyme gene accounting for half the variance of serum enzyme levels. *J. Clin. Invest*. 1990 Oct;86(4):1343-6.
[125] Movva S, Alluri RV, Komandur S, Vattam K, Eppa K, Mukkavali KK, et al. Relationship of angiotensin-converting enzyme gene polymorphism with nephropathy associated with Type 2 diabetes mellitus in Asian Indians. *J. Diabetes Complications*. 2007 Jul-Aug;21(4):237-41.
[126] Boright AP, Paterson AD, Mirea L, Bull SB, Mowjoodi A, Scherer SW, et al; DCCT/EDIC Research Group. Genetic variation at the ACE gene is associated with persistent microalbuminuria and severe nephropathy in type 1 diabetes: the DCCT/EDIC Genetics Study. *Diabetes*. 2005 Apr;54(4):1238-44.
[127] Neamat-Allah M, Feeney SA, Savage DA, Maxwell AP, Hanson RL, Knowler WC, et al. Analysis of the association between diabetic nephropathy and polymorphisms in the aldose reductase gene in Type 1 and Type 2 diabetes mellitus. *Diabet. Med*. 2001 Nov;18(11):906-14.
[128] Liu YF, Wat NM, Chung SS, Ko BC, Lam KS. Diabetic nephropathy is associated with the 5'-end dinucleotide repeat polymorphism of the aldose reductase gene in Chinese subjects with Type 2 diabetes. *Diabet. Med*. 2002 Feb;19(2):113-8.
[129] Tonna S, El-Osta A, Cooper ME, Tikellis C. Metabolic memory and diabetic nephropathy: potential role for epigenetic mechanisms. *Nat. Rev. Nephrol*. 2010 Jun;6(6):332-41.
[130] Fioretto P, Mauer M, Brocco E, Velussi M, Frigato F, Muollo B, et al. Patterns of renal injury in NIDDM patients with microalbuminuria. *Diabetologia*. 1996 Dec;39(12):1569-76.
[131] Mazzucco G, Bertani T, Fortunato M, Bernardi M, Leutner M, Boldorini R, et al. Different patterns of renal damage in type 2 diabetes mellitus: a multicentric study on 393 biopsies. *Am. J. Kidney Dis*. 2002 Apr;39(4):713-20.
[132] Tervaert TW, Mooyaart AL, Amann K, Cohen AH, Cook HT, Drachenberg CB, et al; Renal Pathology Society. Pathologic classification of diabetic nephropathy. *J. Am. Soc. Nephrol*. 2010 Apr;21(4):556-63.
[133] Paueksakon P, Revelo MP, Ma LJ, Marcantoni C, Fogo AB. Microangiopathic injury and augmented PAI-1 in human diabetic nephropathy. *Kidney Int*. 2002 Jun;61(6):2142-8.
[134] Zhu X, Liu F, Peng Y, Liu H, Yuan S, Xu X, et al. [New pathologic classification of diabetic nephropathy (retrospective study of 37 cases)]. Zhong Nan Da Xue Xue Bao Yi Xue Ban. 2012 Feb;37(2):185-9. [Article in Chinese]
[135] Mogensen CE, Vestbo E, Poulsen PL, Christiansen C, Damsgaard EM, Eiskjaer H, et al. Microalbuminuria and potential confounders. A review and some observations on variability of urinary albumin excretion. *Diabetes Care*. 1995 Apr;18(4):572-81.

[136] Vamos EP, Harris M, Millett C, Pape UJ, Khunti K, Curcin V, et al. Association of systolic and diastolic blood pressure and all cause mortality in people with newly diagnosed type 2 diabetes: retrospective cohort study. *BMJ.* 2012 Aug 30;345:e5567.

[137] Kidney Disease: Improving Global. Outcomes (KDIGO) CKD Work Group. KDIGO 2012 Clinical Practice Guideline for the Evaluation and Management of Chronic Kidney Disease. *Kidney inter.,* Suppl. 2013; 3: 1–150.

[138] National Kidney Foundation. KDOQI™Clinical Practice Guidelines and Clinical Practice Recommendations for Diabetes and Chronic Kidney Disease. *Am. J. Kidney Dis.* 49:S1-S180, 2007 (suppl 2)

[139] Giordano M, Lucidi P, Ciarambino T, Gesuè L, Castellino P, Cioffi M, et al. Effects of dietary protein restriction on albumin and fibrinogen synthesis in macroalbuminuric type 2 diabetic patients. *Diabetologia.* 2008 Jan;51(1):21-8.

[140] Pan Y, Guo LL, Jin HM. Low-protein diet for diabetic nephropathy: a meta-analysis of randomized controlled trials. *Am. J. Clin. Nutr.* 2008 Sep;88(3):660-6.

[141] Zheng F, He C, Cai W, Hattori M, Steffes M, Vlassara H. Prevention of diabetic nephropathy in mice by a diet low in glycoxidation products. *Diabetes Metab. Res. Rev.* 2002 May-Jun;18(3):224-37.

[142] Harcourt BE, Sourris KC, Coughlan MT, Walker KZ, Dougherty SL, Andrikopoulos S, et al. Targeted reduction of advanced glycation improves renal function in obesity. *Kidney Int.* 2011 Jul;80(2):190-8.

[143] Hofmann SM, Dong HJ, Li Z, Cai W, Altomonte J, Thung SN, et al. Improved insulin sensitivity is associated with restricted intake of dietary glycoxidation products in the db/db mouse. *Diabetes.* 2002 Jul;51(7):2082-9.

[144] Williams ME, Bolton WK, Khalifah RG, Degenhardt TP, Schotzinger RJ, McGill JB. Effects of pyridoxamine in combined phase 2 studies of patients with type 1 and type 2 diabetes and overt nephropathy. *Am. J. Nephrol.* 2007;27(6):605-14.

[145] Ritz E, Ogata H, Orth SR. Smoking: a factor promoting onset and progression of diabetic nephropathy. *Diabetes Metab.* 2000 Jul;26 Suppl 4:54-63.

[146] Voulgari C, Katsilambros N, Tentolouris N. Smoking cessation predicts amelioration of microalbuminuria in newly diagnosed type 2 diabetes mellitus: a 1-year prospective study. *Metabolism.* 2011 Oct;60(10):1456-64.

[147] Slagman MC, Waanders F, Hemmelder MH, Woittiez AJ, Janssen WM, Lambers Heerspink HJ, et al; HOlland NEphrology STudy Group. Moderate dietary sodium restriction added to angiotensin converting enzyme inhibition compared with dual blockade in lowering proteinuria and blood pressure: randomised controlled trial. *BMJ.* 2011 Jul 26;343:d4366.

[148] Writing Team for the Diabetes Control and Complications Trial/Epidemiology of Diabetes Interventions and Complications Research Group. Sustained effect of intensive treatment of type 1 diabetes mellitus on development and progression of diabetic nephropathy: the Epidemiology of Diabetes Interventions and Complications (EDIC) study. *JAMA.* 2003 Oct 22;290(16):2159-67.

[149] Action to Control Cardiovascular Risk in Diabetes Study Group, Gerstein HC, Miller ME, Byington RP, Goff DC Jr, Bigger JT, et al. Effects of intensive glucose lowering in type 2 diabetes. *N. Engl. J. Med.* 2008 Jun 12;358(24):2545-59.

[150] Shurraw S, Hemmelgarn B, Lin M, Majumdar SR, Klarenbach S, Manns B, et al; Alberta Kidney Disease Network. Association between glycemic control and adverse

outcomes in people with diabetes mellitus and chronic kidney disease: a population-based cohort study. *Arch. Intern. Med.* 2011 Nov 28;171(21):1920-7.

[151] Lipscombe LL, Gomes T, Lévesque LE, Hux JE, Juurlink DN, Alter DA. Thiazolidinediones and cardiovascular outcomes in older patients with diabetes. *JAMA.* 2007 Dec 12;298(22):2634-43.

[152] Butler AE, Campbell-Thompson M, Gurlo T, Dawson DW, Atkinson M, Butler PC. Marked expansion of exocrine and endocrine pancreas with incretin therapy in humans with increased exocrine pancreas dysplasia and the potential for glucagon-producing neuroendocrine tumors. *Diabetes.* 2013 Jul;62(7):2595-604.

[153] Snyder RW, Berns JS. Use of insulin and oral hypoglycemic medications in patients with diabetes mellitus and advanced kidney disease. *Semin. Dial.* 2004 Sep-Oct;17(5):365-70.

[154] Lamos EM, Younk LM, Davis SN. Canagliflozin, an inhibitor of sodium-glucose cotransporter 2, for the treatment of type 2 diabetes mellitus. *Expert Opin. Drug Metab.* Toxicol. 2013 Jun;9(6):763-75.

[155] Young A. Clinical studies. *Adv. Pharmacol.* 2005;52:289-320.

[156] Bretzel RG, Voigt K, Schatz H. The United Kingdom Prospective Diabetes Study (UKPDS) implications for the pharmacotherapy of type 2 diabetes mellitus. *Exp. Clin. Endocrinol. Diabetes.* 1998;106(5):369-72.

[157] ACCORD Study Group, Cushman WC, Evans GW, Byington RP, Goff DC Jr, Grimm RH Jr, et al. Effects of intensive blood-pressure control in type 2 diabetes mellitus. N. *Engl. J. Med.* 2010 Apr 29;362(17):1575-85.

[158] Brown AF, Mangione CM, Saliba D, Sarkisian CA; California Healthcare Foundation/American Geriatrics Society Panel on Improving Care for Elders with Diabetes. Guidelines for improving the care of the older person with diabetes mellitus. *J. Am. Geriatr. Soc.* 2003 May;51(5 Suppl Guidelines):S265-80.

[159] Sinclair AJ, Paolisso G, Castro M, Bourdel-Marchasson I, Gadsby R, Rodriguez Mañas L; European Diabetes Working Party for Older People. European Diabetes Working Party for Older People 2011 clinical guidelines for type 2 diabetes mellitus. Executive summary. *Diabetes Metab.* 2011 Nov;37 Suppl 3:S27-38.

[160] Persson F, Rossing P, Reinhard H, Juhl T, Stehouwer CD, Schalkwijk C, et al. Renal effects of aliskiren compared with and in combination with irbesartan in patients with type 2 diabetes, hypertension, and albuminuria. *Diabetes Care.* 2009 Oct;32(10):1873-9.

[161] Tuomilehto J, Rastenyte D, Birkenhäger WH, Thijs L, Antikainen R, Bulpitt CJ, et al. Effects of calcium-channel blockade in older patients with diabetes and systolic hypertension. Systolic Hypertension in Europe Trial Investigators. *N. Engl. J. Med.* 1999 Mar 4;340(9):677-84.

[162] Bakris GL, Copley JB, Vicknair N, Sadler R, Leurgans S. Calcium channel blockers versus other antihypertensive therapies on progression of NIDDM associated nephropathy. *Kidney Int.* 1996 Nov;50(5):1641-50.

[163] Glenner GG. Amyloid deposits and amyloidosis. The beta-fibrilloses (first of two parts*). N. Engl. J. Med.* 1980 Jun 5;302(23):1283-92.

[164] Westermark P, Benson MD, Buxbaum JN, Cohen AS, Frangione B, Ikeda S, et al; Nomenclature Committee of the International Society of Amyloidosis. Amyloid:

toward terminology clarification. Report from the Nomenclature Committee of the International Society of Amyloidosis. *Amyloid.* 2005 Mar;12(1):1-4.

[165] Dember LM. Amyloidosis-associated kidney disease. *J. Am. Soc. Nephrol.* 2006 Dec;17(12):3458-71.

[166] Westermark P, Benson MD, Buxbaum JN, Cohen AS, Frangione B, Ikeda S, et al. Amyloid fibril protein nomenclature - 2002. Amyloid. 2002 Sep;9(3):197-200.

[167] Merlini G, Bellotti V. Molecular mechanisms of amyloidosis. *N. Engl. J Med.* 2003 Aug 7;349(6):583-96.

[168] D'Sa S, Abildgaard N, Tighe J, Shaw P, Hall-Craggs M. Guidelines for the use of imaging in the management of myeloma. *Br. J. Haematol.* 2007 Apr;137(1):49-63.

[169] Lachmann HJ, Goodman HJ, Gilbertson JA, Gallimore JR, Sabin CA, Gillmore JD, et al. Natural history and outcome in systemic AA amyloidosis. *N. Engl. J. Med.* 2007 Jun 7;356(23):2361-71.

[170] Jacobson DR, Pastore RD, Yaghoubian R, Kane I, Gallo G, Buck FS, et al. Variant-sequence transthyretin (isoleucine 122) in late-onset cardiac amyloidosis in black Americans. *N. Engl. J. Med.* 1997 Feb 13;336(7):466-73.

[171] Benson MD. Ostertag revisited: the inherited systemic amyloidoses without neuropathy. *Amyloid.* 2005 Jun;12(2):75-87.

[172] Teng J, Russell WJ, Gu X, Cardelli J, Jones ML, Herrera GA. Different types of glomerulopathic light chains interact with mesangial cells using a common receptor but exhibit different intracellular trafficking patterns. *Lab. Invest.* 2004 Apr;84(4):440-51.

[173] Keeling J, Teng J, Herrera GA. AL-amyloidosis and light-chain deposition disease light chains induce divergent phenotypic transformations of human mesangial cells. *Lab Invest.* 2004 Oct;84(10):1322-38.

[174] Yamaguchi I, Suda H, Tsuzuike N, Seto K, Seki M, Yamaguchi Y, et al. Glycosaminoglycan and proteoglycan inhibit the depolymerization of beta2-microglobulin amyloid fibrils in vitro. *Kidney Int.* 2003 Sep;64(3):1080-8.

[175] Gregorini G, Izzi C, Obici L, Tardanico R, Röcken C, Viola BF, et al. Renal apolipoprotein A-I amyloidosis: a rare and usually ignored cause of hereditary tubulointerstitial nephritis. *J. Am. Soc. Nephrol.* 2005 Dec;16(12):3680-6.

[176] Palladini G, Lavatelli F, Russo P, Perlini S, Perfetti V, Bosoni T, et al. Circulating amyloidogenic free light chains and serum N-terminal natriuretic peptide type B decrease simultaneously in association with improvement of survival in AL. *Blood.* 2006 May 15;107(10):3854-8.

[177] Brenner DA, Jain M, Pimentel DR, Wang B, Connors LH, Skinner M, et al. Human amyloidogenic light chains directly impair cardiomyocyte function through an increase in cellular oxidant stress. *Circ. Res.* 2004 Apr 30;94(8):1008-10.

[178] Dember LM, Sanchorawala V, Seldin DC, Wright DG, LaValley M, Berk JL, et al. Effect of dose-intensive intravenous melphalan and autologous blood stem-cell transplantation on al amyloidosis-associated renal disease. *Ann. Intern. Med.* 2001 May 1;134(9 Pt 1):746-53.

[179] Kyle RA, Wagoner RD, Holley KE. Primary systemic amyloidosis: resolution of the nephrotic syndrome with melphalan and prednisone. *Arch. Intern. Med.* 1982 Aug;142(8):1445-7.

[180] Zeier M, Perz J, Linke RP, Donini U, Waldherr R, Andrassy K, et al. No regression of renal AL amyloid in monoclonal gammopathy after successful autologous blood stem

cell transplantation and significant clinical improvement. *Nephrol Dial Transplant.* 2003 Dec;18(12):2644-7.

[181] Crowley S, Feinfeld DA, Janis R. Resolution of nephrotic syndrome and lack of progression of heroin-associated renal amyloidosis. *Am. J. Kidney Dis.* 1989 Apr;13(4):333-5.

[182] Desport E, Bridoux F, Sirac C, Delbes S, Bender S, Fernandez B, et al; Centre national de référence pour l'amylose AL et les autres maladies par dépôts d'immunoglobulines monoclonales. Al amyloidosis. *Orphanet. J. Rare Dis.* 2012 Aug 21;7:54.

[183] de Mello RA, Marques Santos DS, Freitas-Silva MP, Andrade JA. Renal failure due to primary amyloidosis: a case report and literature review. *Sao Paulo Med. J.* 2011 May;129(3):176-80.

[184] Simms RW, Prout MN, Cohen AS. The epidemiology of AL and AA amyloidosis. *Baillieres Clin. Rheumatol.* 1994 Aug;8(3):627-34.

[185] Röcken C, Shakespeare A. Pathology, diagnosis and pathogenesis of AA amyloidosis. *Virchows Arch.* 2002 Feb;440(2):111-22.

[186] Lachmann HJ, Booth DR, Booth SE, Bybee A, Gilbertson JA, Gillmore JD, et al. Misdiagnosis of hereditary amyloidosis as AL (primary) amyloidosis. *N. Engl. J. Med.* 2002 Jun 6;346(23):1786-91.

[187] Valderrábano F, Jones EH, Mallick NP. Report on management of renal failure in Europe, XXIV, 1993. *Nephrol. Dial. Transplant.* 1995;10 Suppl 5:1-25.

[188] Davison AM. The United Kingdom Medical Research Council's glomerulonephritis registry. *Contrib. Nephrol.* 1985;48:24-35.

[189] Tanaka F, Migita K, Honda S, Fukuda T, Mine M, Nakamura T, et al. Clinical outcome and survival of secondary (AA) amyloidosis. *Clin. Exp. Rheumatol.* 2003 May-Jun;21(3):343-6.

[190] Joss N, McLaughlin K, Simpson K, Boulton-Jones JM. Presentation, survival and prognostic markers in AA amyloidosis. *QJM.* 2000 Aug;93(8):535-42.

[191] Watanabe T, Saniter T. Morphological and clinical features of renal amyloidosis. *Virchows Arch A Pathol Anat Histol.* 1975;366(2):125-35.

[192] Dikman SH, Churg J, Kahn T. Morphologic and clinical correlates in renal amyloidosis. *Hum. Pathol.* 1981 Feb;12(2):160-9.

[193] Shiiki H, Shimokama T, Yoshikawa Y, Toyoshima H, Kitamoto T, Watanabe T. Renal amyloidosis. Correlations between morphology, chemical types of amyloid protein and clinical features. Virchows Arch. A Pathol. *Anat. Histopathol.* 1988;412(3):197-204.

[194] Sen S, Sarsik B. A proposed histopathologic classification, scoring, and grading system for renal amyloidosis: standardization of renal amyloid biopsy report. *Arch. Pathol. Lab. Med.* 2010 Apr;134(4):532-44.

[195] Verine J. A proposed histopathologic classification, scoring, and grading system for renal amyloidosis. *Arch Pathol Lab Med.* 2011 Feb;135(2):168; author reply 168-9.

[196] Greipp PR, Kyle RA, Bowie EJ. Factor-X deficiency in amyloidosis: a critical review. *Am. J. Hematol.* 1981 Dec;11(4):443-50.

[197] Sucker C, Hetzel GR, Grabensee B, Stockschlaeder M, Scharf RE. Amyloidosis and bleeding: pathophysiology, diagnosis, and therapy. *Am. J. Kidney Dis.* 2006 Jun;47(6):947-55.

[198] Carone FA, Epstein FH. Nephrogenic diabetes insipidus caused by amyloid disease. Evidence in man of the role of the collecting ducts in concentrating urine. *Am. J. Med.* 1960 Sep;29:539-44.

[199] Asmundsson P, Snaedal J. Persistent water diuresis in renal amyloidosis. A case report. *Scand. J. Urol. Nephrol.* 1981;15(1):77-9.

[200] Rikitake O, Sakemi T, Yoshikawa Y, Nagano Y, Watanabe T. Adult Fanconi syndrome in primary amyloidosis with lambda light-chain proteinuria. *Jpn. J. Med.* 1989 Jul-Aug;28(4):523-6.

[201] Libbey CA, Skinner M, Cohen AS. Use of abdominal fat tissue aspirate in the diagnosis of systemic amyloidosis. *Arch. Intern. Med.* 1983 Aug;143(8):1549-52.

[202] Hetzel GR, Uhlig K, Mondry A, Helmchen U, Grabensee B. AL-amyloidosis of the kidney initially presenting as minimal change glomerulonephritis. *Am. J. Kidney Dis.* 2000 Sep;36(3):630-5.

[203] Sen S, Başdemir G. Diagnosis of renal amyloidosis using Congo red fluorescence. *Pathol Int.* 2003 Aug;53(8):534-8.

[204] Picken MM. New insights into systemic amyloidosis: the importance of diagnosis of specific type. *Curr. Opin. Nephrol. Hypertens.* 2007 May;16(3):196-203.

[205] Veeramachaneni R, Gu X, Herrera GA. Atypical amyloidosis: diagnostic challenges and the role of immunoelectron microscopy in *diagnosis. Ultrastruct Pathol.* 2004 Mar-Apr;28(2):75-82.

[206] Westermark P, Davey E, Lindbom K, Enqvist S. Subcutaneous fat tissue for diagnosis and studies of systemic amyloidosis. *Acta Histochem.* 2006;108(3):209-13.

[207] Kyle RA, Gertz MA, Greipp PR, Witzig TE, Lust JA, Lacy MQ, et al. A trial of three regimens for primary amyloidosis: colchicine alone, melphalan and prednisone, and melphalan, prednisone, and colchicine. *N. Engl. J. Med.* 1997 Apr 24;336(17):1202-7.

[208] Skinner M, Anderson J, Simms R, Falk R, Wang M, Libbey C, et al. Treatment of 100 patients with primary amyloidosis: a randomized trial of melphalan, prednisone, and colchicine versus colchicine only. *Am. J. Med.* 1996 Mar;100(3):290-8.

[209] Lachmann HJ, Gallimore R, Gillmore JD, Carr-Smith HD, Bradwell AR, Pepys MB, et al. Outcome in systemic AL amyloidosis in relation to changes in concentration of circulating free immunoglobulin light chains following chemotherapy. *Br. J. Haematol.* 2003 Jul;122(1):78-84.

[210] Palladini G, Perfetti V, Obici L, Caccialanza R, Semino A, Adami F, et al. Association of melphalan and high-dose dexamethasone is effective and well tolerated in patients with AL (primary) amyloidosis who are ineligible for stem cell transplantation. *Blood.* 2004 Apr 15;103(8):2936-8.

[211] Gertz MA, Lacy MQ, Dispenzieri A, Gastineau DA, Chen MG, Ansell SM, et al. Stem cell transplantation for the management of primary systemic amyloidosis. *Am. J. Med.* 2002 Nov;113(7):549-55.

[212] Skinner M, Sanchorawala V, Seldin DC, Dember LM, Falk RH, Berk JL, et al. High-dose melphalan and autologous stem-cell transplantation in patients with AL amyloidosis: an 8-year study. *Ann. Intern. Med.* 2004 Jan 20;140(2):85-93.

[213] Leung N, Dispenzieri A, Fervenza FC, Lacy MQ, Villicana R, Cavalcante JL, et al. Renal response after high-dose melphalan and stem cell transplantation is a favorable marker in patients with primary systemic amyloidosis. *Am. J. Kidney Dis.* 2005 Aug;46(2):270-7.

[214] Fadia A, Casserly LF, Sanchorawala V, Seldin DC, Wright DG, Skinner M, et al. Incidence and outcome of acute renal failure complicating autologous stem cell transplantation for AL amyloidosis. *Kidney Int*. 2003 May;63(5):1868-73.

[215] Yan SD, Zhu H, Zhu A, Golabek A, Du H, Roher A, et al. Receptor-dependent cell stress and amyloid accumulation in systemic amyloidosis. *Nat. Med*. 2000 Jun;6(6):643-51.

[216] Gillmore JD, Lovat LB, Persey MR, Pepys MB, Hawkins PN. Amyloid load and clinical outcome in AA amyloidosis in relation to circulating concentration of serum amyloid A protein. *Lancet*. 2001 Jul 7;358(9275):24-9.

[217] Rumjon A, Coats T, Javaid MM. Review of eprodisate for the treatment of renal disease in AA amyloidosis. *Int. J. Nephrol. Renovasc Dis*. 2012;5:37-43.

[218] Dember LM, Hawkins PN, Hazenberg BP, Gorevic PD, Merlini G, Butrimiene I, et al; Eprodisate for AA Amyloidosis Trial Group. Eprodisate for the treatment of renal disease in AA amyloidosis. *N. Engl. J. Med*. 2007 Jun 7;356(23):2349-60.

[219] Kisilevsky R. The relation of proteoglycans, serum amyloid P and apo E to amyloidosis current status, 2000. *Amyloid*. 2000 Mar;7(1):23-5.

[220] Gandhi NS, Mancera RL. Heparin/heparan sulphate-based drugs. *Drug Discov. Today*. 2010 Dec;15(23-24):1058-69.

Chapter V

Secondary Proliferative Glomerulonephritis

Abstract

Lupus nephritis (LN) is a common complication of systemic lupus erythematosous (SLE), occurring mostly in young females, although in recent years, patients of more advanced age, and males, were reported to be affected. The hallmarks of LN pathology are the immune complex deposition and the proliferative lesions of mesangium and capillaries. This secondary proliferative glomerular disease is classified in 6 distinct classes according to histologic findings on light microscopy.

Renal involvement in hepatitis B and hepatitis C infections is also common. Hepatitis B infection has been associated with different renal pathologic patterns mostly characterized by proliferative lesions such as membranoproliferative glomerulonephritis and membranous nephropathy with mesangial cell proliferation. Hepatitis B infection has been mostly associated with membranoproliferative glomerulonephritis but other glomerular diseases such as mesangioproliferative glomerulonephritis, IgA nephropathy, and postinfectious glomerulonephritis have also been described.

In this chapter, pathogenesis, clinical manifestations, and treatment of the above mentioned diseases are discussed.

1. Lupus Nephritis

Lupus nephritis (LN) is a common severe complication of systemic lupus erythematosous (SLE), presenting at the onset of the disease in more than 50% of patients, or during its course in up to 80% of the patients. [1, 2]

The term lupus nephritis includes different pathologic patterns of renal disease occurring in SLE, comprising a spectrum of vascular, glomerular and tubulointerstitial lesions. The pathogenesis of glomerular injury in LN involves a variety of mechanisms that have not been totally clarified yet, but it is principally related to immune complexes formation *in situ* that induces an inflammatory response. [3, 4]

Typically, LN presents with proteinuria, hypertension, active urine sediment, and in some cases, renal insufficiency. Moreover, cases of asymptomatic lupus nephritis are not lacking. [5]

Presence of LN in SLE patients is a strong predictor of poor outcome [6] therefore early diagnosis and determination of reliable biomarkers for LN, are crucial for evaluating the disease and improving prognosis. [7]

Epidemiology

The overall reported incidence of LN varies from 21.5 to 54.3%. [8-10] These discrepancies on incidence may be a reflection of underdiagnosis or underestimation of SLE cases, however it is estimated around 50% at the onset [9,11,12] and up to 80% during the course of the disease, [2] occurring mostly within 5 years from the onset. [6]

Incidence and prevalence of LN are influenced by age, gender, ethnicity, and socioeconomic status. Most patients develop LN at ages younger than 55 years, with peak incidence in the third decade of life. Yet, it may affect elderly at ages higher than 65 years and children in rates up to 80%, [2] thus children are more likely to develop lupus nephritis than the elderly. [13]

LN affects mostly females, with a female to male ratio of 4:1. [14] It may be more common in women, but affected males present a worse clinical course compared to females. [15, 16] Racial and ethnic groups seem to be disproportionally affected by both SLE and LN, with increased prevalence among Asians, Hispanics, and Native Americans, compared to Caucasians. [17, 18] In a comparison of the incidence of LN after SLE diagnosis in Hispanic, African Americans, and Caucasians, African Americans prevailed with a 50.5% rate over Hispanics (43.1%) and Caucasians (14.3%). [9] Also Asian, African Caribbean, and African Americans present worse clinical course and outcome compared to other ethnic groups. [12]

These differences may be explained by genetic variations between ethnic groups and by a higher prevalence of serologic abnormalities in African-Americans compared to Caucasians. [19, 20] Interestingly, two recent studies showed a lower prevalence of SLE and LN in poorer patients and in areas with a lower average number of rheumatologists, suggesting that access to this subspecialty may significantly reduce underdiagnosis and improve management of these patients. [21, 10] According the USRD 2013, LN accounts for 1% of all ESRD causes. [22] LN patients presenting ESRD at the time of diagnosis are mostly African Americans (48.9%), followed by Caucasians (42.8%), and Hispanics (19%). 9.9% of LN patients will receive renal replacement treatment within the first year from diagnosis. [22]

Pathogenesis

LN is an immune complex glomerulonephritis, which pathogenesis involves extrarenal pathogenic events of the immune system, which compromises the immune tolerance against nuclear autoantibodies and activate innate and adaptive immunity, and intrarenal pathogenic mechanisms that lead to immune complex formation, complement activation and finally tissue damage. Here, both extrarenal and intrarenal pathogenic mechanisms will be briefly discussed.

i. Extrarenal Pathogenic Events

Accumulating data indicate that antiviral immunity plays an important role in the pathogenesis of LN. This concept is based on the observation that lupus autoantigens trigger antiviral immune response and that there are genetic variants associated to LN that compromise apoptosis and dead cell removal, rendering difficult the distinction of self-nucleic acids from viral nucleic acids, triggering antiviral immune responses. [23, 24]

Apoptosis is a complex programmed cell death mechanism that includes chromatin condensation in order to limit chromatin levels in the extracellular compartment and prevents release of nuclear particles in the circulation, [25] opsonization of dead cells by complement and their removal by phagocytes. [26] Genetic defects in these mechanisms allow release of nucleosomes in the circulation that inhibit the activities of DNAse I, an enzyme that demolishes chromatin and nucleic acids, persistently triggering antiviral immune responses that lead to SLE. [27]

The antiviral immune response requires presentation of the nucleic particles by antigen-presenting cells. Normally DNA and RNA submit methylation in order to inhibit their recognition by Toll-like receptors 3, 7, and 9. [28] In case of genetic defects, such as the ones occurring in SLE, the nucleic acids remain unmethylated, and they are recognized by the TLRs as viral nucleic acids. TLRs 7 and 9 are expressed on dendritic and B cells, both antigen-presenting cells. Once nucleic acids are recognized as antigens, TLR signaling activates B cells and plasmacytoid dendritic cells to effectively present these antigens to T cells [29, 30] and induces production of RNA and DNA autoantibodies, [31] suggesting an autoadjuvant effect on antigen presenting cells. [32, 33]

Persistent activation of plasmacytoid dendritic cells by TLR7 and TLR9 prolongs their survival. [34] In addition, TRL9 activation of these cells induces type I interferon release [30, 35, 36] that triggers the autoimmune response and amplifies the recognition of nucleic acids by the TRLs enhancing the entire antiviral response mechanism. [37]

TLR signaling activates proliferation and differentiation of autoreactive B cells to plasma cells that produce autoantibodies. [38] T cell proliferation and hyperactivity induced by the nuclear autoantigens along with B cell activation and production of auto-antibodies are the most important mechanisms underlying immune complex formation within the kidneys that lead to LN.

ii. Intrarenal Pathogenic Events

The hallmark of LN intrarenal pathogenic mechanisms is the deposition or formation *in situ* of immune complexes. In the past, it was believed that immune complexes formed in circulation were deposited in the mesangium, subendothelial, or subepithelial spaces or in peritubular capillaries. [39] Recent data suggests that immune complexes are formed *in situ,* by binding of autoantibodies to glomerular antigens as laminin or annexin. [40, 41]

Another potential mechanism of immune complex formation in the glomeruli is the deposition of circulating DNA nucleosomes in the GBM, and their recognition by anti-DNA autoantibodies to nucleosomes deriving from necrotic glomerular cells. [42, 43] The nucleosomic parts of these immune complexes can be recognized by the TLRs of intrarenal dendritic cells, [44,45] triggering antiviral immunity within the kidney with release of type I interferon, which amplifies expression of nucleic acid receptors, and cytokines that promote intrarenal information and renal damage. [46]

Immune complexes formation in situ activates the alternative pathway of complement cascade with formation of the membrane attack complex (MAC) and release of the anaphylatoxins C3a and C5a. [47] Recently, activation of the lectin pathway of complement cascade was reported to be involved in the pathogenesis of LN. [48, 49] Deposition of C4d and C3 in absence of C1q deposits is considered evidence of the lectin pathway activation. Formation of MAC is followed by activation of the coagulation cascade and platelet aggregation resulting in renal microthrombi. [49]

Inflammatory cells contribute to renal injury by infiltrating the kidney, early in the course of LN, where they produce proinflammatory cytokines that promote inflammation, cell proliferation, immune complex formation, and fibrosis. T cells, especially T helper cells, are predominantly present in the kidney of LN patients where they are activated and release Il-12, IL-8, and IFNγ. These cytokines promote leukocyte infiltration and tubular epithelial cell necrosis. [50-52] Infiltrating B cells secrete antibodies, which contributes to *in situ* immune complex formation. [53] T cell and B cell aggregates may be found in the kidney, secreting nephritogenic antibodies that also contribute to immune complexes formation. [54]

Similarly, neutrophils, monocytes, macrophages, and dendritic cells also release proinflammatory chemokines that participate and promote renal damage.

Pathology and Classification

Given the variety of glomerular, tubulointerstitial and vascular lesions in the course of SLE, the differences in lesions' degree of adjacent glomeruli, and the possibility of transformation of one type of lesion to another, classification of LN has been under discussion for years.

After the first LN classification, known as WHO classification of LN formulated in 1974, different attempts were made of proposing new classifications that provide a more clear distinction between chronic and active lesions, and a better correlation of pathologic findings to clinical symptoms, but revisions of the original WHO classification were difficult to use, due to limitations of reproducibility and predictability. Moreover, the introduction of numerous subcategories in the revisions of the original WHO classification rendered their use more complicated.

The most recent classification of LN proposal was formulated by Weening et al., in 2004 and it is called the "International Society of Nephrology (ISN)/ Renal Pathology Society (RPS) 2003 classification of LN". [55] Superiority on reproducibility and predictive value of this classification, compared to previous classifications, attributes to its worldwide acceptance and diffusion of its use. [56]

The ISN/RPS 2003 classification of LN, as its precursor, is based on light microscopy, immunofluorescence, and electron microscopy. It considers exclusively glomerular lesions, but it is recommended by its authors to report significant vascular and tubulointerstitial pathology, as they are of complementary diagnostic value. [55] Although electron microscopy may be of extreme diagnostic value in some cases of LN, the way ISN-RPS 2003 classification is structured, it permits diagnosis of LN based on light microscopy and immunofluorescence only. [57]

ISN/RPS 2003 class I is defined as minimal mesangial LN. In light microscopy, glomeruli seem normal but immunofluorescence and electron microscopy reveal mesangial electron dense immune complexes.

ISN/RPS 2003 class II is defined as mesangial proliferative LN. Light microscopy reveals mesangial hypercellularity, thus 3 or more mesangial cells per mesangial region in 3μm sections, usually confined to centrilobular areas. On immunofluorescence and electron microscopy, mesangial immune and more rarely paramesangial, subendothelial or subepithelial deposits may be seen. Tubulointerstitial and vascular lesions may be present but they are usually insignificant.

ISN/RPS 2003 class III is defined as focal LN with involvement of less than 50% of the glomeruli who may present proliferative or necrotizing, sclerosing and crescentic (active or chronic) lesions, seen on light microscopy. These lesions may be segmental, involving less than half of the glomerular tuft or global, involving more than 50% of the glomerular tuft. Crescent and diffuse or focal mesangial proliferation and widening may be present. Immunofluorescence reveals irregular granular mesangial deposits, while on electron microscopy, subendothelial deposits accompany mesangial deposits.

Class III is subdivided into 3 subclasses:

- III (A) characterized by active proliferative alternation (focal proliferative LN)
- III (C) characterized by chronic inactive sclerosing lesions with glomerular scars and often crescents.
- III (A/C) with active proliferative and chronic sclerosing lesions

ISN/RPS 2003 class IV is defined as diffuse proliferative LN, with involvement of more than 50% of the glomeruli. Lesions may be diffuse segmental (IV-S) when more than 50% of the glomeruli present segmental lesions, or diffuse global (IV-G) when more than 50% of glomeruli present global lesions. These two subclasses are further subdivided according the activity and the chronicity of the lesions:

- IV-S (A) characterized by diffuse segmental proliferative endocapillary lesions with or without necrosis.
- IV-G (A) presents active diffuse global proliferative endocapillary, extracapillary or mesangiocapillary lesions.
- IV-S and IV-G (A/C) with diffuse segmental or global proliferative and sclerosing lesions.
- IV-S (C) characterized by diffuse segmental sclerosing chronic inactive lesions with glomerular scars.
- IV-G (C) with chronic inactive diffuse global sclerosing lesions with glomerular scars.

Immunofluorescence reveals a rough granular distribution of the immune deposits composed by different types of immunoglobulins in the mesangium and the capillary wall along with deposition of complement components and fibrogen, named the “full-house” immunoglobulin deposition pattern.

The histological picture in electron microscopy is considered a variation of the immunopathologic lesion of class III due their similarities. Immune deposits are observed in mesangial and subendothelial sites, often in a well-organized or crystalline pattern, termed the "fingerprint pattern". Deposits are more numerous and larger than in other classes of LN. Intraendothelial tubular reticular inclusions may be seen.

ISN/RPS 2003 class V is defined as membranous LN characterized by segmental or global subepithelial and intramembranous immune deposits often associated to mesangial deposits and mesangial proliferation. Between the deposits there is thickening of the basement membrane, called spikes, better observed on electron microscopy.

Immunofluorescence shows granular subepithelial and mesangial deposition. Electron microscopy reveals intramembranous electron dense deposits. If subendothelial deposits or glomerular scars are present in more than 50% of the glomeruli on immunofluorescence or electron microscopy, a combined diagnosis of class III or IV and class V should be applied.

ISN/RPS 2003 class VI is defined as advanced sclerosing LN characterized by advanced glomerular sclerosis and interstitial fibrosis in more than 90% of the glomeruli, without evidence of residual activity.

Immunofluorescence and electron microscopy reveal immune deposits. Glomerular immune deposits in all classes detected by immunofluorescence consist mainly of polyclonal IgG and the complement component C3. In some cases C1q, IgA, or IgM may also coexist. If IgA or IgM are the dominant immunoglobulins, other diagnosis should be considered.

Histologic glomerular classes are interconnected between them, as a less proliferative class, such as II or V, may increase activity and transform it to a more proliferative one, such as III and IV. This transformation may have a negative impact on the clinical course, prognosis, and outcome of LN patients.

Finally, SLE patients of class I and II, presenting MCD and FSGS with severe nephrotic syndrome have been reported. [58-60] In these cases, biopsy revealed extensive foot processes effacement without or with minimal mesangial immune deposits and absence of endocapillary proliferation, along with mesangial hypercellularity. This condition is called lupus podocytopathy. The underlying pathogenic mechanism of this condition remains unclear but it has been speculated that T cell activation may be implicated. [58]

It is also believed that the abrupt onset of nephrotic syndrome in these cases is due to podocytopathy provoked by active LN than the result of coexistence of two separate diseases occurring simultaneously. [58]

Clinical Manifestations

Clinical manifestations and their severity are correlated to the histologic findings.

ISN/RPS class I patients are usually asymptomatic with no evidence of renal impairment, inactive urine sediment and suspicion of LN originates from regular follow up laboratory tests showing abnormalities that suggest LN.

ISN/RPS class II patients may be asymptomatic or present mild to moderate proteinuria rarely exceeding 1g/24h with microscopic hematuria. Renal function is usually preserved, but in some cases, there is evidence of mild renal impairment. In rare cases, patients present nephrotic syndrome with proteinuria higher than 3g/24h. [58, 59]

ISN/RPS class III patients show evidence of renal impairment with proteinuria often higher than 3g/24h, microscopic hematuria, and frequently hypertension. In case of glomerular scaring, urinary sediment is typically inactive.

ISN/RPS class IV patients have similar clinical picture to class III patients.

ISN/RPS class V patients present renal impairment with nephrotic syndrome although mild proteinuria lower than 1g/24h may be observed. Clinical manifestations may be similar to class III and IV but prognosis is worse in class V patients. Also, class V patients have a predisposition to thrombotic events that further reduces survival rates.

Class VI patients present as end stage renal disease, with persistent microscopic and hypertension. Proteinuria in this stage is usually mild to moderate. Peripheral edema may be present at all stages but it is observed mostly in cases of excessive proteinuria and hypoalbuminemia. In some cases ascites and pulmonary edema with cardiac decompensation may be seen and pericardial effusion. Other symptoms mostly related to active SLE are fever, fatigue, anemia, skin rashes, alopecia, oral, or nasal ulcers, Raynaud's phenomenon, headaches, dizziness, photosensitivity, visual disturbances and seizures. [61]

SLE and LN women may present worsening of the kidney impairment during pregnancy due to increased workload of the kidney occurring in this condition. Pregnancy may also be complicated with hypertension, nephrotic syndrome, and preeclampsia. Preeclampsia is more frequent in pregnant SLE women presenting antiphospholipid (aPL) antibodies. [62] These women also have a higher incidence of miscarriage, prematurity and fetal loss. [63] SLE with aPL antibodies affects the development of the fetus cardiac tissue and the cardiac conduction system, [64, 65] preventing its complete and appropriate formation, [66] resulting in congenital heart block (CHB) of the first, second and third degree. [67] The third degree CHB corresponds to complete atrioventricular block that has, consequently, fatal loss. CHB may present with severe bradycardia, less than 50 beats per minute while normal fetus heart beats range from 110 to 180 per minute or first heart sound may vary in intensity. [68, 69] Gallops and murmurs may also be present.

In most of the cases that pregnancy comes to term, or there is premature delivery without fetal or perinatal death, immediate placement of a pacemaker is mandatory to the infant survival. Prophylactic treatment for CHB during pregnancy includes glucocorticoids, immunosuppressors, intravenous immunoglobulins, and plasmapheresis. [70] First or second degree CHB may progress to complete heart block, therefore periodic evaluation is of extreme importance. [71]

Diagnosis

Kidney biopsy is the mainstay for LN diagnosis and it should be performed in SLE patients with evidence of active nephritis in order to establish the extent of glomerular damage and the chronicity and activity of the lesions. In most of the cases, SLE is already diagnosed according to the American College of Rheumatology (ACR) diagnostic criteria, [72] but in other cases, renal disease may be the initial clinical manifestation of SLE. [73]

Given the fact that adjacent glomeruli may present differences in lesion degrees, or may transform from one type to another, adequacy of the tissue specimen obtained with biopsy is crucial for a definitive diagnosis. The tissue specimen should contain at least 10 glomeruli, which will be evaluated by light microscopy, immunofluorescence, and electron microscopy in order to be classified. [74]

Along with the biopsy, laboratory tests should be performed to evaluate renal function. As proteinuria is the hallmark of LN, measurement of urinary protein excretion with 24h urine collection is important for estimation of renal impairment, as well as for the screening of the disease and evaluation of response to treatment. A 24h protein to creatinine ratio is also considered a gold standard in the assessment of proteinuria in LN. [75] However, 24h urine collection may be impractical and problematic and may often lead to variable and erroneous results. Alternatively, the protein to creatinine ratio may be measured in a morning or in a random urinary sample, but reliability of this method remains controversial. [76, 77] Clearance of creatinine with 24h urine collection is also mandatory for evaluation of renal function.

Urinary sediment provides information about renal disease activity. Presence of leukocyturia, hematuria, and casts in urine sediment are typical of active disease. [78] Casts are usually hyaline or granular while red cell casts are more rare in LN.

Serology of SLE and LN should include serum antinuclear antibodies (ANA), anti-ds DNA antibodies, complement component C3 and C4 serum levels and aPL and anti C1q antibodies. Although ANA are not specific of SLE or LN, and can be found in different rheumatologic condition, high serum levels have been found in almost all SLE and LN patients, [79] therefore should be always be measured. In contrast, anti-dsDNA antibodies are more specific for SLE and are widely used to evaluate the disease activity. [80]

Serum complement components C3 and C4 are usually decreased in SLE and LN but in some cases, C4 levels are more decreased compared to C3. Complement factor H (CHF), and anti C1q antibodies levels have been well associated with the activity of LN. [81, 82] aPL antibodies are present in up to 50% of lupus patients and their presence have been associated to SLE and LN, to thrombotic events occurring in these patients, and to congenital heart block in the fetus of SLE pregnant mothers.

Recently, different serum and urinary biomarkers helpful in evaluating disease activity, predicting renal histology, and suggesting potential therapeutic targets have been reported. Serum biomarkers include α-proliferation-inducing ligand (APRIL) that has been associated to resistance to treatment, [83] mannose binding lectin (MBL) and soluble interleukin 7 receptor (SIL-7R), which were significantly associated with disease activity in LN. [84, 85]

Novel urinary biomarkers include different proteins of varying molecular weight identified in both SLE adults and children, originating urinary proteomic signatures for LN. [86, 87]

Suzuki et al, showed that urinary levels of transferrin, ceruloplasmin, α1-acid-glycoprotein (AGP), lipocalin-type prostaglandin D sythease (L-PGDS), albumin and albumin-related fragments were significantly higher in SLE children compared to children with juvenile idiopathic arthritis. Of note transferrin, AGP and L-PDGS urinary levels were significantly higher at least 3 months before clinical manifestation of LN progression, suggesting that these proteins are reliable biomarkers in predicting LN flares. [88] Moreover, AGP and L-PGDS may predict diabetic renal disease in adults. [89]

In another study both 20 and 25 aminoacid isoforms of hepcidin urinary levels showed statistically significant variation according to flares. [90] Hepcidin 20 levels increase 4 months before flare while hepcidin 25 decreased during flares and normalized 4 months after resolution of the flare, suggesting that hepcidin 20 could be used as a reliable predictor of flares while hepcidin 25 may be used as an indicator of treatment responsiveness.

Also levels of vascular cell adhesion molecule 1 (VCAM-1), that promote adhesion of leukocytes to endothelial cells were found to be correlated with increased disease activity in LN patients but its association to LN flares remains to be evaluated. [91]

Finally, IL-6 and Il-8 urinary levels were found to be increased in patients with active LN and decreased within 6 months after treatment with cyclophosphamide, suggesting that these cytokines may be used as biomarkers of both disease activity and treatment responsiveness. [92]

Although all these biomarkers are promising in predicting disease activity and response to treatment, more clinical studies and RCTs are required to determine their predictive power and their effectiveness in early diagnosis and prognosis of LN.

Treatment

Treatment of LN varies according to the classification of the histopathologic findings and focuses in obtaining remission, preventing disease flares, and treating extrarenal manifestations that may affect kidney function.

Definition of remission and flares in LN has long been under discussion, but the Lupus Nephritis Terminology Advisory Group in 2009 developed a consensus statement that clarified divergences on this subject. [93] According this statement, remission is defined as reduction of proteinuria below 500mg/24h or protein to creatinine ratio below 500mg/g, absence of hematuria and normalization or stabilization of GFR. Flares are defined as increased disease activity with isolated proteinuria higher than 1g/24h, or proteinuria and hematuria along with decrease of GFR. [93] In this context, the term relapse will be used instead of flares in order to avoid potential confusion.

Responsiveness to treatment, relapse, and remission rates may be influenced by gender, ethnicity, renal function, chronicity, and activity of the disease, lesion histology and socioeconomic status. [94] Although conventional therapeutic agents, such as corticosteroids, cyclophosphamide, mycophenolate mofetil (MMF), and azathioprine have significantly improved outcomes, treatment of LN remains suboptimal. Accumulating data on the pathogenic mechanisms of the disease allowed and stimulated the development of new therapeutic strategies. Here, therapeutic options will be discussed according the ISN/RPS classification. New therapeutic strategies will be briefly reported.

ISN/RPS class I or minimal mesangial LN is asymptomatic in 90% of the cases and only extrarenal manifestations of lupus may be observed. [95] In these cases, no specific treatment is required for lupus nephritis, but there may be need for immunosuppressive treatment for the extrarenal symptomatology and SLE activity. [8] However, class I patients should be monitored periodically and carefully because of the risk of transition of class I to a more aggressive class of LN. [96]

ISN/RPS class II or mesangial proliferative LN usually presents with hematuria and mild proteinuria. Nephrotic range proteinuria is usually observed in patients with class II LN and concomitant podocytopathy. For patients with proteinuria below 1g/24h there is no need for specific treatment. Treatment considerations should be made only for extrarenal manifestations. In case of nephrotic range proteinuria over 3g/24h, patients should be treated as in case of MCD, thus with corticosteroids or CNIs. [8] Oral prednisone's suggested doses are 1mg/kg/day up to a maximum of 80mg or 2mg/kg every other day up to a maximum of 120mg, administered for 4 to 16 weeks and followed by tapering for 6 or more months after complete remission. Cyclosporine A should be administered at doses of 4 to 5mg/kg/day in 2 divided doses for at least 12 months. Tacrolimus' suggested doses are 0.05 to 0.1 mg/kg/day in 2 divided doses for 1 to 2 years. Supportive therapy with ACE inhibitors along with low doses of prednisone can also be useful in reducing proteinuria in patients with non-nephrotic range proteinuria higher than 1g/24h.

Additionally, treatment with hydroxychloroquine, an antimalarial agent that antagonizes histamine and serotonin and inhibits prostaglandin synthesis, can also be considered, unless contraindicated, in all LN patients, as there is evidence that it protects from relapse, vascular thrombosis, and progression to ESRD. Suggested doses are 6 to 6.5mg/kg/day. [97]

ISN/RPS classes III and IV or focal and diffuse proliferative LN presents with microscopic hematuria, proteinuria mostly of nephrotic range and impairment of renal function. Treatment of these classes is subdivided in two phases, the induction, and the maintenance phase.

Induction phase aims at the reduction of kidney inflammation and obtainment of complete remission, while maintenance treatment goals to the prevention of relapses or as usually referred to, of SLE and LN flares. [98]

ISN/RPS Classes III and IV

Induction Treatment

i. Corticosteroids

Corticosteroids are used in all SLE patients for controlling both extrarenal and renal manifestations. As monotherapy, they can be used in class I /II and in early stages of class III LN. In patients of class III who do not respond to steroid monotherapy, and in class IV LN patients, corticosteroids should be combined with immunosuppressive agents such as cyclophospamide or MMF. However, KDIGO 2012 guidelines, suggest combined therapy in all class II and IV LN patients. Suggested doses of oral prednisone are 1mg/kg/day for at least 4 weeks, followed by tapering for 6 to 12 months. Alternatively, or in cases of more severe disease, intravenous methylprednisolone at doses up to 1g/day in monthly pulses for 3 consecutive days and then flowed by oral prednisone may be used. [8]

ii. Cyclophosphamide

Cyclophosphamide in oral or intravenous administration, in combination with corticosteroids, has been found to be effective in obtaining remission, preserving renal function and preventing progression to ESRD in proliferative class III and IV LN. [99] However, intravenous administration is usually preferred by nephrologists, given that cumulative doses are higher in oral administration, increasing the risk for adverse events.

Optimal dosage of cyclophosphamide and treatment duration in LN have for long been under discussion. Currently, 2 regimens are widely used; the National Institute of Health

(NIH) regimen and the Euro-Lupus regimen, named after the respective controlled trials that provided strong evidence of efficacy and safety.

The NIH regimen consists in intravenous administration of cyclophosphamide at doses of 0.5 to $1g/m^2$ in monthly pulses for 6 months.

This regimen resulted by evidence obtained by 3 RCTs sponsored by the US National Institute of Health (NIH). [100-103]

The first trial demonstrated the superiority of intravenous cyclophosphamide in preventing ESRD, compared to oral corticosteroids and azathioprine. [100,101] The second NIH trial showed that 6 monthly pulses of intravenous cyclophosphamide at doses of 0.5 to $1g/m^2$ followed by every-3-month pulses of this agent for 2 years, were associated with lower risk for ESRD and relapses of LN compared to the 6 month regimen. [102] The third NIH trial showed that combined treatment with intravenous methylprednisolone and intravenous cyclophosphamide had higher remission rates (85%) compared to cyclophosphamide (62%) or methylprednisolone (29%) alone. [103]

Follow up of the patients included in these trials showed that there were no differences in frequency and intensity of adverse events of the combined treatment compared to cyclophosphamide alone. Additionally, after 10 years of follow up, none of these patients had progressed to ESRD.

The Euro-Lupus regimen consists in cyclophosphamide combined to prednisone, administered in intravenous pulses of 500mg every two weeks for 3 months, followed by maintenance therapy with azathioprine at doses of 2mg/kg/day. [104]

In the Euro-Lupus trial, patients were randomized to either receiving the NIH regimen or 500mg of IV cyclophosphamide every 2 weeks for 6 months.

After 73 months of follow up, the two groups showed similar results in reducing proteinuria and preserving renal function.

Although both regimens are efficient in severe class III/IV LN, superiority of one over the other regimen is hard to establish, given that the Euro-Lupus regimen has not been tested in ethnicities other than Caucasians.

iii. Azathioprine

Azathioprine is used as maintenance therapy in the Euro-Lupus regimen at doses of 2mg/kg/day, but it can also be used as a second-line therapy in moderate to severe LN. Azathioprine is effective in both maintaining remission and preventing progression to ESRD but appears to be not as effective as cyclophosphamide. [105]

An RCT conducted by the Dutch Working Party of SLE that included 87 SLE patients with proliferative LN, compared results of therapy with azathioprine at dose of 2mg/kg/day combined to IV methylprednisolone followed by oral prednisone, to cyclophosphamide pulse therapy ($750mg/m^2$) combined with oral prednisone. Although remission rates were similar in both groups, [105] repeated biopsies performed after two years from recruitment, showed a more pronounced chronicity of the lesions at the tissue specimens of the azathioprine group compared to the cyclophosphamide group, proving the superiority in efficacy of cyclophosphamide. [106]

However, the azathioprine/methylprednisolone regimen may be used as induction therapy to patients intolerant of other therapeutic regimens or in women who wish to preserve fertility.

iv. Mycophenolate Mofetil

Mycophenolate mofetil (MMF) is considered an effective alternative treatment option for LN class III/IV patients. Equivalence of MMF's effectiveness compared to cyclophosphamide was first reported by Chan et al, [98] who randomized 42 patients with LN class IV to either oral MMF at doses of 2g/day for 6 months, tapered to 1g/day or to oral cyclophosphamide 2.5mg/kg/day, followed by azathioprine at doses of 1.5mg/kg/day. Both groups showed complete remission rates of 80% with no significant differences in partial remission and relapsing rates. Therefore, authors concluded that MMF was as effective as oral cyclophosphamide. Of note, the MMF group presented less infectious events, suggesting superiority in safety of MMF compared to cyclophosphamide.

In another multicentered RCT, Ginzler et al., randomized 140 patients, 55% of whom were African Americans, presenting WHO classes III, IV and V LN, to either 500-00mg/m^2 of iv monthly pulses of cyclophosphamide or oral MMF at doses of 1 to 3g/day. [107] After a median follow up of 6 months, MMF was proved superior to IV cyclophosphamide in remission rates, with fewer adverse events and treatment withdrawals.

In 2009, Appel et al., conducted the Aspreva Lupus Management Study (ALMS), a large RCT that included 370 SLE patients of different races, with WHO classes III/IV and V LN. [108] These patients were randomized to either oral MMF (1 to 3 g/day) or monthly IV pulses of cyclophosphamide (0.5 to 1g/m^2) for 24 weeks. Both groups showed similar remission rates, as well as similar frequency and severity of adverse events. Of note, a post-hoc analysis of the ALMS study showed that Hispanics, Africans Americans and mixed races have better outcomes with MMF than IV cyclophosphamide, [109] therefore the American College of Rheumatology recommend MMF for African American and Hispanic LN patients as induction therapy.

MMF has also been administrated in combination with tacrolimus at doses of 4mg/day and oral steroids (multitarget therapy) in a small RCT, and results were compared to monthly IV pulses of cyclophosphamide at doses of 750mg/m^2 combined with steroids. After 6 months of treatment, 90% of the patients receiving the multitarget therapy obtained complete or partial remission while only 45% of the patients in the cyclophosphamide group responded. [110] Although this multitarget therapy seems promising, its use is limited by the fact that only Chinese patients were included in this study and its results on other ethnicities are unknown.

Maintenance Treatment

Most of the class III/IV LN patients require more than 6 months of induction treatment to achieve remission, partial or complete. Complete remission rates at 6 to 12 months range between 8 to 30%, rates quite low compared to partial remission, especially if at the time of diagnosis serum creatinine levels are increased, proteinuria is higher than 1g/day and most importantly if there is a delay in treatment initiation of more than 3 months from diagnosis. [111, 112]

Even if complete remission is achieved and proteinuria and serum creatinine levels are normalized, repeated biopsies show that tissue lesions are rarely reverted to a less severe class of LN or completely resolved. [106] Therefore, it is crucial once remission is achieved, to maintain this result, to prevent flares of SLE activity and relapses of LN. All class III and IV patients should receive maintenance therapy after remission is achieved, especially those treated with short-term regimens as they are at greater risk for kidney relapses. [102]

KDIGO 2012 guidelines recommend azathioprine at doses of 1.5 to 2.5mg/kg/day in divided doses and corticosteroids in limited doses as maintenance therapy. [8] Cyclosporine or tacrolimus in combination with low dose corticosteroids could be used as an alternative in patients intolerant of MMF and azathioprine.

Long-term administration of cyclophosphamide has been considered for maintenance therapy, but numerous adverse events due to high cumulative doses as infertility, cystitis and bladder cancer limited its use. In addition, a study that included 59 patients, mostly African Americans and Hispanics with class III/IV LN and compared azathioprine or MMF to every-3-months administration of IV cyclophosphamide for 1 years, showed that cyclophosphamide maintenance group patients presented significantly higher risk of developing CKD, experience more adverse events such as amenorrhea, gastrointestinal complications, and infections and had higher mortality rates compared to the MMF or azathioprine group. [113] Relapse-free survival was higher in the MMF group (87%) followed by azathioprine (58%) compared to cyclophosphamide (43%).

The choice between azathioprine and MMF as maintenance treatment has been under investigation, although there is evidence provided by two RCTs, the MAINTAIN and the ALMS trial, that MMF is superior to azathioprine. In the MAINTAIN Nephritis trial, [114] 105 patients were involved, mostly Caucasians with proliferative LN that received the Euro Lupus regimen, thus 500mg of IV cyclophosphamide and then randomized to either azathioprine (2mg/kg/day) or MMF (2mg/kg/day) as maintenance therapy. After a median follow up of 4 years, authors found no significant difference between the 2 groups in remission or relapsing rates. A limitation of this trial was that only patients with not severe renal dysfunction and mostly Caucasians were included.

In the maintenance phase of the ALMS trial, 227 patients were treated for 36 months with either azathioprine at doses of 2mg/kg/day or MMF (2mg/kg/day), after the 6-month induction treatment with MMF at doses of 1 to 3mg/kg/day and achievement of complete or partial remission. [115] MMF was found to be superior compared to azathioprine in preventing relapses, preventing progression to ESRD and showing lower mortality risk rates. Moreover, serious adverse events and treatment withdrawals were more common in the azathioprine group. Of note, superiority of MMF was independent from racial differences.

Cyclosporine A has also been used as monotherapy in the maintenance phase of LN treatment in class IV LN patients. [116] In this randomized pilot trial, 69 patients were randomized after induction therapy to either cyclosporine A (n=36) at doses of 2.5 to 4mg/kg/day or azathioprine at doses of 1.5 to 2mg/kg/day for 2 years. After 4 years of follow up there were no significant differences in mean creatinine clearance levels and proteinuria, and efficacy in preventing ESRD. Relapses were more common in the azathioprine group (13.4%) compared to the cyclosporine A group (10.6%), but the difference was not of extreme importance. These data suggest that cyclosporine A may be considered as an alternative option in the maintenance arm or LN treatment. However, further investigations are required for confirmation.

Although there are no clear indications for the duration of the maintenance treatment, KDIGO guidelines recommend continuation for at least 1 year after partial or complete remission is achieved. If complete remission is not achieved after 1 year of maintenance therapy or if kidney function deteriorates, it is rational and cautious to perform a repeat biopsy before change of treatment is decided. [8]

ISN/RPS class V or membranous LN comprises approximately 10 to 40% of LN cases. [117]. It clinically manifests with nephrotic range proteinuria with or without hematuria and edema. Kidney function is usually preserved. Spontaneous remissions are rare, and prognosis is less favorable if membranous and proliferative lesions coexist. [118] 8 to 28% of class V LN patients will reach ESRD within 12 years from the onset. [119]

In pure class V LN patients with non-range proteinuria, corticosteroids, and immunosuppression is not necessary and it should be administrated only for the management of extrarenal manifestations of SLE. [8] However, these patients should receive antiproteinuric and antihypertensive treatment in order to reduce proteinuria. Patients with nephrotic range proteinuria should receive coritcosteroids and immunosuppressive treatment, often in association with antihypertensive and antiproteinuric medication.

The optimal treatment remains controversial and challenging as RCTs for pure membranous LN are lacking. Clinical evidence indicates that azathioprine, cyclophosphamide, cyclosporine A, and MMF are effective agents in reducing proteinuria. Superiority of one of these agents over another is under investigation.

In a recent RCT by Austin et al, 42 class V LN patients of different racial groups (Caucasians, Hispanics, African American) with nephrotic range proteinuria, were randomized to either cyclosporine A for or IV cyclophosphamide at every-other-month pulses for 6 doses or alternate day oral steroids. [120] After 1 year of follow up, cyclosporine prevailed in cumulative probability of remission (83%) over cyclophosphamide (60%) and prednisone (27%). Relapses were more frequent in the cyclosporine A group compared to cyclophosphamide.

Efficacy of MMF was compared to IV cyclosporine A in 2 different RCTs and results were then analyzed by Rahakrishnan et al. [121] In this pooled analysis, 87 class V LN patients who were included in the 2 RCTs were considered. The end points were reduction of proteinuria and serum creatinine levels and were evaluated after 24 weeks of treatment. Both agents were efficient in reducing proteinuria with no difference in remission rates, but serum creatinine levels remained unchanged. This analysis suggests that cyclosporine A and cyclophosphamides are equivalent in the short term, but long-term results are lacking.

Tacrolimus was also considered in various studies for the treatment of pure memebranous LN. [122] Szeto et al, recruited 18 SLE patients with biopsy proven V LN and treated them with oral prednisone and 0.1 to 0.2mg/kg/day of tacrolimus for 6 months. Patients received maintenance treatment with azathioprine and prednisolone. Results were then compared with those of 19 controls receiving oral cyclophosphamide or azathioprine. All patients were followed for 1 year. At 12 weeks from the treatment initiation, complete and partial remission rates were 27.8% and 50% respectively for the tacrolimus group and 15.8% and 47.4% respectively for the control group. Based on this study, tacrolimus may be considered a safe and effective option for class V LN treatment, but long-term results require further investigation.

Azathioprine can be used as maintenance therapy in pure membranous LN. In a small open labeled study, 38 patients with membranous LN received azathioprine and prednisone for 12 months as induction therapy and continued with azathioprine and low prednisone as maintenance therapy. [123] After a mean follow up of 90 months, complete and partial remissions rates were 67% and 22%, respectively.

ISN/RPS class VI presents global glomerular sclerosis with interstitial fibrosis and tubular atrophy. At this stage, kidney function is severely impaired and it is usually accompanied by proteinuria or more rarely hematuria. These lesions are chronic and extent, therefore immunosuppressive treatment at this point would be futile. Antiproteinuric and antihypertensive treatment, are indicated and should be administered in order to preserve residual renal function and delay progression to ESRD. [8]

In case of relapses after partial or complete remission, the induction treatment should be repeated. If there is risk of high cumulative doses of cyclophosphamide, a non-cyclophosphamide regimen should be considered. If there is suspicion of transformation to a more severe class of LN, repeated biopsy is indicated. In case of patients of any ISN/RPS class resistant to the treatment, that haven't obtained remission despite repeated coursed of the induction treatment, administration of rituximab (see below), IV immunoglobulins, tacrolimus or cyclosporine A should be considered. [8]

New Treatment Options in LN

Although the introduction of immunosuppressive agents in the therapy of LN reduced the five-year mortality rates by 60% and the risk of progressing to ESRD, these rates remained unchanged for more than 10 years, indicating that the conventional immunosuppressive therapies are not able to provide better results than the ones already provided. [124] To achieve better outcomes, in the past 15 years interest was addressed in new treatment strategies, based on the improved understanding of the pathogenic mechanism underlying the disease.

Once the role of B and T cells on the pathogenesis of LN has been established, it seemed quite reasonable for investigators to consider depletion of these cells as an important therapeutic target. Different agents have been and still are under investigation.

Rituximab is a chimeric monoclonal antibody against CD20, a cell surface protein implicated in the differentiation and activation of B cells. This biological agent induces an antibody-dependent cell-mediated toxicity that leads to B cells depletion in the peripheral blood. Accumulating data from case reports and uncontrolled trials suggest the use of rituximab as induction therapy or in cases of refractory and relapsing LN. [125] Contrarily, in the Lupus Nephritis assessment for Rituximab (LUNAR), [126] a randomized double-blind placebo controlled phase III trial, where 144 patients of different races with proliferative LN were included and randomized to either rituximab (1000mg) or placebo administered on days 1, 15, 168 and 182 in addition to MMF at doses of 1.5 to 3gm/day, there were no statistically significant differences in partial or complete remission between the 2 groups. Of note, in this study African Americans had a stronger response compared to other races.

In some studies, relapses occurred with the normalization at number of B cells. [125] This happens probably because CD20 is absent from the hemopoietic stem cells and from plasma cells, thus rituximab is not able to prevent regeneration of B cells from B precursors. [127]

Retreatment with rituximab may be effective but before restarting administration, the possibility of adverse events such as multifocal encephalopathy should be considered. As efficacy and safety of rituximab in the treatment of LN remains controversial, further RCTs are required.

Ocrelizumab is a humanized monoclonal antibody against CD20 that binds to a different epitope and presents different pharmacodynamics than rituximab. In a recent RCT that included 378 patients with biopsy proven class III/IV LN receiving placebo or 400mg of ocrelizumab or 1000mg of ocrelizumab, administered on days 1 and 15, followed by an infusion at weeks 16 and 32, in all cases in addition to MMF or the Euro Lupus regimen, the ocrelizumab treated patients showed reduction of proteinuria higher than 50% compared to controls. [128] Response rates were numerically greater than in controls but difference was not statistically significant. Despite the good results, unfortunately this trial had to stop prematurely due to serious infections. Remarkably, infections occurred in patients receiving MMF but not in the Euro Lupus regimen patients.

Epratuzumab is a humanized monoclonal anti-CD22 antibody that mediates an antibody-dependent cellular toxicity with subsequent depletion of B cells and inhibition of their activation and proliferation. [129, 130] Dörner et al., administrated intravenously epratuzumab to 14 SLE patients at doses of 360mg/m^2 every two weeks for 4 doses, associated with analgesics or antihistamines. [129] 93% of these patients showed improvement of disease activity within 18 weeks. However, RCTs confirming effectiveness and safety in the treatment of LN are lacking.

Belimumab is a fully humanized monoclonal antibody against B lymphocyte stimulator (BlyS) or BAFF receptor on B cells, a cytokine essential for B cell differentiation and survival. Belimumab induces B depletion but its effect is not as strong as rituximab's. This immunomodulator has been used with success in SLE patients in 2 clinical trials (BLISS-52, BLISS-76), [131] but patients with active LN were excluded from both trials. However, in a post-hoc analysis on the recruited patients of BLISS-52 and BLISS-76, with active LN that received belimumab or placebo in addition to MMF showed superiority of belimumab on increasing remission rates, improving renal organ disease, reducing proteinuria and relapsing rates. [132]

Abatacept is a recombinant fusion protein containing the Fc region of IgG1 fused to extacellular domain of cytotoxic T lymphocyte antigen 4 (CTLA-4), known also as CD152. CD152 is a homologue of CD28 that binds CD80 and CD86 and inhibits costimulation of T cells. In a recent phase II/III multicentered double-blind RCT, [133] 298 LN patients were treated with placebo, or 10mg/kg of abatacept or 30mg/kg of abatacept for 3 months and were followed for 52 weeks. Patients treated with abatacept showed greater reduction in mean urinary protein to creatinine ratio and greater improvement in C3, C4, and anti-ds DNA antibody serum levels. Adverse events were similar in all three arms, with exception gastroenteritis and herpes zoster infections, occurring more frequently in the abatacept arms. An ongoing phase II multicentered double-blind randomized trial of the National Institute of Health, called Abatacept and Cyclophosphamide Combination Therapy for Lupus Nephritis trial or ACCESS trial (NCT00774852), is evaluating the effectiveness of a combined treatment of abatacept with Euro Lupus regimen versus cyclophosphamide alone. Patients were treated with IV abatacept at doses of 500 to 1000mg at weeks 0,2 and 4, and then every 4 weeks until week 24 if complete remission is obtained, or 48 if only partial remission is achieved. Cyclophosphamide was administrated at doses of 500mg IV every 2 weeks for 12 weeks. Positive results might be expected from this trial, but currently data on both effectiveness and safety are limited. In conclusion, B cell depleting agents could be an alternative or an adjuvant on the conservative treatments.

2. Hepatitis B Associated Glomerulonephritis

Hepatitis B virus (HBV) infection, despite prevention strategies through immunization with HBV vaccination, remains a significant public health problem worldwide as almost 350 million people are chronically infected. [134]

Renal involvement in HBV infection was first described by Combes et al., in a case report, published in 1971, of a patient with persistent HBsAg viremia associated with membranous nephropathy (MGN). Since then, different pathological patterns have been reported to be associated with HBV infection such as membranoproliferative GN (MPGN), [135] mesangial proliferative GN (MsPGN), [136] minimal change disease (MCD), [137] FSGS, [138] lupus nephritis (LN), [139] IgA nephropathy (IgAN) [140] and rarely IgM nephropathy (IgMN). [141] MGN is the commonest histopathological type associated with HBV, particularly in children. [142]

Although MGN belongs to the non-proliferative glomerular diseases, HBV-associated MGN differs from the idiopathic form as mesangial cell proliferation is usually observed in light microscopy. [143]

Given that glomerular disease associated with HBV infection, demonstrate proliferative lesions with the only exception being the FSGS and minimal change disease, in this context HBV-associated GN will be considered as a secondary proliferative glomerulonephritis.

Epidemiology

Prevalence of HBVAGN varies according the geographic distribution of HBV infection. Developing countries such as Eastern Europe, Central and Southeast Asia, China and North America are endemic areas with prevalence rates of HBV infection up to 10%. [142, 144, 145] China is the most endemic area with high incidence of HBV infection and poor prognosis especially in adults. In endemic areas transmission of HBV is mainly vertical, thus mother to infant perinatal transmission, and horizontal due to continuous contact with familial carriers and exposure to the pathogen.

Infants and children are more likely to become chronic carriers of HBV virus, thus are more likely to develop HBVAGN. In these patients, HBVAGN presents between 2 and 12 years of age with nephritic or nephrotic syndrome and more rarely with microscopic or macroscopic hematuria or non-nephrotic range proteinuria. Hypertension is usually absent, but it may be observed in children with renal insufficiency. Both genders may be affected, but HBVAGN mainly occurs in male children, prevailing over females with rates up to 80%. [146]

Children rarely present HBVAGN associated with acute hepatitis in contrast to adults.

In adults transmission is usually horizontal, via direct contact with blood or body fluids of infected subjects or percutaneously, in case of needle sharing between drug abusers. In the USA, transmission is mostly horizontal, between intravenous drug abusers and heterosexuals with multiple partners, affecting mainly African Americans. [147,148] However, in developed countries, such as the USA and Europe, incidence rates are quite low due to early immunization against the HBV virus.

Adults may present active chronic hepatitis and cirrhosis, acute hepatitis and in rare cases, fulminant hepatitis. HBVAGN in adults presents with nephrotic syndrome and hematuria, and about 30% of these patients progress to renal failure. [142] 10% of them will necessitate renal replacement therapy. [142]

The most common type of glomerulonephritis in HBV children is MGN. [149] In HBVAGN patients, membranous glomerulonephritis remains one of the most common histological patterns. However, IgA nephropathy seems to be the most common glomerulonephritis in adults, especially in endemic areas such as China. [150-153] Lai et al., suggested that HBV viremia might play an important role in the pathogenesis of IgA nephropathy. [151-153]

Additionally in a recent international data analysis, including 119 patients from 10 articles published on Pubmed, [138] authors found that 50.4% of kidney biopsy specimens presented IgAN, prevailing over MGN (34.5%). FSGS, MsPGN, MCD, and crescentic nephropathy followed with lower incidence rates. Authors suggested that HBV children are more likely to develop MGN, while adults are more likely to develop IgAN, [138] but this finding remains controversial. Most of the reports included in the aforementioned analysis were conducted in endemic areas, especially China where IgA is the most common glomerular disease. [154] It is therefore believed that prevalence of IgAN in HBV patients may be the result of coexistence of both diseases in areas where both IgAN and HBV infection are common. [149]

Spontaneous remissions of HBVAGN may occur in pediatric patients, but to date, reports on spontaneous remissions in adults are lacking. [155] Also, prognosis is usually more favorable in children that may be asymptomatic for many years and rarely progress to renal failure, in contrast to adults that develop ESRD more frequently. [142]

Although introduction of HBV immunization in endemic areas has significantly decreased incidence of HBV infection and HBVAGN, HBV infection is responsible for up to 700,000 deaths annually. [156]

Pathogenesis

The pathogenic mechanism underlying the development of HBVAGN is not totally clarified yet and different pathogenic routes have been described through the years. [138] However, data collected from animal models and human subjects, made of deposition of immune complexes formed by HBV antigens and host antibodies, offer the most widely accepted mechanism associated with HBVAGN.

Three HBV antigens, HBsAg, HBcAg and HBeAg have been found in kidney biopsy specimens with HBVAGN. KBsAg and HBcAg are anionic and have high molecular weight (2.5 to 3.6 x 10^6 Da) while HBeAg, also anionic, have small molecular weight (2.5 x 10^5 Da). [157] Therefore, it is difficult for HBsAg and HBcAg to penetrate the GBM and reach the subepithelial space, while it seems easier for HBeAg. [158] For these reasons, HBeAg is thought to be the antigen mainly responsible for the subepithelial deposits and development of HBVAGN. [142] However, contemporaneous presence of mesangial HBsAg and capillary HBeAg deposits in HBVAGN patients have also been reported, [152,159] suggesting a different distribution of HBV antigens according to their molecular weight.

Formation of immune complexes requires the presence of anti-HBe antibodies that are cationic. According to Takekoshi et al, [160] presence of IgG that can be cationic is essential in the pathogenesis of HBVAGN.

Remarkably, not all patients with HBV infection develop HBVAGN. This observation can be explained by the presence of HBV DNA in patients' renal tissue. [161,162] HBV DNA has been found in the nucleus and cytoplasm of epithelial and mesangial cells of glomeruli, in epithelial cells of renal tubules and in renal interstitial tissue. [161] HBV DNA localization in glomerular and tubular epithelium takes place with in situ hybridization. [163, 164] Detention of active transcriptional HBV genome and mRNA in the glomeruli of HBVAGN patients, strongly advocate the *in situ* hybridization and *in situ* immune complex formation. [164] Existence of HBV genome in the kidney induces expression of HBV antigens leading to *in situ* formation of immune complexes that provoke immunological responses with consecutive renal tissue damage.

In conclusion, it is more plausible that immune complexes in renal tissue of HBVAGN patients consist of both circulating and *in situ* formed immune complexes.

Inflammation and innate immunity are mechanisms implicated in the pathogenic process of HBVAGN development, activated by the immune complex formation. Absent melanoma 2 inflammasome (AIM2) is a protein belonging to the family of HIN-200 proteins, [165] seems to play an important role in the inflammation-associated renal damage in HBVAGN. [166, 167] AIM2 acts as a cytosolic sensor that senses and binds infective cytoplasmic dsDNA through its C-terminal HIN domain, [165, 168, 169] inducing formation of containing apoptosis-associated speck-like protein (CARD) or ASC inflassome that in its turn activates caspase-1 and releases IL-16 and IL-8, causing tissue damage. [166]

In two recent studies, expression of AIM2 in renal tissue was found to be higher in HBVAGN patients when compared to patients with other glomerular diseases. [166, 167] In these patients, AIM2 expression was strongly correlated to caspase-1, IL-1β and IL-18, [167] but not significantly correlated to HbeAg serum levels or other HBV antigens deposited in renal tissue. [166, 167] Importantly, there were no significant differences in AIM2 expression between different pathologic types of HBVAGN. [166]

Based on this finding one can conclude that AIM2 elevation in HBV infection contributes to inflammation that promotes renal damage.

Finally, it is believed that a genetic predisposition underlies the development of HBVAGN, as not all HBV carriers, with or without chronic or acute hepatitis, present the disease.

In fact, in a immunogenetic study conducted by Bhimma et al, [170] including 30 African American children with biopsy proven HBV-MGN, where HLA class I and II antigens, frequencies were compared to healthy controls, HLA DQB*0603 was more frequently present in HBV-MGN patients. HLA DRB1*07 and HLA DRB1*02 were also higher, but the difference was not statistically significant.

In another study, HLA-DRB and DQB1 alleles' frequencies were compared between HBV-MGN Caucasian children, healthy controls, and HBV carriers without renal abnormalities. [171] HLA DQB1*0303 frequency was significantly higher in HBV-MGN patients. HLADRB1*301 and HLA DQB1*0603 also showed increased frequency but were not statistically significant. The authors postulated that increased HLA DQB1*0603 may have been due to poor clearance of HBV antigens with their consecutive deposition in the GBM and immune complex formation.

Pathology

i. HBV-MGN

On light microscopy, there is diffuse thickening of the glomerular capillary walls with protrusions of the GBM between immune complexes, called spikes. In contrast to idiopathic MGN, there may be mesangial proliferation and focal mesangiocapillary changes.

Immunofluorescence shows positive staining for HBeAg and HBcAg. Electron microscopy shows subepithelial and subendothelial deposits.

ii. HBV-MsPGN

On light microscopy, MsPGN demonstrates mesangial hypercellularity and increased mesangial matrix. On immunofluorescence, deposits may be confined to the mesangium or extend to subendothelial areas. On electron microscopy, increased mesangial matrix and cellularity are observed. Subendothelial deposits and endocapillary proliferation may also be seen.

iii. HBV-MPGN

MPGN is characterized by increased mesangial matrix and hypercellularity with thickening of the glomerular capillary wall. On electron microscopy, there is immune complex deposition in subedothelial and mesangial areas. The subendothelial depositis are more often within the GBM, under the lamina densa giving it a double contour appearance.

Clinical Manifestations

HBVAGN occurs more often in children and presents with nephrotic syndrome. Some of the pediatric patients may present microscopic hematuria. Renal function is usually preserved, but in some cases, there may be mildly impaired renal function.

In adults, nephrotic syndrome is usually accompanied by hypertension and renal dysfunction.

Children have a more favorable prognosis, presenting in some cases spontaneous remission. On the other hand, adults are more likely to progress in renal failure and ESRD.

Treatment

Treatment of HBVAGN aims in remission of nephrotic syndrome and concomitant complications such as edema, thrombotic tendency, and infections, preservation of renal and hepatic function, by reducing serum HBV DNA titers and removing the immune complexes, and finally eradication of the virus itself.

Corticosteroids, [172] adenine arabinoside, [173] thymic extracts, [173] acyclovir, [174] interferon-α (IFN-α), [142] lamivudine, [142] and newer antiviral drugs as entecavir, tenofovir, adefovir, and clevudine have been used as therapeutic approaches in HBVAGN. Effectiveness of these drugs has been established only by small clinical trials and case reports, but large RCTs are lacking.

Use of corticosteroids has been proposed as a potential therapeutic regimen in patients with HBV-MGN presenting normal serum ALT levels, [155] at doses of 60mg of oral prednisone daily, halved after eight weeks and then tapered over 4 months, or at doses of 2mg/kg/day. [175]

Despite good results in obtaining remission of nephrotic syndrome in some HBV-MGN cases, its use has been controversial, as there is evidence that steroids induce transient viral replication and increase serum concentrations of HBeAg and HBV DNA, [176] leading to deterioration of liver and kidney function. In addition, a recent metanalysis showed that corticosteroids are not superior in achieving proteinuria remission than non-specific symptomatic treatment. [177]

Therefore, use of steroids should not be recommended for HBVAGN patients, especially if viral load and antigens haven't previously been evaluated.

Antiviral drugs have been recommended as the most important therapy for HBVAGN, as they can effectively inhibit HBV replication and decrease proteinuria, with remission rates reaching up to 60%. [178]

IFN-α is a natural cytokine produced by lymphocytes and macrophages, implicated in innate immune response against viral infections due to its antiviral, antiproliferative and immunomodulatory effects. Also, it induces proliferation of natural killer cells, which is important for the clearance of virally infected cells. [179]

Monotherapy with IFN-α, leads to HBeAg seroconversion in 30-40% of patients with hepatitis B. [180, 181] Different case reports have shown the effectiveness of IFN in remitting nephrotic syndrome in HBVAGN. [135, 182] Suggested doses are 5 million IU daily or more for 3 times per week, for at least 6 months. [183] Others suggest 5 to 8 million IU/day. [184]

Transitory elevation of serum ALT levels and increased protein excretion may be observed before antigen/antibody seroconversion due to increased activity in both liver and kidney. [185] IFN-α therapy seems to be more successful in adults. [177] In a recent metanalysis where patients included were mostly children, only 25% of the patients receiving IFN-α showed remission, partial or complete. [177]

On the other hand, others reported good results in children but disappointing results in adults. [186]

Also, IFN-α treatment has been proven to be less successful in obtaining remission than lamivudine. [184, 138]

Lamivudine is a potent nucleoside analog reverse transcriptase inhibitor that improves seroconversion of HBeAg. This antiviral drug has been proven as safe and effective against hepatitis B as IFN-α in both adults and children. [187] Commonly administered doses are 100mg/day pos for 12 months.

Lamivudine gas been used as treatment in HBV nephrotic patients with good results. [188]. It has also been suggested that lamivudine could be used as first line treatment in HBVAGN. [138]

Long-term lamivudine therapy should be used only for patients who do not respond to supportive treatment and in patients who relapse after lamivudine treatment withdrawal. [183, 189] However, long-term use of lamivudine may induce emergences of drug resistant strains due to mutation in the tyrosine-methiotine-aspartate-aspartate (YMDD) locus of the HBV reverse transcriptase gene, mostly resistance mutations M204I and M204V of the C domain of the HBV polymerase region, which decrease the efficacy of the antiviral therapy. [184,188-190] Incidence of lamivudine resistant HBV strains reaches up to 20% per year. [184]

Combination therapy of lamivudine and corticosteroids has also been used in HBVAGN patients and although remission was obtained rapidly, authors noticed a more frequent reactivation of HBV DNA after the treatment compared to lamivudine monotherapy, [191] probably due to steroids and not to the lamivudine-steroids combination. [172]

Combination of lamivudine and adefovir has also been effective in obtaining remission in a case of HBV-MGN. [192] Addition of adefovir to lemivudine is recommended by the American Association For The Study Of Liver Disease (AASLD) guidelines for lamivudine-resistant patients. [193]

Additionally, a recent study showed that *de novo* combination therapy with lamivudine and adefovir gives better results in Child-Pugh score, viral inhibition, and renal function, compared to addition of adefovir in the course of lamivudine treatment. [194]

Adefovir is an orally administered acyclic nucleotide analog that inhibits the reverse transcriptase of HBV, used in chronic HBV adult patients with evidence of active viral replication. Suggested doses are 10mg/day pos, but dosage needs adjustment according to kidney function due to potential nephrotoxicity. [8, 195, 196] However, the recommended dose of 10mg is associated with low risk of nephrotoxicity.

Adefovir resistance has also been described recently, most likely due to rtl233V mutation of HBV polymerase gene. [197]

Entecavir is an orally administrated guanosine analog that inhibits reverse transcriptase, used in chronic hepatitis B and in patients with HIV/HBV infection. Of note, entecavir is not effective against HIV but it prevents HBV replication and infection of healthy hepatic cells. Entecavir has been successfully used in HBV-MGN patients, showing HbeAg seroconversion, HBV clearance, and consecutive complete remission of proteinuria. [198, 199]

It has been suggested as a first line therapy for HBV-MGN due to its strong HBV suppressive effect, the good renal outcomes and effectiveness in obtaining remission and finally, because of its low rates of resistance. [200]

Suggested doses are 0.5mg pos daily, with dose adjustment according to renal function. [8] It may also be administrated in lamivudine-resistant patients and in this case, dose may reach 1mg pos daily. [201]

Although all these antiviral drugs are effective in HBV infection, data on their effectiveness and safety in HBVAGN patients are limited and result mostly by case reports and small clinical trials. Therefore, guidelines on the management of HBV chronic infection do not include specific indications for HBVAGN treatment. [134, 202] RCTs are needed to establish clear recommendations for both adult and children HBVAGN patients.

3. Hepatitis C Associated GN

Hepatitis C virus (HCV) is a positive-stranded RNA virus belonging to the family of Flaviviridae, which affects 3 to 4 million people worldwide annually, 80% of whom present chronic hepatitis. [203].

The World Health organization estimates that 210 million people, corresponding to 3% of the worlds' population, are infected with HCV. More than 350,000 people die from cirrhosis and hepatocellular carcinoma every year. [204,205] In the USA, approximately 4 million people are infected, thus 2% of the population. [206]

Although chronic HCV mainly affects livers and causes chronic hepatitis, a variety of extrahepatic manifestations may also occur, such as mixed cryoglobulinemia (MC), lymphoproliferative disorders, porphyria cutanea tarda, lichen planus, type II diabetes mellitus, seronegative arthritis, and renal disease. [207] Forty to 75% of chronic HCV patients present at least one extrahepatic manifestation. [203, 207] Both glomerular and tubulointerstitial alternations associated to chronic HCV infection have been described. [208]

The most common renal manifestations of HCV infection are cryoglobulinemic MPGN and non-cryoglobulinemic MPGN, followed by membranous nephropathy (MN). [209] Other forms of kidney disease related to HCV infection include FSGS, [210] fibrillary glomerulonephritis, [211] immunotactoid glomerulopathy, [211] renal thrombotic microangiopathy associated with anticardiolipin antibodies, [212] mesangioproliferative glomerulonephritis (MsPGN), [213] IgA nephropathy (IgAN), [214] postinfectious glomerulonephritis, [215] IgM nephropathy (IgMN) [215] and interstitial nephritis. [216]

Typical clinical manifestations of glomerular disease include proteinuria, microscopic hematuria, hypertension, acute nephritis, or nephrotic syndrome, with or without impairment of renal function.

Clinical course is characterized by remission and relapsing phases and prognosis is generally poor, due to high risk of progression to ESRD, but also because of high incidence of hepatic failure, infections, and cardiovascular events.

Herein, immunopathogenesis, clinical manifestations, and current therapeutic approaches of HCV associated glomerulonephritis (HCVAGN) will be reviewed.

Pathogenesis

Glomerular injury due to HCV occurs because of immunological mechanisms, including both cellular and humoral pathways. Humoral response to HCV infection induces production of antibodies against HCV antigens and monoclonal and polyclonal antibodies due to chronic antigenic stimulation. Anti-HCV-IgG and HCV lipoprotein complexes act as B-cells superantigens leading to production of non-HCV reactive IGM that presents activity similar to rheumatoid factor.

In most HCV cases, antibodies have properties of cryoglobulins, thus are monoclonal, mixed or polyclonal immunoglobulins that reversibly precipitate in vitro at temperatures lower that 37°C.

According to the Brouet classification system, [217] cryoglobulinemia is grouped into 3 types. Type 1 cryoglobulinemia is composed of monoclonal IgM, usually associated with lymphoproliferative diseases; type 2 or mixed cryoglobulinemia (MC), which consists of a complex of polyclonal IgG and monoclonal IgM with anti-γ-globulin that has a rheumatoid factor-like activity.

MC type 2 has been associated to HCV, HBV and cytomegalovirus infections, in SLE, Sjögren's syndrome and rheumatoid arthritis, and is the most frequently reported MC. [205]

Type 3 MC consists of mixed immune complexes formed by polyclonal IgM and polyclonal IgG, usually observed in SLE and rheumatoid arthritis. [205]

Type 2 is the most commonly associated MC with chronic HCV infection; however, association of type 3 MC to HCV infection has also been reported. [218] Up to 90% of patients with MC present anti-HCV antibodies and HCV-RNA, [219] but only 10 to 15% of HCV patients develop MC, [220] suggesting that HCV infection is not mandatory for the development of MC.

The pathophysiologic mechanism underlying HCV related MC development is not totally clarified yet, but it has been suggested that specific HCV proteins, the KCV envelope E2 proteins, interact with CD81, a cellular receptor for HCV, expressed on hepatocytes and B lymphocytes, [221] inducing monoclonal proliferation and clonal expansion of B lymphocytes secreting IgM-RF. [221, 222]

The HCVE2- CD81 interaction makes B-cells more susceptible to stimulation, with consecutive aberrant secretion of IgM-RF, [221] thus cryoglobulinemia. IgMκ is the most expressed IgM component of type 2 MC. [223]

Cryoglobulins are deposited in the mesangium and in subendothelial areas, where they exert their nephrotoxic activity by interaction of IgMκ-RF with cellular fibronectin present in the mesangial matrix. [224, 225]

In an experimental mouse model, MPGN was induced by intravenous administration of type 2 cryoglobulins obtained by patients with HCV associated MPGN. In this model, monoclonal IgMκ-RF was isolated from other cryoglobulins and separately injected into mice. It has been demonstrated that IgMκ-RF had affinity for fibronectin, while other monoclonal RF weren't able to fix fibronectin, [226] suggesting a special affinity of IgMκ-RF for glomerular structures.

Cryoglobulins may also induce endotheliitis by activating antibodies against the endothelium and the complement cascade that lead to increased expression of VCAM-1 and platelet aggregation. [227]

Innate immune response mechanism may also be implicated in the pathogenesis of HCVAGN. Presence of microbial antigens such as HCV core protein and HCV non-structural protein 3 and HCV-RNA are recognized by Toll-like receptors, with subsequent intracellular signaling and activation of mesangial cells to produce growth factors and cytokines, such as TNF-a and chemokine IP-10, triggering inflammatory pathways. [228-230] TRL3 was found to be overexpressed in the mesangial cells of HCV–related MPGN patients. [229]

Finally, activation of the complement cascade due to immune complex deposition induces glomerular cell proliferation, mesangial matrix expansion, and recruitment of inflammatory cells, particularly monocytes, [231] directly damaging the glomeruli.

Pathology

i. HCV Associated MPGN Type I

MPGN type I is the most common presentation of renal involvement in chronic HCV infection, especially if associated to type 2 MC.

Histologically, glomeruli present deposition of immune complexes on the capillary walls, mesangial hypercellularity due to increased mesangial proliferation and mesangial interposition of monocytes, and diffuse endocapillary proliferation. Capillary walls are thickened due to immune complexes deposition and infiltration of inflammatory cells between the endothelium and GBM, resulting in a double contoured basement membrane.

Large eosinophilic and periodic acid-Schiff (PAS) positive intraluminal deposits called hyaline thrombi may also be observed. Vasculitic changes on small and medium size arteries may occasionally be present. Interstitial fibrosis and tubular atrophy in various degrees are often present.

On immunofluorescence, staining, granular deposits of IgG, IGM, C3, and more rarely IgA are visualized along the capillary walls and in the mesangium. Occasionally, intraluminal immune deposits forming hyaline thrombi may be seen in cases of cryoglobulinemia.

On electron microscopy, mesangial and subendothelial immune deposits are observed. Cryoglobulins seem like microtubular, annular, cylindrical, or crystalloid deposits. [232, 233] More rarely, intramembranous and subendothelial deposits may be observed.

ii. HCV Associated MN

Histological findings are similar to idiopathic MN; showing by electron microscopy, diffuse global subepithelial electron dense deposits. On light microscopy, glomeruli seem normal or in some cases present thickening of the GBM. There may be protrusions of the GBM between immune deposits, the so-called spikes. Typically, there is no evidence of endocapillary proliferation. Mild mesangial hypercellularity may be present.

On immunofluorescence, subepithelial electron dense deposits, mostly represented by IgG, [234] appear like granular formations. Cryoglobulins are lacking. In advanced stages of the disease, electron dense deposits are reabsorbed, leaving behind lucent areas, called holes, seen on Jones silver staining. Foot processes effacement is observed even in early stages of the disease. In more advanced stages, interstitial fibrosis, tubular atrophy and segmental sclerosis may be present.

iii. IgA Nephropathy

HCV associated IgAN presents histological features similar to idiopathic IgAN. Light microscopy reveals mesangial proliferation and mesangial matrix expansion, usually focal and segmental, or in more severe cases, diffuse or global. Occasionally, focal segmental sclerosis with tubular atrophy and more rarely crescents may be present.

By immunofluorescence, dominant IgA deposits confined in diffuse granular pattern or extended to subendothelial and subepithelial sites, mostly polymeric IgA of the IgA1 subclasses are observed. Co-dominant C3 complement deposits may also be present.

By electron microscopy, mesangial, and paramesangial granular deposits are identified, accompanied by subendothelial and subepithelial granular deposits in cases of endocapillary proliferation. Foot processes effacement may be observed in areas of sclerosis.

Clinical Manifestations

Manifestations of renal involvement may occur several years from the infection with HCV. Given that the most common renal manifestation of HCV infection is cryoglobulinemic MPGN type I, patients may present the characteristic clinical triad of MC, thus purpura, arthralgias and weakness, or other symptoms of cryoglobulinemia including peripheral neuropathy, abdominal pain and intestinal bleeding along with renal signs.

In some cases, renal disease is the only clinical manifestation of cryoglobulinemia.

Renal manifestations include proteinuria of nephrotic or non-nephrotic range, and/or hematuria. Renal function may be mildly or moderately decreased and in only 5% of the cases, acute renal failure may occur, with oliguria or anuria. [235] Arterial hypertension is almost always present, occurring in more than 80% of the patients. In most of the cases, hypertension is quite severe and difficult to control. Malignant hypertension is usually observed in patients with rapidly progressive nephritis. [236]

Diagnosis

Diagnosis of HCVAGN may be suspected by positive test of HCV-RNA and antibodies in the serum, but it can be confirmed only with renal biopsy. Of note, cases of HCVAGN in patients with negative HCV-RNA tests have been reported. [237]

Serology usually reveals positive rheumatoid factor. Complement components C1q, C3 and C4 serum concentrations are typically low. [222, 235] Serum cryoglobulins are measured as cryocrit, showing various levels, but in MC-related HCVAGN are usually elevated. Serum aminotransferase levels are increased in the majority of the patients.

Prognosis

HCV patients with cryoglobulinemic MPGN have poor prognosis and negative outcomes, although ESRD requiring renal replacement therapy is quite rare (<10%). The overall poor prognosis is due to cardiovascular events, infections, or progression of the hepatic disease into cirrhosis. In a study conducted by Rocatello et al., in 2007, including 146 patients with cryoglobulinemic nephritis, 87% of whom where HCV positive, cardiovascular events were the most common cause of death (60%), followed by hepatic failure (19%), and infections (10%). [238].

These data suggest that ESRD in these patients rarely occurs, as they die before renal failure is established, due to cardiovascular events, liver failure, and infections.

Treatment

Recently acquired knowledge on the pathophysiologic mechanisms underlying HCVAGN and the association with MC allowed novel treatment considerations. Currently three different therapeutic approaches are suggested:

- antiviral therapy, to reduce or eliminate HCV replication, immune complexes formation and further renal damage
- B-cell depletion therapy to prevent production of cryoglobulins and immune complexes formation
- Non-specific immunosuppressive therapy targeting inflammatory cells, in order to limit or prevent immune complexes formation and to treat cryoglobulin associated vasculitis. [215, 239, 240]

i. Antiviral Therapy

The aim of antiviral therapy is the elimination of the virus and the reduction of circulating HCV-related immune complexes. Sustained virologic response (SVR) is the best long-term prognostic indicator of HCVAGN and corresponds to the clearance of HCV-RNA from serum, maintained for at least 6 months after treatment discontinuance. Although RCTs regarding antiviral treatment of HCVAGN are lacking, different small uncontrolled studies, case reports and experts' opinions suggest interferon-α (IFN-α) combined to ribavirin as a first line treatment, as it provides higher SVR due to a better HCV-RNA clearance and subsequent reduction of circulating cryoglobulin levels.

Initially, monotherapy with conventional or pegylated IFN-α was used. Despite good results in HCV-RNA clearance and reduction of proteinuria, serum creatinine levels were more likely to stabilize than decrease. [241-243]

Also, recurrence of viremia and relapse of kidney disease after IFN-α cessation were quite common. Furthermore, treatment with IFN-α has been associated with deterioration of the glomerular disease and exacerbation of cryoglobulinemic vasculitis. [244, 245]

In a comparison of antiviral versus immunosuppressive therapy for HCVAGN, IFN-α was more effective in lowering proteinuria, whereas serum creatinine levels remained unchanged; [246] both treatments failed to improve kidney function.

Combined therapy of IFN-α, conventional or pegylated, and ribavirin provides better outcomes. [247-250] Responsiveness to IFN-a-based treatment depends on HCV genotype. Patients infected by genotype 1 and 4 HCV show poor outcomes, with SVR rates of 45 to 50%, while genotypes 2 and 3 are more responsive, with SVR rates reaching up to 80%. [240] Therefore, determination of HCV genotype has an important prognostic value and it should be performed before treatment initiation. [240]

According to the most recent guidelines, triple therapy consisted of pegylated IFN-α (pegIFN-a) plus ribavirin and direct-acting agents (DAA) such as telaprevir or boceprevir, is considered the gold standard approach for the management of chronic HCV. [251] This combination was found to be highly effective in HCV-induced MC, in both reducing viremia and improving renal function. [252] However, telaprevir or boceprevir should be administered with caution, always considering levels of renal function and patients' tolerance, as both have been associated with significant decrease of GFR. [253]

KDIGO guidelines recommend combined antiviral treatment with pegIFN-α and ribavirin. [8] Suggested doses vary according renal function. CKD stage 1 and CKD stage 2 patients should receive 180μg/week of IFN-α-2a or 1.5μg/week of IFN-α-2b subcutaneously and 800 to 1200mg/day of ribavirin in two divided doses, orally or intravenously. CKD stage 3 and 4 patients should be treated with 135μg/week of IFN-α-2a or 1μg/week of IFN-α-2b subcutaneously. Ribavirin in these patients should be administered with caution, at doses of 200 to 800mg/day in divided doses; [8] oral administration should be avoided and if necessary doses should be reduced, especially if GFR is lower than 50ml/min. [8] Serum ribavirin levels should be monitored in order to avoid hemolytic anemia. [215] If serum creatinine levels are higher than 2 mg/dL IFN-α and ribavirin should be discontinued. [254]

Duration of the treatment depends on the genotype; interferon therapy in patients with genotypes 1 and 4 should last 48 weeks while genotypes 2 and 3, usually more responsive, should be treated for 24 weeks.

Patients with MC related HCV, nephrotic range proteinuria, and/or rapidly progressive renal disease should receive additional therapy with immunosuppressive agents, B-cell depletion therapy with rituximab or plasmapheresis, each one associated with intravenous methyprednisolone. [240]

ii. Immunosuppressive Agents

In patients with nephrotic syndrome and severe renal disease, immunosuppressive therapy administrated in order to obtain remission and improvement of renal function, should be considered a priority and antiviral therapy should be temporarily disregarded.

Cyclophosphamide, administrated orally at a dose of 2mg/kg/day combined to 3 pulses of intravenous methylprednisolone at dose of 1mg/kg/day, followed by oral prednisolone 1mg/kg/day and then tapered, has been successful in decreasing production of cryoglobulins and improving renal function. [255, 256]

However, cyclophosphamide treatment may increase viral replication and HCV-RNA levels, worsening cryoglobulinemic symptoms and renal function. [255, 257, 258] Corticosteroids may also increase viral load. [222] MMF could be used as an alternative to cyclophosphamide as it seems to be less toxic and more selective in inhibiting lymphocyte proliferation that cyclophosphamide. [259]

iii. B-Cell Depletion Therapy

Given that HCV related MC is caused by chronic stimulation of B-lymphocytes by HCV, it seems reasonable to consider MC patients as appropriate candidates for B cell depletion therapy.

Rituximab is a chimeric monoclonal CD20 antibody that targets and depletes B-cells, inhibiting the production of pathogenic cryoglobulins. Rituximab proved to be efficient in the management of symptomatic mixed cryoglobulinemia and in the treatment of HVAGN with or without cryoglobulinemia. [260, 261]

Sansonno et al, [262] administered rituximab at dose of 375mg/m^2 weekly for 4 weeks, to 20 HCV-positive patients with mixed cryoglobulinemia and observed them for a follow-up period of 12 months. Complete remission of proteinuria was obtained by 80% of the patients. Authors reported a significant reduction of cryoglobulins and rheumatoid factor. Importantly, they observed a deep impact of rituximab on HCV viremia; HCV-RNA levels were almost reduplicated in responders, whereas they remained unchanged in non-responders. In the view of increased viremia, authors suggested combination of rituximab with antiviral agents as a possible solution to this complication.

In 2008, Saadoun et al., [263] treated 16 patients with severe HCV-related MC vasculitis with rituximab plus pegIFN-α with good results. Ten of 16 patients achieved complete remission. Relapses occurred only in 2 patients, in concomitance with increase of B-cells numbers and cryoglobulins levels.

In 2003 Rocatello et al, [261] treated 6 patients with HCV-associated MC vasculitis, five of whom presented renal involvement, with rituximab at a dose of 375mg/m^2 for 4 weekly doses. All patients showed reduction of proteinuria. In contrast to Saadoun et al., findings, HCV viral load decreased or remained unchanged.

In another study conducted by Quartuccio et al, [260] including 5 HCVAGN patients with mixed cryoglobulinemia receiving 4 weekly doses of rituximab 375mg/m^2, renal function improved within 2 months in all cases, but 3 of the patients relapsed within 12 months. After a repeated cycle of rituximab, only 2 patients achieved remission.

Concomitant reduction of rheumatoid factor levels was found in both studies and no adverse effects, acute or delayed, were observed.

Rituximab was also found to be efficient in treating de novo cryoglobulinemic HCVAGN in renal transplant patients but its association with high incidence of infectious complications may limit its use. [264] Also, rituximab rarely forms complexes with IgM-RF, increasing cryoprecipitation. [265] In order to avoid this complication, rituximab should be administered after plasma exchange, especially in patients with high baseline cryoglobulin levels. [246]

Although treatment with rituximab seems promising, exact indications on dosage are lacking and knowledge on its long-term efficacy and safety is limited. Further investigation and RCTs are required to define optimal dosage and frequency of rituximab administration and to evaluate long term results.

iv. Plasmapheresis

Plasma exchange therapy is performed in the acute phase of the disease as it offers the advantage of removing cryoglobulins and immune complexes from the circulation, preventing their deposition into the kidney. [266] It is usually combined with immunosuppressive and HCV antiviral treatment, in order to reduce viral load and prevent reaccumulation of cryoglobulins and immune complexes. Typically, plasma exchange sessions take place 2 times a week and exchanged plasma volumes are usually 3 lt. However, a relatively recent study showed that association of plasma exchange therapy to IFN-α, administrated after the sessions, has not modified viral response in HCV-associated systemic vasculitis patients. [267]

Recently, double filtration plasmapheresis (DFPP) combined to pegIFN-α/ribavirin was successfully used to treat chronic genotype 1b HCV patients. [268]

In a recent case report, IFN-α therapy combined to DFPP was performed to treat a patient with HCV associated MPGN presenting genotype 1b HCV-RNA. The treatment reduced viral load and induced clinical remission of MPGN. [269].

Efficacy and safety of this regimen haven't been confirmed by RCTs however; it is believed that DFPP may be more favorable than classic plasmapheresis and that it may represent an effective therapeutic method for refractory HCVAGN.

References

[1] Cervera R, Abarca-Costalago M, Abramovicz D, Allegri F, Annunziata P, Aydintug AO, et al; European Working Party on Systemic Lupus Erythematosus. Systemic lupus erythematosus in Europe at the change of the millennium: lessons from the "Euro-Lupus Project". *Autoimmun. Rev.* 2006 Mar;5(3):180-6.

[2] Cameron JS. Lupus nephritis: an historical perspective 1968-1998. *J. Nephrol.* 1999 Jul-Aug;12 Suppl 2:S29-41.

[3] Apostolidis SA, Crispín JC, Tsokos GC. IL-17-producing T cells in lupus nephritis. *Lupus.* 2011 Feb;20(2):120-4.

[4] Miyake K, Akahoshi M, Nakashima H. Th subset balance in lupus nephritis. *J. Biomed Biotechnol.* 2011;2011:980286.

[5] Christopher-Stine L, Siedner M, Lin J, Haas M, Parekh H, Petri M, et al. Renal biopsy in lupus patients with low levels of proteinuria. *J. Rheumatol.* 2007 Feb;34(2):332-5.

[6] Alba P, Bento L, Cuadrado MJ, Karim Y, Tungekar MF, Abbs I, et al. Anti-dsDNA, anti-Sm antibodies, and the lupus anticoagulant: significant factors associated with lupus nephritis. *Ann. Rheum. Dis.* 2003 Jun;62(6):556-60.

[7] Liu CC, Manzi S, Ahearn JM. Biomarkers for systemic lupus erythematosus: a review and perspective. *Curr. Opin. Rheumatol.* 2005 Sep;17(5):543-9.

[8] Kidney Disease: Improving Global Outcomes (KDIGO) Glomerulonephritis Work Group. KDIGO Clinical Practice Guideline for Glomerulonephritis. *Kidney inter.,* Suppl. 2012; 2: 139–274.

[9] Bastian HM, Roseman JM, McGwin G Jr, Alarcón GS, Friedman AW, Fessler BJ, et al; LUMINA Study Group. LUpus in MInority populations: NAture vs nurture. Systemic lupus erythematosus in three ethnic groups. XII. Risk factors for lupus nephritis after diagnosis. *Lupus.* 2002;11(3):152-60.

[10] Feldman CH, Hiraki LT, Liu J, Fischer MA, Solomon DH, Alarcón GS, et al. Epidemiology and sociodemographics of systemic lupus erythematosus and lupus nephritis among US adults with Medicaid coverage, 2000-2004. *Arthritis. Rheum.* 2013 Mar;65(3):753-63.

[11] Al Arfaj AS, Khalil N. Clinical and immunological manifestations in 624 SLE patients in Saudi *Arabia. Lupus.* 2009 Apr;18(5):465-73.

[12] Seligman VA, Lum RF, Olson JL, Li H, Criswell LA. Demographic differences in the development of lupus nephritis: a retrospective analysis. *Am. J. Med.* 2002 Jun 15;112(9):726-9.

[13] Mak A, Mok CC, Chu WP, To CH, Wong SN, Au TC. Renal damage in systemic lupus erythematosus: a comparative analysis of different age groups. *Lupus.* 2007;16(1):28-34.

[14] Saxena R, Mahajan T, Mohan C. Lupus nephritis: current update. Arthritis. Res. Ther. 2011;13(5):240.

[15] Soni SS, Gowrishankar S, Adikey GK, Raman A. Sex-based differences in lupus nephritis: a study of 235 Indian patients. *J. Nephrol.* 2008 Jul-Aug;21(4):570-5.

[16] de Carvalho JF, do Nascimento AP, Testagrossa LA, Barros RT, Bonfá E. Male gender results in more severe lupus nephritis. *Rheumatol Int.* 2010 Aug;30(10):1311-5.

[17] Balluz L, Philen R, Ortega L, Rosales C, Brock J, Barr D, et al. Investigation of systemic lupus erythematosus in Nogales, Arizona. *Am. J. Epidemiol.* 2001 Dec 1;154(11):1029-36.

[18] Fernández M, Alarcón GS, Calvo-Alén J, Andrade R, McGwin G Jr, Vilá LM, et al; LUMINA Study Group. A multiethnic, multicenter cohort of patients with systemic lupus erythematosus (SLE) as a model for the study of ethnic disparities in SLE. *Arthritis. Rheum.* 2007 May 15;57(4):576-84.

[19] McCarty DJ, Manzi S, Medsger TA Jr, Ramsey-Goldman R, LaPorte RE, Kwoh CK. Incidence of systemic lupus erythematosus. Race and gender differences. *Arthritis Rheum.* 1995 Sep;38(9):1260-70.

[20] Ward MM, Studenski S. Clinical manifestations of systemic lupus erythematosus. Identification of racial and socioeconomic influences. *Arch. Intern. Med.* 1990 Apr;150(4):849-53.

[21] Yazdany J, Gillis JZ, Trupin L, Katz P, Panopalis P, Criswell LA, et al. Association of socioeconomic and demographic factors with utilization of rheumatology subspecialty care in systemic lupus erythematosus. *Arthritis Rheum*. 2007 May 15;57(4):593-600.

[22] US Renal Data System: Annual Data Report 2013, Reference Tables: ESRD, Vol. 2 : 335-358.

[23] Hof D, Raats JM, Pruijn GJ. Apoptotic modifications affect the autoreactivity of the U1 snRNP autoantigen. *Autoimmun Rev*. 2005 Jul;4(6):380-8. Epub 2005 Mar 23.

[24] Huck S, Deveaud E, Namane A, Zouali M. Abnormal DNA methylation and deoxycytosine-deoxyguanine content in nucleosomes from lymphocytes undergoing apoptosis. *FASEB J*. 1999 Aug;13(11):1415-22.

[25] Hotchkiss RS, Strasser A, McDunn JE, Swanson PE. Cell death. *N. Engl. J. Med*. 2009 Oct 15;361(16):1570-83.

[26] Muñoz LE, Lauber K, Schiller M, Manfredi AA, Herrmann M. The role of defective clearance of apoptotic cells in systemic autoimmunity. *Nat. Rev. Rheumatol*. 2010 May;6(5):280-9.

[27] Yasutomo K, Horiuchi T, Kagami S, Tsukamoto H, Hashimura C, Urushihara M, et al. Mutation of DNASE1 in people with systemic lupus erythematosus. *Nat. Genet*. 2001 Aug;28(4):313-4.

[28] Karikó K, Ni H, Capodici J, Lamphier M, Weissman D. mRNA is an endogenous ligand for Toll-like receptor 3. *J. Biol. Chem*. 2004 Mar 26;279(13):12542-50.

[29] Leadbetter EA, Rifkin IR, Hohlbaum AM, Beaudette BC, Shlomchik MJ, Marshak-Rothstein A. Chromatin-IgG complexes activate B cells by dual engagement of IgM and Toll-like receptors. *Nature*. 2002 Apr 11;416(6881):603-7.

[30] Means TK, Latz E, Hayashi F, Murali MR, Golenbock DT, Luster AD. Human lupus autoantibody-DNA complexes activate DCs through cooperation of CD32 and TLR9. *J. Clin. Invest*. 2005 Feb;115(2):407-17.

[31] Chan OT, Hannum LG, Haberman AM, Madaio MP, Shlomchik MJ. A novel mouse with B cells but lacking serum antibody reveals an antibody-independent role for B cells in murine lupus. *J. Exp. Med*. 1999 May 17;189(10):1639-48.

[32] Anders HJ. Pseudoviral immunity - a novel concept for lupus. *Trends Mol. Med*. 2009 Dec;15(12):553-61.

[33] Christensen SR, Shupe J, Nickerson K, Kashgarian M, Flavell RA, Shlomchik MJ. Toll-like receptor 7 and TLR9 dictate autoantibody specificity and have opposing inflammatory and regulatory roles in a murine model of lupus. *Immunity*. 2006 Sep;25(3):417-28.

[34] Guiducci C, Gong M, Xu Z, Gill M, Chaussabel D, Meeker T, et al. TLR recognition of self nucleic acids hampers glucocorticoid activity in lupus. *Nature*. 2010 Jun 17;465(7300):937-41.

[35] Migliorini A, Anders HJ. A novel pathogenetic concept-antiviral immunity in lupus nephritis. *Nat. Rev. Nephrol*. 2012 Jan 17;8(3):183-9.

[36] Teichmann LL, Ols ML, Kashgarian M, Reizis B, Kaplan DH, Shlomchik MJ. Dendritic cells in lupus are not required for activation of T and B cells but promote their expansion, resulting in tissue damage. *Immunity*. 2010 Dec 14;33(6):967-78.

[37] Bekeredjian-Ding IB, Wagner M, Hornung V, Giese T, Schnurr M, Endres S, Hartmann G. Plasmacytoid dendritic cells control TLR7 sensitivity of naive B cells via type I IFN. *J Immunol*. 2005 Apr 1;174(7):4043-50.

[38] Rönnblom L, Alm GV, Eloranta ML. Type I interferon and lupus. *Curr Opin Rheumatol.* 2009 Sep;21(5):471-7.

[39] Yu F, Wu LH, Tan Y, Li LH, Wang CL, Wang WK, et al. Tubulointerstitial lesions of patients with lupus nephritis classified by the 2003 International Society of Nephrology and Renal Pathology Society system. *Kidney Int.* 2010 May;77(9):820-9.

[40] Yung S, Cheung KF, Zhang Q, Chan TM. Anti-dsDNA antibodies bind to mesangial annexin II in lupus nephritis. *J Am Soc Nephrol.* 2010 Nov;21(11):1912-27.

[41] Zhao Z, Deocharan B, Scherer PE, Ozelius LJ, Putterman C. Differential binding of cross-reactive anti-DNA antibodies to mesangial cells: the role of alpha-actinin. *J. Immunol.* 2006 Jun 15;176(12):7704-14.

[42] Fenton KA, Rekvig OP. A central role of nucleosomes in lupus nephritis. *Ann. N. Y. Acad Sci.* 2007 Jun;1108:104-13.

[43] Kalaaji M, Mortensen E, Jørgensen L, Olsen R, Rekvig OP. Nephritogenic lupus antibodies recognize glomerular basement membrane-associated chromatin fragments released from apoptotic intraglomerular cells. *Am. J. Pathol.* 2006 Jun;168(6):1779-92.

[44] Pawar RD, Patole PS, Ellwart A, Lech M, Segerer S, Schlondorff D, et al. Ligands to nucleic acid-specific toll-like receptors and the onset of lupus nephritis. *J. Am. Soc. Nephrol.* 2006 Dec;17(12):3365-73.

[45] Allam R, Lichtnekert J, Moll AG, Taubitz A, Vielhauer V, Anders HJ. Viral RNA and DNA trigger common antiviral responses in mesangial cells. *J. Am. Soc. Nephrol.* 2009 Sep;20(9):1986-96.

[46] Flür K, Allam R, Zecher D, Kulkarni OP, Lichtnekert J, Schwarz M, et al. Viral RNA induces type I interferon-dependent cytokine release and cell death in mesangial cells via melanoma-differentiation-associated gene-5: Implications for viral infection-associated glomerulonephritis. *Am. J. Pathol.* 2009 Nov;175(5):2014-22.

[47] Elliott MK, Jarmi T, Ruiz P, Xu Y, Holers VM, Gilkeson GS. Effects of complement factor D deficiency on the renal disease of MRL/lpr mice. *Kidney Int.* 2004 Jan;65(1):129-38.\

[48] Sato N, Ohsawa I, Nagamachi S, Ishii M, Kusaba G, Inoshita H, et al. Significance of glomerular activation of the alternative pathway and lectin pathway in lupus nephritis. Lupus. 2011 Nov;20(13):1378-86.

[49] Murata K, Baldwin WM 3rd. Mechanisms of complement activation, C4d deposition, and their contribution to the pathogenesis of antibody-mediated rejection. *Transplant Rev* (Orlando). 2009 Jul;23(3):139-50.

[50] Menke J, Bork T, Kutska B, Byrne KT, Blanfeld M, Relle M, et al. Targeting transcription factor Stat4 uncovers a role for interleukin-18 in the pathogenesis of severe lupus nephritis in mice. *Kidney Int.* 2011 Feb;79(4):452-63.

[51] Tucci M, Lombardi L, Richards HB, Dammacco F, Silvestris F. Overexpression of interleukin-12 and T helper 1 predominance in lupus nephritis. *Clin. Exp. Immunol.* 2008 Nov;154(2):247-54.

[52] Tucci M, Quatraro C, Lombardi L, Pellegrino C, Dammacco F, Silvestris F. Glomerular accumulation of plasmacytoid dendritic cells in active lupus nephritis: role of interleukin-18. *Arthritis. Rheum.* 2008 Jan;58(1):251-62.

[53] Espeli M, Bökers S, Giannico G, Dickinson HA, Bardsley V, Fogo AB, et al. Local renal autoantibody production in lupus nephritis. *J. Am. Soc. Nephrol.* 2011 Feb;22(2):296-305.

[54] Chang A, Henderson SG, Brandt D, Liu N, Guttikonda R, Hsieh C, et al. In situ B cell-mediated immune responses and tubulointerstitial inflammation in human lupus nephritis. *J. Immunol.* 2011 Feb 1;186(3):1849-60.

[55] Weening JJ, D'Agati VD, Schwartz MM, Seshan SV, Alpers CE, Appel GB, et al. The classification of glomerulonephritis in systemic lupus erythematosus revisited. *J. Am. Soc. Nephrol.* 2004 Feb;15(2):241-50.

[56] Furness PN, Taub N. Interobserver reproducibility and application of the ISN/RPS classification of lupus nephritis-a UK-wide study. *Am. J. Surg. Pathol.* 2006 Aug;30(8):1030-5.

[57] Markowitz GS, D'Agati VD. Classification of lupus nephritis. Curr. Opin. Nephrol. Hypertens. 2009 May;18(3):220-5.

[58] Dube G, Markowitz GS, Radhakrishnan J, Appel GB, D'Agati VD. Minimal change disease in systemic lupus erythematosus. *Clin. Nephrol.* 2002 Feb;57(2):120-6.

[59] Hertig A, Droz D, Lesavre P, Grünfeld JP, Rieu P. SLE and idiopathic nephrotic syndrome: coincidence or not? *Am. J. Kidney Dis.* 2002 Dec;40(6):1179-84.

[60] Kraft SW, Schwartz MM, Korbet SM, Lewis EJ. Glomerular podocytopathy in patients with systemic lupus erythematosus. *J. Am. Soc. Nephrol.* 2005 Jan;16(1):175-9.

[61] Khamashta MA. Systemic lupus erythematosus and pregnancy. *Best Pract Res Clin Rheumatol.* 2006 Aug;20(4):685-94.

[62] Repke JT. Hypertensive disorders of pregnancy. Differentiating preeclampsia from active systemic lupus erythematosus. *J. Reprod. Med.* 1998 Apr;43(4):350-4.

[63] Clark CA, Spitzer KA, Laskin CA. Decrease in pregnancy loss rates in patients with systemic lupus erythematosus over a 40-year period. *J. Rheumatol.* 2005 Sep;32(9):1709-12.

[64] Miranda-Carús ME, Askanase AD, Clancy RM, Di Donato F, Chou TM, Libera MR, et al. Anti-SSA/Ro and anti-SSB/La autoantibodies bind the surface of apoptotic fetal cardiocytes and promote secretion of TNF-alpha by macrophages. *J. Immunol.* 2000 Nov 1;165(9):5345-51.

[65] Buyon JP, Hiebert R, Copel J, Craft J, Friedman D, Katholi M, et al. Autoimmune-associated congenital heart block: demographics, mortality, morbidity and recurrence rates obtained from a national neonatal lupus registry. *J. Am. Coll Cardiol.* 1998 Jun;31(7):1658-66.

[66] Garcia S, Campos-de-Carvalho AC. Neonatal lupus syndrome: the heart as a target of the immune system. An. *Acad. Bras. Cienc.* 2000;72(1):83-9.

[67] Brucato A, Cimaz R, Stramba-Badiale M. Neonatal lupus. *Clin Rev Allergy Immunol.* 2002 Dec;23(3):279-99.

[68] Matsushita H, Higashino M, Sekizuka N, Kurabayashi T, Takakuwa K, Tanaka K. Successful prenatal treatment of congenital heart block with ritodrine administered transplacentally. *Arch. Gynecol. Obstet.* 2002 Nov;267(1):51-3.

[69] Friedman DM, Llanos C, Izmirly PM, Brock B, Byron J, Copel J, et al. Evaluation of fetuses in a study of intravenous immunoglobulin as preventive therapy for congenital heart block: Results of a multicenter, prospective, open-label clinical trial. *Arthritis Rheum.* 2010 Apr;62(4):1138-46. doi: 10.1002/art.27308.

[70] Yang CH, Chen JY, Lee SC, Luo SF. Successful preventive treatment of congenital heart block during pregnancy in a woman with systemic lupus erythematosus and anti-

Sjögren's syndrome A/Ro antibody. *J. Microbiol. Immunol. Infect*. 2005 Oct;38(5): 365-9.

[71] Jaeggi ET, Hamilton RM, Silverman ED, Zamora SA, Hornberger LK. Outcome of children with fetal, neonatal or childhood diagnosis of isolated congenital atrioventricular block. A single institution's experience of 30 years. *J. Am. Coll.* Cardiol. 2002 Jan 2;39(1):130-7.

[72] Hochberg MC. Updating the American College of Rheumatology revised criteria for the classification of systemic lupus erythematosus. *Arthritis Rheum*. 1997 Sep;40(9):1725.

[73] Cameron JS. Lupus nephritis. *J. Am. Soc. Nephrol*. 1999 Feb;10(2):413-24.

[74] Corwin HL, Schwartz MM, Lewis EJ. The importance of sample size in the interpretation of the renal biopsy. *Am. J. Nephrol*. 1988;8(2):85-9.

[75] Christopher-Stine L, Petri M, Astor BC, Fine D. Urine protein-to-creatinine ratio is a reliable measure of proteinuria in lupus nephritis. *J. Rheumatol*. 2004 Aug;31(8): 1557-9.

[76] Liang MH, Schur PH, Fortin P, St. Clair W.E, Balow JE, Costenbader K, et al; Renal Disease Subcommittee of the American College of Rheumatology Ad Hoc Committee on Systemic Lupus Erythematosus Response Criteria. The American College of Rheumatology response criteria for proliferative and membranous renal disease in systemic lupus erythematosus clinical trials. *Arthritis. Rheum*. 2006 Feb;54(2):421-32.

[77] Birmingham DJ, Rovin BH, Shidham G, Nagaraja HN, Zou X, Bissell M, et al. Spot urine protein/creatinine ratios are unreliable estimates of 24 h proteinuria in most systemic lupus erythematosus nephritis flares. *Kidney Int*. 2007 Oct;72(7):865-70.

[78] Austin HA. Clinical evaluation and monitoring of lupus kidney disease. *Lupus*. 1998;7(9):618-21.

[79] Waldman M, Madaio MP. Pathogenic autoantibodies in lupus nephritis. *Lupus*. 2005;14(1):19-24.

[80] Gualtierotti R, Biggioggero M, Penatti AE, Meroni PL. Updating on the pathogenesis of systemic lupus erythematosus. *Autoimmun. Rev*. 2010 Nov;10(1):3-7.

[81] Chen Z, Wang GS, Wang GH, Li XP. Anti-C1q antibody is a valuable biological marker for prediction of renal pathological characteristics in lupus nephritis. *Clin. Rheumatol.* 2012 Sep;31(9):1323-9.

[82] Wang FM, Yu F, Tan Y, Song D, Zhao MH. Serum complement factor H is associated with clinical and pathological activities of patients with lupus nephritis. *Rheumatology* (Oxford). 2012 Dec;51(12):2269-77.

[83] Treamtrakanpon W, Tantivitayakul P, Benjachat T, Somparn P, Kittikowit W, Eiam-Ong S, et al. APRIL, a proliferation-inducing ligand, as a potential marker of lupus nephritis. *Arthritis. Res. Ther*. 2012 Nov 21;14(6):R252.

[84] Panda AK, Parida JR, Tripathy R, Pattanaik SS, Ravindran B, Das BK. Mannose binding lectin: a biomarker of systemic lupus erythematosus disease activity. *Arthritis. Res. Ther.* 2012 Oct 15;14(5):R218.

[85] Badot V, Luijten RK, van Roon JA, Depresseux G, Aydin S, Van den Eynde BJ, et al. Serum soluble interleukin 7 receptor is strongly associated with lupus nephritis in patients with systemic lupus erythematosus. *Ann. Rheum. Dis*. 2013 Mar;72(3):453-6.

[86] Miyake K, Nakashima H, Akahoshi M, Inoue Y, Nagano S, Tanaka Y, et al. Genetically determined interferon-gamma production influences the histological phenotype of lupus nephritis. *Rheumatology* (Oxford). 2002 May;41(5):518-24.

[87] Sunahori K, Juang YT, Kyttaris VC, Tsokos GC. Promoter hypomethylation results in increased expression of protein phosphatase 2A in T cells from patients with systemic lupus erythematosus. *J. Immunol.* 2011 Apr 1;186(7):4508-17.

[88] Suzuki M, Wiers K, Brooks EB, Greis KD, Haines K, Klein-Gitelman MS, et al. Initial validation of a novel protein biomarker panel for active pediatric lupus nephritis. *Pediatr. Res.* 2009 May;65(5):530-6.

[89] Uehara Y, Makino H, Seiki K, Urade Y; L-PGDS Clinical Research Group of Kidney. Urinary excretions of lipocalin-type prostaglandin D synthase predict renal injury in type-2 diabetes: a cross-sectional and prospective multicentre study. *Nephrol. Dial. Transplant.* 2009 Feb;24(2):475-82.

[90] Zhang X, Jin M, Wu H, Nadasdy T, Nadasdy G, Harris N, et al. Biomarkers of lupus nephritis determined by serial urine proteomics. *Kidney Int.* 2008 Sep;74(6):799-807.

[91] Kiani A, Mohan C, Wu T, Magder L, Petri M; VCAM-1 Is a Better Measure of SLE Renal Activity Than NGAL and CXCL16 [abstract]. *Arthritis. Rheum.* 2009;60 Suppl 10 :919.

[92] Tsai CY, Wu TH, Yu CL, Lu JY, Tsai YY. Increased excretions of beta2-microglobulin, IL-6, and IL-8 and decreased excretion of Tamm-Horsfall glycoprotein in urine of patients with active lupus nephritis. *Nephron.* 2000 Jul;85(3):207-14.

[93] Gordon C, Jayne D, Pusey C, Adu D, Amoura Z, Aringer M, et al. European consensus statement on the terminology used in the management of lupus glomerulonephritis. *Lupus.* 2009 Mar;18(3):257-63.

[94] Tesar V, Hruskova Z. Treatment of proliferative lupus nephritis: a slowly changing landscape. *Nat. Rev. Nephrol.* 2011 Feb;7(2):96-109.

[95] Gonzalez-Crespo MR, Lopez-Fernandez JI, Usera G, Poveda MJ, Gomez-Reino JJ. Outcome of silent lupus nephritis. *Semin Arthritis Rheum.* 1996 Aug;26(1):468-76.

[96] Zabaleta-Lanz ME, Muñoz LE, Tapanes FJ, Vargas-Arenas RE, Daboin I, Barrios Y, et al. Further description of early clinically silent lupus nephritis. *Lupus.* 2006;15(12):845-51.

[97] Ruiz-Irastorza G, Ramos-Casals M, Brito-Zeron P, Khamashta MA. Clinical efficacy and side effects of antimalarials in systemic lupus erythematosus: a systematic review. *Ann. Rheum. Dis.* 2010 Jan;69(1):20-8.

[98] Grootscholten C, Berden JH. Discontinuation of immunosuppression in proliferative lupus nephritis: is it possible? *Nephrol. Dial. Transplant.* 2006 Jun;21(6):1465-9.

[99] Houssiau FA, Vasconcelos C, D'Cruz D, Sebastiani GD, de Ramon Garrido E, Danieli MG, et al. The 10-year follow-up data of the Euro-Lupus Nephritis Trial comparing low-dose and high-dose intravenous cyclophosphamide. *Ann. Rheum. Dis.* 2010 Jan;69(1):61-4.

[100] Austin HA 3rd, Klippel JH, Balow JE, le Riche NG, Steinberg AD, Plotz PH, et al. Therapy of lupus nephritis. Controlled trial of prednisone and cytotoxic drugs. *N. Engl. J. Med.* 1986 Mar 6;314(10):614-9.

[101] Steinberg AD, Steinberg SC. Long-term preservation of renal function in patients with lupus nephritis receiving treatment that includes cyclophosphamide versus those treated with prednisone only. *Arthritis. Rheum.* 1991 Aug;34(8):945-50.

[102] Boumpas DT, Austin HA 3rd, Vaughn EM, Klippel JH, Steinberg AD, Yarboro CH, et al. Controlled trial of pulse methylprednisolone versus two regimens of pulse cyclophosphamide in severe lupus nephritis. *Lancet.* 1992 Sep 26;340(8822):741-5.

[103] Gourley MF, Austin HA 3rd, Scott D, Yarboro CH, Vaughan EM, Muir J, et al. Methylprednisolone and cyclophosphamide, alone or in combination, in patients with lupus nephritis. A randomized, controlled trial. *Ann. Intern. Med.* 1996 Oct 1;125(7):549-57.

[104] Houssiau FA, Vasconcelos C, D'Cruz D, Sebastiani GD, Garrido Ed Ede R, Danieli MG, et al. Immunosuppressive therapy in lupus nephritis: the Euro-Lupus Nephritis Trial, a randomized trial of low-dose versus high-dose intravenous cyclophosphamide. *Arthritis. Rheum.* 2002 Aug;46(8):2121-31.

[105] Grootscholten C, Ligtenberg G, Hagen EC, van den Wall Bake AW, de Glas-Vos JW, Bijl M, et al; Dutch Working Party on Systemic Lupus Erythematosus. Azathioprine/methylprednisolone versus cyclophosphamide in proliferative lupus nephritis. A randomized controlled trial. *Kidney Int.* 2006 Aug;70(4):732-42.

[106] Grootscholten C, Bajema IM, Florquin S, Steenbergen EJ, Peutz-Kootstra CJ, Goldschmeding R, et al; Dutch Working Party on Systemic Lupus Erythematosus. Treatment with cyclophosphamide delays the progression of chronic lesions more effectively than does treatment with azathioprine plus methylprednisolone in patients with proliferative lupus nephritis. *Arthritis. Rheum.* 2007 Mar;56(3):924-37.

[107] Ginzler EM, Dooley MA, Aranow C, Kim MY, Buyon J, Merrill JT, et al. Mycophenolate mofetil or intravenous cyclophosphamide for lupus nephritis. *N. Engl. J. Med.* 2005 Nov 24;353(21):2219-28.

[108] Appel GB, Contreras G, Dooley MA, Ginzler EM, Isenberg D, Jayne D, et al; Aspreva Lupus Management Study Group. Mycophenolate mofetil versus cyclophosphamide for induction treatment of lupus nephritis. *J. Am. Soc. Nephrol.* 2009 May;20(5):1103-12.

[109] Isenberg D, Appel GB, Contreras G, Dooley MA, Ginzler EM, Jayne D, et al. Influence of race/ethnicity on response to lupus nephritis treatment: the ALMS study. *Rheumatology* (Oxford). 2010 Jan;49(1):128-40.

[110] Bao H, Liu ZH, Xie HL, Hu WX, Zhang HT, Li LS. Successful treatment of class V+IV lupus nephritis with multitarget therapy. *J. Am. Soc. Nephrol.* 2008 Oct;19(10):2001-10.

[111] Korbet SM, Schwartz MM, Evans J, Lewis EJ; Collaborative Study Group. Severe lupus nephritis: racial differences in presentation and outcome. *J. Am. Soc. Nephrol.* 2007 Jan;18(1):244-54.

[112] Ioannidis JP, Boki KA, Katsorida ME, Drosos AA, Skopouli FN, Boletis JN, et al. Remission, relapse, and re-remission of proliferative lupus nephritis treated with cyclophosphamide. *Kidney Int.* 2000 Jan;57(1):258-64.

[113] Contreras G, Pardo V, Leclercq B, Lenz O, Tozman E, O'Nan P, et al. Sequential therapies for proliferative lupus nephritis. *N. Engl. J. Med.* 2004 Mar 4;350(10):971-80.

[114] Houssiau FA, D'Cruz D, Sangle S, Remy P, Vasconcelos C, Petrovic R, et al; MAINTAIN Nephritis Trial Group. Azathioprine versus mycophenolate mofetil for long-term immunosuppression in lupus nephritis: results from the MAINTAIN Nephritis Trial. *Ann Rheum Dis.* 2010 Dec;69(12):2083-9.

[115] Dooley MA, Jayne D, Ginzler EM, Isenberg D, Olsen NJ, Wofsy D, et al; ALMS Group. Mycophenolate versus azathioprine as maintenance therapy for lupus nephritis. *N Engl J Med.* 2011 Nov 17;365(20):1886-95.

[116] Moroni G, Doria A, Mosca M, Alberighi OD, Ferraccioli G, Todesco S, et al. A randomized pilot trial comparing cyclosporine and azathioprine for maintenance therapy in diffuse lupus nephritis over four years. *Clin. J. Am. Soc. Nephrol.* 2006 Sep;1(5):925-32.

[117] Bhinder S, Singh A, Majithia V. Membranous (class V) renal disease in systemic lupus erythematosus may be more common than previously reported: results of a 6-year retrospective analysis. *Am. J. Med. Sci.* 2010 Mar;339(3):230-2.

[118] Gonzalez-Dettoni H, Tron F. Membranous glomerulopathy in systemic lupus erythematosus. *Adv Nephrol Necker Hosp.* 1985;14:347-64.

[119] Mok CC, Ying KY, Yim CW, Ng WL, Wong WS. Very long-term outcome of pure lupus membranous nephropathy treated with glucocorticoid and azathioprine. *Lupus.* 2009 Oct;18(12):1091-5.

[120] Austin HA 3rd, Illei GG, Braun MJ, Balow JE. Randomized, controlled trial of prednisone, cyclophosphamide, and cyclosporine in lupus membranous nephropathy. *J. Am. Soc. Nephrol.* 2009 Apr;20(4):901-11.

[121] Radhakrishnan J, Moutzouris DA, Ginzler EM, Solomons N, Siempos II, Appel GB. Mycophenolate mofetil and intravenous cyclophosphamide are similar as induction therapy for class V lupus nephritis. *Kidney Int.* 2010 Jan;77(2):152-60.

[122] Szeto CC, Kwan BC, Lai FM, Tam LS, Li EK, Chow KM, et al. Tacrolimus for the treatment of systemic lupus erythematosus with pure class V nephritis. *Rheumatology* (Oxford). 2008 Nov;47(11):1678-81.

[123] Mok CC, Ying KY, Lau CS, Yim CW, Ng WL, Wong WS, et al. Treatment of pure membranous lupus nephropathy with prednisone and azathioprine: an open-label trial. *Am. J. Kidney Dis.* 2004 Feb;43(2):269-76.

[124] Croca SC, Rodrigues T, Isenberg DA. Assessment of a lupus nephritis cohort over a 30-year period. *Rheumatology* (Oxford). 2011 Aug;50(8):1424-30.

[125] Catapano F, Chaudhry AN, Jones RB, Smith KG, Jayne DW. Long-term efficacy and safety of rituximab in refractory and relapsing systemic lupus erythematosus. *Nephrol Dial. Transplant.* 2010 Nov;25(11):3586-92.

[126] Rovin BH, Furie R, Latinis K, Looney RJ, Fervenza FC, Sanchez-Guerrero J, et al; LUNAR Investigator Group. Efficacy and safety of rituximab in patients with active proliferative lupus nephritis: the Lupus Nephritis Assessment with Rituximab study. *Arthritis Rheum.* 2012 Apr;64(4):1215-26.

[127] Rezvani AR, Maloney DG. Rituximab resistance. *Best Pract. Res. Clin. Haematol.* 2011 Jun;24(2):203-16.

[128] Genovese MC, Kaine JL, Lowenstein MB, Del Giudice J, Baldassare A, Schechtman J, et al; ACTION Study Group. Ocrelizumab, a humanized anti-CD20 monoclonal antibody, in the treatment of patients with rheumatoid arthritis: a phase I/II randomized, blinded, placebo-controlled, dose-ranging study. Arthritis Rheum. 2008 Sep;58(9):2652-61.

[129] Dörner T, Kaufmann J, Wegener WA, Teoh N, Goldenberg DM, Burmester GR. Initial clinical trial of epratuzumab (humanized anti-CD22 antibody) for immunotherapy of systemic lupus erythematosus. *Arthritis. Res. Ther.* 2006;8(3):R74.

[130] Jacobi AM, Goldenberg DM, Hiepe F, Radbruch A, Burmester GR, Dörner T. Differential effects of epratuzumab on peripheral blood B cells of patients with systemic lupus erythematosus versus normal controls. *Ann. Rheum. Dis*. 2008 Apr;67(4):450-7.

[131] Lateef A, Petri M. Biologics in the treatment of systemic lupus erythematosus. *Curr. Opin. Rheumatol*. 2010 Sep;22(5):504-9.

[132] Dooley MA, Houssiau F, Aranow C, D'Cruz DP, Askanase A, Roth DA, et al; BLISS-52 and -76 Study Groups. Effect of belimumab treatment on renal outcomes: results from the phase 3 belimumab clinical trials in patients with SLE. *Lupus*. 2013 Jan;22(1):63-72.

[133] Furie R, Nicholls K, Cheng TT, Houssiau F, Burgos-Vargas R, Chen SL, et al. Efficacy and safety of abatacept in lupus nephritis: a twelve-month, randomized, double-blind study. *Arthritis. Rheumatol*. 2014 Feb;66(2):379-89.

[134] European Association For The Study Of The Liver. EASL Clinical Practice Guidelines: management of chronic hepatitis *B. J Hepatol*. 2009 Feb;50(2):227-42.

[135] Abbas NA, Pitt MA, Green AT, Solomon LR. Successful treatment of hepatitis B virus (HBV)-associated membranoproliferative glomerulonephritis (MPGN) with alpha interferon. *Nephrol. Dial. Transplant*. 1999 May;14(5):1272-5.

[136] Zhang L, Meng H, Han X, Han C, Sun C, Ye F, et al. The relationship between HBV serum markers and the clinicopathological characteristics of hepatitis B virus-associated glomerulonephritis (HBV-GN) in the northeastern Chinese population. *Virol. J*. 2012 Sep 14;9:200.

[137] Lai KN, Lai FM, Tam JS, Chow CB, Au TC. High prevalence of hepatitis B surface antigenaemia in nephrotic syndrome in Hong Kong. *Ann. Trop. Paediatr*. 1989 Mar;9(1):45-8.

[138] Khedmat H, Taheri S. Hepatitis B virus-associated nephropathy: an International Data Analysis. Iran J Kidney Dis. 2010 Apr;4(2):101-5.

[139] Safadi R, Almog Y, Dranitzki-Elhalel M, Rosenmann E, Tur-Kaspa R. Glomerulonephritis associated with acute hepatitis B. *Am. J. Gastroenterol*. 1996 Jan;91(1):138-9.

[140] Lai KN, Lai FM, Lo S, Ho CP, Chan KW. IgA nephropathy associated with hepatitis B virus antigenemia. *Nephron*. 1987;47(2):141-3.

[141] Du W, Zheng Z, Han S, Ma S, Chen S. HBV reactivation in an occult HBV infection patient treated with prednisone for nephrotic syndrome: case report and literature review. *BMC Infect. Dis*. 2013 Aug 27;13:394.

[142] Bhimma R, Coovadia HM. Hepatitis B virus-associated nephropathy. *Am. J. Nephrol*. 2004 Mar-Apr;24(2):198-211.

[143] Liu XR, Shen Y, Yang YH. Membranous Glomerulonephropathy Associated with Hepatitis B Virus Infection *HK J Paediatr* (New Series) 2008;13:23-29 [Abstract in Chinese]

[144] Alavian SM, Fallahian F, Lankarani KB. The changing epidemiology of viral hepatitis B in Iran. *J. Gastrointestin. Liver. Dis*. 2007 Dec;16(4):403-6.

[145] André F. Hepatitis B epidemiology in Asia, the Middle East, and Africa. *Vaccine*. 2000 Feb 18;18 Suppl 1:S20-2.

[146] Levy M, Gagnadoux MF. Membranous nephropathy following perinatal transmission of hepatitis B virus infection-long-term follow-up study. *Pediatr. Nephrol.* 1996 Feb;10(1):76-8.

[147] Southwest Pediatric Nephrology Study Group. Hepatitis B surface antigenemia in North American children with membranous glomerulonephropathy. *J. Pediatr.* 1985 Apr;106(4):571-8. [No authors listed]

[148] McMahon BJ, Alberts SR, Wainwright RB, Bulkow L, Lanier AP. Hepatitis B-related sequelae. Prospective study in 1400 hepatitis B surface antigen-positive Alaska native carriers. *Arch. Intern. Med.* 1990 May;150(5):1051-4.

[149] Elewa U, Sandri AM, Kim WR, Fervenza FC. Treatment of hepatitis B virus-associated nephropathy. *Nephron. Clin. Pract.* 2011;119(1):c41-9; discussion c49.

[150] Wang NS, Wu ZL, Zhang YE, Guo MY, Liao LT. Role of hepatitis B virus infection in pathogenesis of IgA nephropathy. *World J Gastroenterol.* 2003 Sep;9(9):2004-8.

[151] Lai KN, Lai FM, Tam JS. IgA nephropathy associated with chronic hepatitis B virus infection in adults: the pathogenetic role of HBsAG. *J. Pathol.* 1989 Apr;157(4):321-7.

[152] Lai KN, Lai FM, Lo ST, Lam CW. IgA nephropathy and membranous nephropathy associated with hepatitis B surface antigenemia. *Hum. Pathol.* 1987 Apr;18(4):411-4.

[153] Lai KN, Lai FM, Tam JS, Vallance-Owen J. Strong association between IgA nephropathy and hepatitis B surface antigenemia in endemic areas. *Clin. Nephrol.* 1988 May;29(5):229-34.

[154] Zhou FD, Zhao MH, Zou WZ, Liu G, Wang H. The changing spectrum of primary glomerular diseases within 15 years: a survey of 3331 patients in a single Chinese centre. *Nephrol. Dial. Transplant.* 2009 Mar;24(3):870-6.

[155] Lai KN, Li PK, Lui SF, Au TC, Tam JS, Tong KL, et al. Membranous nephropathy related to hepatitis B virus in adults. *N. Engl. J. Med.* 1991 May 23;324(21):1457-63.

[156] Kowdley KV. The cost of managing chronic hepatitis B infection: a global perspective. *J Clin Gastroenterol.* 2004 Nov-Dec;38(10 Suppl 3):S132-3.

[157] Gregorek H, Jung H, Ułanowicz G, Madaliński K. Immune complexes in sera of children with HBV-mediated glomerulonephritis. *Arch. Immunol. Ther. Exp.* (Warsz). 1986;34(1):73-83.

[158] Johnson RJ, Couser WG. Hepatitis B infection and renal disease: clinical, immunopathogenetic and therapeutic considerations. *Kidney Int.* 1990 Feb;37(2):663-76.

[159] Ohba S, Kimura K, Mise N, Konno Y, Suzuki N, Miyashita K, et al. Differential localization of s and e antigens in hepatitis B virus-associated glomerulonephritis. *Clin. Nephrol.* 1997 Jul;48(1):44-7.

[160] Takekoshi Y, Tanaka M, Shida N, Satake Y, Saheki Y, Matsumoto S. Strong association between membranous nephropathy and hepatitis-B surface antigenaemia in Japanese children. *Lancet.* 1978 Nov 18;2(8099):1065-8.

[161] He XY, Fang LJ, Zhang YE, Sheng FY, Zhang XR, Guo MY. In situ hybridization of hepatitis B DNA in hepatitis B-associated glomerulonephritis. *Pediatr. Nephrol.* 1998 Feb;12(2):117-20.

[162] Zhou S, Zhang Y, Fang L. A study on the appearance of hepatitis B virus markers in renal tissue of glomerulonephritis. *Zhonghua Bing Li Xue Za Zhi.* 1995 Oct;24(5):296-9. [Article in Chinese]

[163] Lin CY. Hepatitis B virus deoxyribonucleic acid in kidney cells probably leading to viral pathogenesis among hepatitis B virus associated membranous nephropathy patients. *Nephron.* 1993;63(1):58-64.

[164] Lai KN, Ho RT, Tam JS, Lai FM. Detection of hepatitis B virus DNA and RNA in kidneys of HBV related glomerulonephritis. *Kidney Int.* 1996 Dec;50(6):1965-77.

[165] Hornung V, Ablasser A, Charrel-Dennis M, Bauernfeind F, Horvath G, Caffrey DR, et al. AIM2 recognizes cytosolic dsDNA and forms a caspase-1-activating inflammasome with ASC. *Nature.* 2009 Mar 26;458(7237):514-8.

[166] Du W, Zhen J, Zheng Z, Ma S, Chen S. Expression of AIM2 is high and correlated with inflammation in hepatitis B virus associated glomerulonephritis. *J. Inflamm* (Lond). 2013 Dec 10;10(1):37.

[167] Zhen J, Zhang L, Pan J, Ma S, Yu X, Li X, et al. AIM2 mediates inflammation-associated renal damage in hepatitis B virus-associated glomerulonephritis by regulating caspase-1, IL-1β, and IL-18. *Mediators Inflamm.* 2014;2014:190860.

[168] Bürckstümmer T, Baumann C, Blüml S, Dixit E, Dürnberger G, Jahn H, et al. An orthogonal proteomic-genomic screen identifies AIM2 as a cytoplasmic DNA sensor for the inflammasome. *Nat. Immunol.* 2009 Mar;10(3):266-72.

[169] Roberts TL, Idris A, Dunn JA, Kelly GM, Burnton CM, Hodgson S, et al. HIN-200 proteins regulate caspase activation in response to foreign cytoplasmic DNA. *Science.* 2009 Feb 20;323(5917):1057-60.

[170] Bhimma R, Coovadia M, Hammond MG, Kramvis A, Adhikari M, Kew MC. HLA associations with HBV carriage and proteinuria. *Pediatr. Nephrol.* 2002 Sep;17(9): 724-9.

[171] Vaughan RW, Zurowska A, Moszkowska G, Kondeatis E, Clark AG. HLA-DRB and -DQB1 alleles in Polish patients with hepatitis B associated membranous nephropathy. *Tissue Antigens.* 1998 Aug;52(2):130-4.

[172] Lai KN, Tam JS, Lin HJ, Lai FM. The therapeutic dilemma of the usage of corticosteroid in patients with membranous nephropathy and persistent hepatitis B virus surface antigenaemia. Nephron. 1990;54(1):12-7.

[173] Lin CY, Lo SC. Treatment of hepatitis B virus-associated membranous nephropathy with adenine arabinoside and thymic extract. *Kidney Int.* 1991 Feb;39(2):301-6.

[174] de Man RA, Schalm SW, van der Heijden AJ, ten Kate FW, Wolff ED, Heijtink RA. Improvement of hepatitis B-associated glomerulonephritis after antiviral combination therapy. *J. Hepatol.* 1989 May;8(3):367-72.

[175] Dhingra S, Kanitkar M, Sengupta P. Steroid resistant nephrotic syndrome in a child with chronic hepatitis B infection. *Med. J. Armed. Forces India.* 2012 Oct;68(4):376-8.

[176] Chung DR, Yang WS, Kim SB, Yu E, Chung YH, Lee Y, et al. Treatment of hepatitis B virus associated glomerulonephritis with recombinant human alpha interferon. *Am. J. Nephrol.* 1997;17(2):112-7.

[177] Zhang Y, Zhou JH, Yin XL, Wang FY. Treatment of hepatitis B virus-associated glomerulonephritis: a meta-analysis. *World J. Gastroenterol.* 2010 Feb 14;16(6):770-7.

[178] Fabrizi F, Dixit V, Martin P. Meta-analysis: anti-viral therapy of hepatitis B virus-associated glomerulonephritis. *Aliment. Pharmacol. Ther.* 2006 Sep 1;24(5):781-8.

[179] Haria M, Benfield P. Interferon-alpha-2a. A review of its pharmacological properties and therapeutic use in the management of viral hepatitis. *Drugs.* 1995 Nov;50(5): 873-96.

[180] Wong DK, Cheung AM, O'Rourke K, Naylor CD, Detsky AS, Heathcote J. Effect of alpha-interferon treatment in patients with hepatitis B e antigen-positive chronic hepatitis B. A meta-analysis. *Ann. Intern. Med.* 1993 Aug 15;119(4):312-23.

[181] Di Bisceglie AM. Long-term outcome of interferon-alpha therapy for chronic hepatitis B. *J Hepatol.* 1995;22(1 Suppl):65-7.

[182] Dhiman RK, Kohli HS, Das G, Joshi K, Chawla Y, Sakhuja V. Remission of HBV-related mesangioproliferative glomerulonephritis after interferon therapy. *Nephrol. Dial. Transplant.* 1999 Jan;14(1):176-8.

[183] Mesquita M, Lasser L, Langlet P. Long-term (7-year-) treatment with lamivudine monotherapy in HBV-associated glomerulonephritis. *Clin. Nephrol.* 2008 Jul;70(1): 69-71.

[184] Yi Z, Jie YW, Nan Z. The efficacy of anti-viral therapy on hepatitis B virus-associated glomerulonephritis: A systematic review and meta-analysis. *Ann. Hepatol.* 2011 Apr-Jun;10(2):165-73.

[185] Lopes Neto EP, Lopes LV, Kirsztajn GM, Cruz CN, Ferraz ML, Silva AE. alpha-Interferon therapy for HBV-related glomerulonephritis. *Sao Paulo Med. J.* 1998 Sep-Oct;116(5):1823-5.

[186] Lin CY. Treatment of hepatitis B virus-associated membranous nephropathy with recombinant alpha-interferon. *Kidney Int.* 1995 Jan;47(1):225-30.

[187] Khaira A, Upadhyay BK, Sharma A, Das P, Mahajan S, Makhariya G, et al. Hepatitis B virus associated focal and segmental glomerular sclerosis: report of two cases and review of literature. *Clin. Exp. Nephrol.* 2009 Aug;13(4):373-7.

[188] Chayama K, Suzuki Y, Kobayashi M, Kobayashi M, Tsubota A, Hashimoto M, et al. Emergence and takeover of YMDD motif mutant hepatitis B virus during long-term lamivudine therapy and re-takeover by wild type after cessation of therapy. *Hepatology.* 1998 Jun;27(6):1711-6.

[189] Lai MY, Yang WC, Lee SD, Ng YY. Long-term lamivudine therapy is not reasonable for HBV-associated nephropathy. *Nephrol. Dial Transplant.* 2006 Jun;21(6):1740-1.

[190] Ntziora F, Paraskevis D, Haida C, Magiorkinis E, Manesis E, Papatheodoridis G, et al. Quantitative detection of the M204V hepatitis B virus minor variants by amplification refractory mutation system real-time PCR combined with molecular beacon technology. *J Clin Microbiol.* 2009 Aug;47(8):2544-50.

[191] Shin SK, Ryu DR, Hwang JH, Song HY, Noh HJ, Kang SW, et al. Comparison between Lamivudine alone and Lamivudine and Steroid Combination in Treatment of Nephrotic Syndrome Associated with Hepatitis B. *Korean J. Nephrol.* 1999 Jul;18(4):550-559. Korean.

[192] Sun IO, Hong YA, Park HS, Choi SR, Chung BH, Park CW, et al. Experience of anti-viral therapy in hepatitis B-associated membranous nephropathy, including Lamivudine-resistant strains. *Korean J. Intern. Med.* 2012 Dec;27(4):411-6.

[193] Lok AS, McMahon BJ. Chronic hepatitis B. Hepatology. 2007 Feb;45(2):507-39.

[194] Du QW, Ding JG, Sun QF, Hong L, Cai FJ, Zhou QQ, et al. Combination lamivudine and adefovir versus entecavir for the treatment of naïve chronic hepatitis B patients: a pilot study. *Med. Sci. Monit.* 2013 Sep 9;19:751-6.

[195] Yuen MF, Lai CL. Adefovir dipivoxil in chronic hepatitis B infection. *Expert Opin Pharmacother.* 2004 Nov;5(11):2361-7.

[196] Marcellin P, Chang TT, Lim SG, Tong MJ, Sievert W, Shiffman ML, et al; Adefovir Dipivoxil 437 Study Group. Adefovir dipivoxil for the treatment of hepatitis B e antigen-positive chronic hepatitis B. *N. Engl. J. Med*. 2003 Feb 27;348(9):808-16.

[197] Schildgen O, Olotu C, Funk A, Zöllner B, Helm M, Rockstroh JK, et al. Selection and counterselection of the rtI233V adefovir resistance mutation during antiviral therapy. *J. Clin. Microbiol*. 2010 Feb;48(2):631-4.

[198] Ikee R, Ishioka K, Oka M, Maesato K, Moriya H, Hidaka S, et al. Hepatitis B virus-related membranous nephropathy treated with entecavir. *Nephrology* (Carlton). 2010 Mar;15(2):266.

[199] Tenney DJ, Rose RE, Baldick CJ, Pokornowski KA, Eggers BJ, Fang J, et al. Long-term monitoring shows hepatitis B virus resistance to entecavir in nucleoside-naïve patients is rare through 5 years of therapy. *Hepatology*. 2009 May;49(5):1503-14.

[200] Chang TT, Gish RG, de Man R, Gadano A, Sollano J, Chao YC, et al; BEHoLD AI463022 Study Group. A comparison of entecavir and lamivudine for HBeAg-positive chronic hepatitis B. *N. Engl. J. Med.* 2006 Mar 9;354(10):1001-10.

[201] Pawłowska M, Halota W, Smukalska E, Woźniakowska-Gęsicka T, Kupś J. HBV DNA suppression during entecavir treatment in previously treated children with chronic hepatitis B. *Eur. J. Clin. Microbiol Infect. Dis*. 2012 Apr;31(4):571-4.

[202] Sorrell MF, Belongia EA, Costa J, Gareen IF, Grem JL, Inadomi JM, et al. National Institutes of Health Consensus Development Conference Statement: management of hepatitis B. *Ann. Intern. Med.* 2009 Jan 20;150(2):104-10.

[203] Cacoub P, Renou C, Rosenthal E, Cohen P, Loury I, Loustaud-Ratti V, et al. Extrahepatic manifestations associated with hepatitis C virus infection. A prospective multicenter study of 321 patients. The GERMIVIC. Groupe d'Etude et de Recherche en Medecine Interne et Maladies Infectieuses sur le Virus de l'Hepatite C. Medicine (Baltimore). 2000 Jan;79(1):47-56.

[204] Lauer GM, Walker BD. Hepatitis C virus infection. *N. Engl. J. Med*. 2001 Jul 5;345(1):41-52.

[205] Latt N, Alachkar N, Gurakar A. Hepatitis C virus, and its renal manifestations: a review and update. *Gastroenterol. Hepatol* (N Y). 2012 Jul;8(7):434-45.

[206] Armstrong GL, Wasley A, Simard EP, McQuillan GM, Kuhnert WL, Alter MJ. The prevalence of hepatitis C virus infection in the United States, 1999 through 2002. *Ann. Intern. Med.* 2006 May 16;144(10):705-14.

[207] Galossi A, Guarisco R, Bellis L, Puoti C. Extrahepatic manifestations of chronic HCV infection. *J Gastrointestin Liver Dis*. 2007 Mar;16(1):65-73.

[208] Kasuno K, Ono T, Matsumori A, Nogaki F, Kusano H, Watanabe H, et al. Hepatitis C virus-associated tubulointerstitial injury. *Am. J. Kidney Dis*. 2003 Apr;41(4):767-75.

[209] Dammacco F, Lauletta G, Montrone M, Sansonno D. Mixed cryoglobulinemia: a model of virus-related disease in internal medicine. *Dig. Liver. Dis*. 2007 Sep;39 Suppl 1:S8-S12.

[210] Stehman-Breen C, Alpers CE, Fleet WP, Johnson RJ. Focal segmental glomerular sclerosis among patients infected with hepatitis C virus. *Nephron*. 1999 Jan;81(1): 37-40.

[211] Markowitz GS, Cheng JT, Colvin RB, Trebbin WM, D'Agati VD. Hepatitis C viral infection is associated with fibrillary glomerulonephritis and immunotactoid glomerulopathy. *J. Am. Soc. Nephrol*. 1998 Dec;9(12):2244-52.

[212] Baid S, Pascual M, Williams WW Jr, Tolkoff-Rubin N, Johnson SM, Collins B, et al. Renal thrombotic microangiopathy associated with anticardiolipin antibodies in hepatitis C-positive renal allograft recipients. *J. Am. Soc. Nephrol.* 1999 Jan;10(1): 146-53.

[213] Tsui JI, Vittinghoff E, Shlipak MG, Bertenthal D, Inadomi J, Rodriguez RA, et al. Association of hepatitis C seropositivity with increased risk for developing end-stage renal disease. *Arch. Intern. Med.* 2007 Jun 25;167(12):1271-6.

[214] Kitamura T, Nakase H, Iizuka H. Henoch-Schönlein purpura after postoperative Staphylococcus aureus infection with hepatic IgA nephropathy. *J. Nephrol.* 2006 Sep-Oct;19(5):687-90.

[215] Perico N, Cattaneo D, Bikbov B, Remuzzi G. Hepatitis C infection and chronic renal diseases. Clin. J. Am. Soc. Nephrol. 2009 Jan;4(1):207-20.

[216] Ozkok A, Yildiz A. Hepatitis C virus associated glomerulopathies. *World J. Gastroenterol.* 2014 Jun 28;20(24):7544-7554.

[217] Brouet JC, Clauvel JP, Danon F, Klein M, Seligmann M. Biologic and clinical significance of cryoglobulins. A report of 86 cases. *Am. J. Med.* 1974 Nov;57(5): 775-88.

[218] Trejo O, Ramos-Casals M, García-Carrasco M, Yagüe J, Jiménez S, de la Red G, Cervera R, et al. Cryoglobulinemia: study of etiologic factors and clinical and immunologic features in 443 patients from a single center. *Medicine* (Baltimore). 2001 Jul;80(4):252-62.

[219] Ferri C, Greco F, Longombardo G, Palla P, Moretti A, Marzo E, et al. Association between hepatitis C virus and mixed cryoglobulinemia [see comment*]. Clin. Exp. Rheumatol.* 1991 Nov-Dec;9(6):621-4.

[220] Sene D, Ghillani-Dalbin P, Thibault V, Guis L, Musset L, Duhaut P, et al. Longterm course of mixed cryoglobulinemia in patients infected with hepatitis C virus. *J. Rheumatol.* 2004 Nov;31(11):2199-206.

[221] Rosa D, Saletti G, De Gregorio E, Zorat F, Comar C, D'Oro U, et al. Activation of naïve B lymphocytes via CD81, a pathogenetic mechanism for hepatitis C virus-associated B lymphocyte disorders. *Proc. Natl. Acad. Sci. U S A.* 2005 Dec 20;102(51):18544-9.

[222] Charles ED, Dustin LB. Hepatitis C virus-induced cryoglobulinemia. *Kidney Int.* 2009 Oct;76(8):818-24.

[223] Choo QL, Kuo G, Weiner AJ, Overby LR, Bradley DW, Houghton M. Isolation of a cDNA clone derived from a blood-borne non-A, non-B viral hepatitis genome. *Science.* 1989 Apr 21;244(4902):359-62.

[224] Gordon CE, Uhlig K, Lau J, Schmid CH, Levey AS, Wong JB. Interferon treatment in hemodialysis patients with chronic hepatitis C virus infection: a systematic review of the literature and meta-analysis of treatment efficacy and harms. *Am. J. Kidney Dis.* 2008 Feb;51(2):263-77.

[225] Fabrizi F, Takkouche B, Lunghi G, Dixit V, Messa P, Martin P. The impact of hepatitis C virus infection on survival in dialysis patients: meta-analysis of observational studies. *J. Viral. Hepat.* 2007 Oct;14(10):697-703.

[226] Fornasieri A, Li M, Armelloni S, de Septis CP, Schiaffino E, Sinico RA, et al. Glomerulonephritis induced by human IgMK-IgG cryoglobulins in mice. *Lab. Invest.* 1993 Nov;69(5):531-40.

[227] Barsoum RS. Hepatitis C virus: from entry to renal injury-facts and potentials. *Nephrol. Dial Transplant.* 2007 Jul;22(7):1840-8.

[228] Dolganiuc A, Oak S, Kodys K, Golenbock DT, Finberg RW, Kurt-Jones E, et al. Hepatitis C core and nonstructural 3 proteins trigger toll-like receptor 2-mediated pathways and inflammatory activation. *Gastroenterology.* 2004 Nov;127(5):1513-24.

[229] Wörnle M, Schmid H, Banas B, Merkle M, Henger A, Roeder M, et al. Novel role of toll-like receptor 3 in hepatitis C-associated glomerulonephritis. *Am. J. Pathol.* 2006 Feb;168(2):370-85.

[230] Merkle M, Ribeiro A, Wörnle M. TLR3-dependent regulation of cytokines in human mesangial cells: a novel role for IP-10 and TNF-alpha in hepatitis C-associated glomerulonephritis. *Am. J. Physiol. Renal. Physiol.* 2011 Jul;301(1):F57-69.

[231] Alpers CE, Kowalewska J. Emerging paradigms in the renal pathology of viral diseases. *Clin. J. Am. Soc. Nephrol.* 2007 Jul;2 Suppl 1:S6-12.

[232] Iskandar SS, Herrera GA. Glomerulopathies with organized deposits. *Semin. Diagn. Pathol.* 2002 Aug;19(3):116-32.

[233] Szymanski IO, Pullman JM, Underwood JM. Electron microscopic and immunochemical studies in a patient with hepatitis C virus infection and mixed cryoglobulinemia type II. *Am. J. Clin. Pathol.* 1994 Sep;102(3):278-83.

[234] Davda R, Peterson J, Weiner R, Croker B, Lau JY. Membranous glomerulonephritis in association with hepatitis C virus infection. *Am J Kidney Dis.* 1993 Sep;22(3):452-5.

[235] Meyers CM, Seeff LB, Stehman-Breen CO, Hoofnagle JH. Hepatitis C and renal disease: an update. *Am. J. Kidney Dis.* 2003 Oct;42(4):631-57.

[236] Tarantino A, Campise M, Banfi G, Confalonieri R, Bucci A, Montoli A, et al. Long-term predictors of survival in essential mixed cryoglobulinemic glomerulonephritis. *Kidney Int.* 1995 Feb;47(2):618-23.

[237] Yamabe H, Johnson RJ, Gretch DR, Fukushi K, Osawa H, Miyata M, et al. Hepatitis C virus infection and membranoproliferative glomerulonephritis in Japan. *J. Am. Soc. Nephrol.* 1995 Aug;6(2):220-3.

[238] Roccatello D, Fornasieri A, Giachino O, Rossi D, Beltrame A, Banfi G, et al. Multicenter study on hepatitis C virus-related cryoglobulinemic glomerulonephritis. *Am J Kidney Dis.* 2007 Jan;49(1):69-82.

[239] Fabrizi F, Lunghi G, Messa P, Martin P. Therapy of hepatitis C virus-associated glomerulonephritis: current approaches. *J Nephrol.* 2008 Nov-Dec;21(6):813-25.

[240] Kidney Disease: Improving Global Outcomes (KDIGO). KDIGO clinical practice guidelines for the prevention, diagnosis, evaluation, and treatment of hepatitis C in chronic kidney disease. *Kidney Int Suppl.* 2008 Apr;(109):S1-99.

[241] Feng B, Eknoyan G, Guo ZS, Jadoul M, Rao HY, Zhang W, et al. Effect of interferon-alpha-based antiviral therapy on hepatitis C virus-associated glomerulonephritis: a meta-analysis. *Nephrol Dial Transplant.* 2012 Feb;27(2):640-6.

[242] Sabry AA, Sobh MA, Irving WL, Grabowska A, Wagner BE, Fox S, et al. A comprehensive study of the association between hepatitis C virus and glomerulopathy. *Nephrol Dial Transplant.* 2002 Feb;17(2):239-45.

[243] Abbas G, Hussain S, Shafi T. Effect of antiviral therapy on hepatitis C virus related glomerulopathy. *Saudi J. Kidney Dis. Transpl.* 2008 Sep;19(5):775-80.

[244] Suzuki T, Yonemura K, Miyaji T, Suzuki H, Takahira R, Fujigaki Y, et al. Progressive renal failure and blindness due to retinal hemorrhage after interferon therapy for

hepatitis C virus-associated membranoproliferative glomerulonephritis. *Intern. Med.* 2001 Aug;40(8):708-12.

[245] Boonyapisit K, Katirji B. Severe exacerbation of hepatitis C-associated vasculitic neuropathy following treatment with interferon alpha: a case report and literature review. *Muscle Nerve.* 2002 Jun;25(6):909-13.

[246] Fabrizi F, Bruchfeld A, Mangano S, Dixit V, Messa P, Martin P. Interferon therapy for HCV-associated glomerulonephritis: meta-analysis of controlled trials. *Int. J. Artif. Organs.* 2007 Mar;30(3):212-9.

[247] Garini G, Allegri L, Lannuzzella F, Vaglio A, Buzio C. HCV-related cryoglobulinemic glomerulonephritis: implications of antiviral and immunosuppressive therapies. *Acta. Biomed.* 2007;78(1):51-9.

[248] Alric L, Plaisier E, Thébault S, Péron JM, Rostaing L, Pourrat J, et al. Influence of antiviral therapy in hepatitis C virus-associated cryoglobulinemic MPGN. *Am. J. Kidney Dis.* 2004 Apr;43(4):617-23.

[249] Saadoun D, Resche-Rigon M, Thibault V, Piette JC, Cacoub P. Antiviral therapy for hepatitis C virus--associated mixed cryoglobulinemia vasculitis: a long-term followup study. *Arthritis. Rheum.* 2006 Nov;54(11):3696-706.

[250] Bruchfeld A, Lindahl K, Ståhle L, Söderberg M, Schvarcz R. Interferon and ribavirin treatment in patients with hepatitis C-associated renal disease and renal insufficiency. *Nephrol. Dial Transplant.* 2003 Aug;18(8):1573-80.

[251] Ghany MG, Nelson DR, Strader DB, Thomas DL, Seeff LB; American Association for Study of Liver Diseases. An update on treatment of genotype 1 chronic hepatitis C virus infection: 2011 practice guideline by the American Association for the Study of Liver Diseases. *Hepatology.* 2011 Oct;54(4):1433-44.

[252] Saadoun D, Resche Rigon M, Thibault V, Longuet M, Pol S, Blanc F, et al. Peg-IFNα/ribavirin/protease inhibitor combination in hepatitis C virus associated mixed cryoglobulinemia vasculitis: results at week 24. *Ann. Rheum Dis.* 2014 May;73(5): 831-7.

[253] Mauss S, Hueppe D, Alshuth U. Renal impairment is frequent in chronic hepatitis C patients under triple therapy with telaprevir or boceprevir. *Hepatology.* 2014 Jan;59(1):46-8.

[254] Dammacco F, Sansonno D. Therapy for hepatitis C virus-related cryoglobulinemic vasculitis. *N. Engl. J. Med.* 2013 Sep 12;369(11):1035-45.

[255] D'Amico G. Renal involvement in hepatitis C infection: cryoglobulinemic glomerulonephritis. *Kidney Int.* 1998 Aug;54(2):650-71.

[256] Vassilopoulos D, Calabrese LH. Hepatitis C virus infection and vasculitis: implications of antiviral and immunosuppressive therapies. *Arthritis Rheum.* 2002 Mar;46(3): 585-97.

[257] Johnson RJ, Gretch DR, Yamabe H, Hart J, Bacchi CE, Hartwell P, et al. Membranoproliferative glomerulonephritis associated with hepatitis C virus infection. *N. Engl. J. Med.* 1993 Feb 18;328(7):465-70.

[258] Fong TL, Valinluck B, Govindarajan S, Charboneau F, Adkins RH, Redeker AG. Short-term prednisone therapy affects aminotransferase activity and hepatitis C virus RNA levels in chronic hepatitis C. *Gastroenterology.* 1994 Jul;107(1):196-9.

[259] Reed MJ, Alexander GJ, Thiru S, Smith KG. Hepatitis C-associated glomerulonephritis-a novel therapeutic approach. *Nephrol Dial Transplant.* 2001 Apr;16(4):869-71.

[260] Quartuccio L, Soardo G, Romano G, Zaja F, Scott CA, De Marchi G, et al. Rituximab treatment for glomerulonephritis in HCV-associated mixed cryoglobulinaemia: efficacy and safety in the absence of steroids. *Rheumatology* (Oxford). 2006 Jul;45(7):842-6.

[261] Roccatello D, Baldovino S, Rossi D, Mansouri M, Naretto C, Gennaro M, et al. Long-term effects of anti-CD20 monoclonal antibody treatment of cryoglobulinaemic glomerulonephritis. *Nephrol Dial Transplant.* 2004 Dec;19(12):3054-61.

[262] Sansonno D, De Re V, Lauletta G, Tucci FA, Boiocchi M, Dammacco F. Monoclonal antibody treatment of mixed cryoglobulinemia resistant to interferon alpha with an anti-CD20. *Blood.* 2003 May 15;101(10):3818-26.

[263] Saadoun D, Resche-Rigon M, Sene D, Perard L, Karras A, Cacoub P. Rituximab combined with Peg-interferon-ribavirin in refractory hepatitis C virus-associated cryoglobulinaemia vasculitis. *Ann. Rheum. Dis.* 2008 Oct;67(10):1431-6.

[264] Basse G, Ribes D, Kamar N, Mehrenberger M, Sallusto F, Esposito L, et al. Rituximab therapy for mixed cryoglobulinemia in seven renal transplant patients. *Transplant Proc.* 2006 Sep;38(7):2308-10.

[265] Sène D, Ghillani-Dalbin P, Amoura Z, Musset L, Cacoub P. Rituximab may form a complex with IgMkappa mixed cryoglobulin and induce severe systemic reactions in patients with hepatitis C virus-induced vasculitis. *Arthritis. Rheum.* 2009 Dec;60(12):3848-55.

[266] Koziolek MJ, Scheel A, Bramlage C, Groene HJ, Mueller GA, Strutz F. Effective treatment of hepatitis C-associated immune-complex nephritis with cryoprecipitate apheresis and antiviral therapy. *Clin. Nephrol.* 2007 Apr;67(4):245-9.

[267] Hausfater P, Cacoub P, Assogba U, Lebon P, Piette JC. Plasma exchange and interferon-alpha pharmacokinetics in patients with hepatitis C virus-associated systemic vasculitis. *Nephron.* 2002 Aug;91(4):627-30.

[268] Fujiwara K, Kaneko S, Kakumu S, Sata M, Hige S, Tomita E, et al; Virus Reduction Therapy Study Group. Double filtration plasmapheresis and interferon combination therapy for chronic hepatitis C patients with genotype 1 and high viral load. *Hepatol Res.* 2007 Sep;37(9):701-10.

[269] Namba T, Shiba R, Yamamoto T, Hirai Y, Moriwaki T, Matsuda J, et al. Successful treatment of HCV-related cryoglobulinemic glomerulonephritis with double-filtration plasmapheresis and interferon combination therapy. *Clin. Exp. Nephrol.* 2010 Aug;14(4):372-6.

Section D.
Inherited Glomerular Diseases

Chapter VI

Inherited Glomerular Diseases

Abstract

Fabry's disease is a rare X-linked systemic inherited disease characterized by accumulation of glycosphingolipids in the lysosomes. Approximately 50% of Fabry's patients present renal involvement with non-proliferative mesangial, epithelial and endothelial lesions. Fabry's disease may present a "heart variant" manifesting with left ventricular hypertrophy arrhythmias, coronary artery disease, myocardial infarction and aortic root dilatation, and a "kidney variant", manifesting with proteinuria, and progressive renal failure leading to ESRD.

In Alport's syndrome, also an inherited disorder caused by mutations of type IV collagen genes, renal involvement consists of non-proliferative lesions of the glomerular basement membrane (GBM) due to deposition of type IV collagen α chains. In this chapter, pathogenesis, pathology, clinical manifestations and treatment of these diseases will be discussed.

1. Fabry's Disease

Fabry's disease is a rare X-linked hereditary disorder of the catabolism of glycosphingolipids caused by mutations in the gene (GLA gene) encoding the lysosomal enzyme α-galactosidase A (α-GAL A), leading to deficiency or impaired function of the enzyme.

α-GAL A normally degradates sphyngolipids, predominantly globotriaosylceramide (Gb3 or GL3). Deficiency or defective function of this enzyme leads to reduced degradation and subsequent accumulation of Gb3 in lysosomes of a wide range of cells and increases circulating levels of globotriaosylsphingosine (Lyso-Gb3). [1]

According to the Human Gene Mutation Database, there are 655 mutations of GLA and more than 400 of them have been associated to Fabry's disease. [1] Affected patients present mainly missense mutations but nonsense and spicing mutations with deletions and insertions are observed. [2] Partial gene duplication associated with Fabry's disease has also been reported. [3]

Vascular endothelial, renal, cardiac, and neural cells are the cells mainly affected, but any type of cells in the human body is a potential target.

Given that Fabry's disease is an X-linked disorder, hemizygote males are more frequently affected, presenting earlier onset of the disease and a more severe clinical picture. In the past, women were considered as carriers of recessively transmitted mutation of Fabry's disease. Clinical manifestations on women were considered a result of random inactivation of the X chromosomes (lyonization). [4] Others suggested that women might present less severe mutations that cause partial enzymatic deficits resulting in a non-classical phenotype of the disease. [5-7]

The classical form of Fabry's disease is characterized by severe deficit of the enzymatic activity, with less than 1% of α-GAL A being operative. Initial signs may appear in childhood or adolescence, [8] including anhidrosis or hypohidrosis, acroparaesthesia, muscle pain, diarrhea, abdominal pain, angiokeratomas and recurrent fever but with absence of major organ involvement. [9]

Multisystemic involvement manifests by the 3rd or 4th decade of life showing high phenotypic variability. [10, 11] Late onset variants of Fabry's disease include the "heart variant", manifesting with left ventricular hypertrophy arrhythmias due to involvement of the conduction system often requiring a pacemaker, coronary artery disease and myocardial infarction and aortic root dilatation, [12, 13] and the "kidney variant", manifesting with proteinuria, and progressive renal failure leading to ESRD. [14-16]

Cerebrovascular involvement rarely presents in young ages as microvascular ischemic brain, [14, 17, 18] but mostly occurs in males in the 4th decade of life, as transient ischemic attacks (TIA) and stroke. [14, 18] Dysarthria, memory loss, ataxia, and hemiparesis may also occur.

The earliest visible skin lesion of Fabry's disease is angiokeratomas typically located on lower trunk, umbilicus, and upper thighs, and rarely on mucosal areas such as mouth. Telangiectasias may also be observed. [19, 20]

Corneal opacities, vessel tortuosity, and cataract are frequently encountered. [21] Sensorineural hearing loss and tinnitus is quite frequent, occurring in both adults and children. [22]

Epidemiology

Incidence of Fabry's disease was estimated to be 1:40,000 to 1:60,000 born males, [23] but the worldwide incidence remains unknown, as there is significant variation of incidence rates among different countries. In the USA, incidence was estimated to range between 1:40,000 to 1:117,000, [23] in Australia 1:833, [23] while in a recent Italian study incidence was estimated at 1:3,100 newborn males. [24]

In Taiwan, Fabry's disease seem to be much more common, as incidence rates were estimated at 1 per every 1,600 newborns, males and females. [25]

Approximately 50% of all Fabry's patients present renal involvement with overt proteinuria and progressive renal failure, reaching to ESRD before 50 years of age. [26]

Pathogenesis of Fabry's Nephropathy

In patients with Fabry's disease, accumulation of glycosphingolipids in the kidney, especially globotriaosylceramide (Gb3), begins in prenatal life, mainly with deposits within the podocytes. [27] Even in patients with normal renal function and absence of proteinuria, deposits in renal tissue could be observed by electron microscopy. [28]

Podocytes, mesangium, glomerular capillary endothelium, tubular epithelium, endothelial, and interstitial cells are all potential sites of Gb3 deposition. [29] Gb3 synthease and Gb3 are strongly expressed in the human kidney, [30, 31] suggesting endogenous production of Gb3, as Gb3 is a normal constituent of cell membranes and the membranes of intracellular organelles, and its expression in cultured human glomerular and tubular epithelial cells was found to be inversely related to α-GAL A expression. [32]

Defective expression of lysosomal α-GAL A, leads to a progressive accumulation of Gb3 in kidney tissue, causing cellular damage and disruption of normal kidney architecture. Vacuolization of podocytes, of parietal epithelial cells of Bowman's capsule, Henles's Loop, and distal tubules, with mesangial expansion, progressive glomerulosclerosis, and interstitial fibrosis are the most characteristic findings of Fabry's nephropathy that can be seen even in early stages of the disease. [28, 29, 33] Although the exact pathogenesis of Fabry's nephropathy is not fully understood, multiple studies agree that podocyte damage plays a key role in the development of proteinuria and progression of the disease. Podocytes present the largest amount of glycolipid accumulation within the glomerulus in Fabry's disease, followed by parietal epithelial mesangial and glomerular epithelial cells. [34] This accumulation is thought to be not only due to increased podocytic Gb3 uptake but also due to endogenous production and accumulation. [35] Also, expression of α-GAL A in podocytes is impaired, supporting the hypothesis of endogenous accumulation. [35]

Accumulation of Gb3 is associated with increase of autophagosomes in Fabry podocytes. [35] Activation of autophagy occurs in different lysosomal storage disorders including sphingolipid accumulation. [36-38] Additionally, in a human podocyte model of Fabry's disease, podocytes showed a decreased activity of mTOR and of the serine/threonine kinase Akt, activation of which is known to decrease autophagy. [39]

Finally, lyso-Gb3, which circulating levels are increased in Fabry's disease, increases the CD74-related apoptosis in human cultured Fabry podocytes. [40]

Podocyte Gb3 inclusions volume and density, and foot processes width increases with the advancing of age and progression of the disease, till loss of podocytes in the urine. Endothelial damage can also contribute to progression of the disease. In addition to the direct damage, it has been demonstrated in cultured endothelial cells, that Gb3 accumulation increases oxidative stress by increasing reactive oxygen species and upregulating expression of cell adhesion molecules. [41] Also, accumulation of Gb3 in the tubular cells has a direct toxic effect, contributing to development of proteinuria and CKD progression. [29, 42]

Pathology of Fabry's Nephropathy

Renal biopsy should be performed in all Fabry patients with proteinuria and/or renal dysfunction in order to evaluate the degree of renal impairment. However, diagnosis of Fabry's disease may be missed in cases that standard light microscopy is performed.

Staining with methylene blue or toluidine blue of semi-thin section of epoxy-embedded tissue designates better histopathologic features of Fabry's nephropathy. [29, 43-45]

On light microscopy, podocytes and tubular epithelial cells present intense vacuolization. Mesangial, endothelial and parietal epithelial cells may also present vacuoles in advanced stages of the disease. Mesangial expansion, glomerular sclerosis (initial focal and segmental and later global) with interstitial fibrosis and tubular atrophy may be seen even in early stages of the disease. Inclusions may also be present in Henle's Loop, distal tubules and rarely in proximal tubules. Sclerosis and collapse of capillaries can also be seen in early stages of the disease along with hyaline or fibrinoid deposits in the media of arterioles.

Immunofluorescence may show deposition of IgM and C3 in mesangial areas.

On electron microscopy, there are several inclusions, mainly in podocytes, but also in cells of distal and proximal tubules and Henle's Loop, as well as in interstitial cells. The inclusions can be rounded, whorled, or present as parallel lamella called "zebra bodies". In advanced stages of the disease, there is fusion of the podocyte with widening of slit diaphragms. Rarely there is also focal duplication of the GBM that can also be observed in light microscopy.

Clinical Manifestations

The earliest clinical manifestations of renal involvement in Fabry's disease are microalbuminuria and signs of tubular dysfunction. Isosthenuria can be seen even in patients with normal GFR reflecting renal tubular damage that leads to urinary concentration defects. Isosthenuria may lead to polyuria, nocturia, and polydipsia. [15]

Proximal tubular dysfunction may also lead to decreased glucose reabsorption with distal tubules dysfunction, defective acidification mechanism, and consecutive formation of alkaline urine reflecting decreased urinary ammonium excretion.

Glycosphingolipid deposition in the cells of collecting ducts interferes with tubular potassium reabsorption, increasing its secretion and causing hypokaliemia. [46, 47] Urinary sediment may present lipid globules with a "Maltese cross" configuration under polarized light microscopy, along with red blood cells, white blood cells, and hyaline casts, reflecting the glycosphingolipids deposition and tubular damage.

Microalbuminuria may be observed in young Fabry's patients, especially males, even younger than 18 years old and in some cases in childhood. [48] Most of Fabry's patients develop proteinuria in the second, but mainly in the third decade of life, and more than 50% of urine protein content is albumin. In 20% of the cases proteinuria is of nephrotic range (>3g/24h) and is usually observed in more advanced stages of the disease, when CKD is already established. [15] A full-blown nephrotic syndrome with nephrotic range proteinuria, hypoalbuminemia, and hyperlipidemia rarely occurs. [26]

Proteinuria is considered as an independent factor for the severity of renal dysfunction and progression of the disease in both treated and untreated Fabry's patients, as well as for the outcome of the enzyme replacement treatment. [49] Therefore, monitoring proteinuria in these patients is of extreme importance.

Hypertension may also be observed in more advanced Fabry's nephropathy and its severity and responsiveness to treatment are associated with serum creatinine levels and eGFR. [15, 50, 51] Hypotension predominates over hypertension in Fabry's patients especially in cases of cardiovascular involvement and autonomic dysfunction. [52]

Diagnosis of Fabry's Nephropathy

Diagnosis of Fabry's disease is confirmed by measurement of α-GAL A enzyme in leukocytes, plasma and dried blood spots (DBS). [4, 11, 53]

Use of leukocytes as sample is usually preferred and it has become a gold standard for diagnosis of Fabry's disease, as use of plasma has been associated with a higher rate of false negative test results. [4, 53] Use of DBS may show similar accuracy to leukocytes, but its use may result cumbersome, given that it requires large volumes of blood, particular storage processing, and analysis in specialized laboratories.

Alternatively to α-GAL A enzyme activity assays, molecular genetic analysis of the GLA gene mutations, also called "pedigree analysis" may also be performed, even for prenatal diagnosis. [2] Renal biopsy confirms renal involvement, and assesses the extent of renal damage and it should be performed even in patients with pre-established diagnosis of Fabry's disease. In undiagnosed patients, diagnosis of Fabry's disease may be missed if standard light microscopy is performed.

Renal biopsy should also be performed in Fabry's patients showing rapid progression of renal disease in order to exclude concomitant renal disease other than Fabry's nephropathy.

Evaluation of renal impairment with periodic 24 hour urine collections for proteinuria with assessment and estimation of GFR as well as plasma creatinine levels during follow up is necessary not only for valuation of the disease progression but also for assessment of response to enzyme replacement treatment (ERT).

Treatment

Until 2001, management of Fabry's nephropathy aimed on relief of symptoms and delay of progression of renal disease, adopting the general measured used for CKD. Since 2001, two recombinant enzymes α-agalsidase produced from human fibroblasts, and β-agalsidase produced from ovary cells of Chinese hamsters able to reduce tissue deposition of GB3, are available. [54, 55]

These enzyme replacement treatments have significantly improved the clinical outcome of Fabry's nephropathy patients by stabilizing renal function, [8, 54, 56, 57] although they don't seem to improve proteinuria and GFR. [54] It has been reported that ERT may reduce microalbuminuria. [58] Both enzymes were found to improve renal structure as they decrease deposition of GB3, reduce progressive decline of renal function and stabilize the degree of proteinuria. [54, 59, 60]

It is not known if α-agalsidase prevails over β-agalsidase, and vice versa, in efficacy and safety. In a clinical comparative study of the two recombinant enzymes, published by Vedder et al, [61] no differences were observed between the two treatments, but RCTs are required to confirm this finding.

Recommended doses are 0.2mg/kg/2 weeks for α-agalsidase and 1mg/kg/2 weeks for β-agalsidase. ERT should be initiated as soon as diagnosis of Fabry's disease is confirmed, in order to prevent the irreversible glomerular and interstitial lesions of GB3 deposition and proteinuria. Guidelines for the assessment and management of Fabry's disease recommend initiation of ERT in patients with proteinuria >300mg/24h and GFR< 80ml/min /1.73m^2. [62] Others suggest that ERT should be administered to all male patients older than 16 years old diagnosed with Fabry's disease independently from the extent of renal involvement and in children and women when symptoms occur. [63]

ESRD patients with Fabry's disease undergoing dialysis should also receive ERT in order to prevent multisystemic involvement. ERT can be administered during hemodialysis sessions, as the enzyme is not lost in the dialysate and enzymatic activity remains unchanged. [64]

Renal transplantation is an effective treatment for patients with Fabry's disease and ESRD, and it should be considered as a first line option. Indeed, in grafted kidneys, typical lesions of Fabry's disease do not occur. [65, 66] However, these patients should continue to receive ERT for the prevention and/or treatment of extrarenal complications of the disease. [65]

Adverse events of ERT are mostly related to the infusion and include fever, rigor, flushing, pruritus, acroparaesthesia, headaches, nausea, and vomiting. Preventative medications are usually efficient in reducing frequency of these events and withdrawal of ERT is rarely required. Most of these effects decrease after some repeat infusions. [67, 68]

An important adverse event that may impair effectiveness of the treatment is the generation of anti-agalsidase antibodies, mainly IgG. It occurs mostly in men with no residual α-agalsidase activity, but rarely in women with residual α-agalsidase activity. [69] IgE may also be detected, in case of β-agalsidase. [70]

α-agalsidase and β-agalsidase seem to have identical immunogenicity. [71] In a comparison of the two recombinant enzymes there were no differences observed in prevalence of neutralizing antibodies. [72] Changing from α-agalsidase το β-agalsidase and vice versa would be futile as there is complete cross-reaction between them. [71]

Chaperon molecules are under investigation as another Fabry's disease therapeutic approach. These molecules can selectively bind to residual α-agalsidase, prolonging its half-life and correctly directing it to the lysosomes. [73, 74] Use of 1-deoxygalactojirimycin hydrochloride seems to increase activity of α-GAL A, and reduce urinary levels of Gb3 in patients with missense mutations. [75] However, knowledge on safety and long-term efficacy of these molecules is limited and to date no licensed chaperon drugs are available. [76]

2. Alport's Syndrome

Alport's syndrome (AS) is a generalized heterogeneous, inherited disorder of the basement membranes caused by mutations of type IV collagen genes COL4A3, COL4A4 and COL4A5, which manifests with hematuria, progressive nephritis with proteinuria, and progressive decline of renal function, sensonrineural deafness and ocular abnormalities.

This syndrome was first described in 1927 by A. Cecil Alport as association of deafness with hereditary familial hemorrhagic nephritis, where male members of a family developed nephritis and deafness, with rapid progression to ESRD and death, while females presented hematuria and deafness and lived longer. [77]

Alport's syndrome is mainly transmitted as an X-linked disorder, accounting for 80-85% of the cases. X-linked AS (XLAS) results from mutations in the COL4A5 gene located in the Xq22.3 of chromosome X, encoding for the α5 chain of type IV collagen [α5(IV)]. More than 300 mutations of COL4A5 have been described, including deletions, nonsense, missense, and splice-site mutations. Males with COL4A5 deletions and nonsense mutation present higher risk of progressing to ESRD before the age of 30 years, while splicing and missense mutation are associated with late-onset of ESRD. [78, 79]

Autosomal recessive transmission of AS (ARAS) accounts for approximately 15% of the cases and is the result of mutations of COL4A3 and COL4A4 located in chromosome 2 and encoding for α3 and α4 chains of type IV collagen [α4(IV)]. These patients present a high risk of developing ESRD before the age of 30, independently from the gender. [80, 81]

Autosomal dominant AS (ADAS) is more rare, corresponding to only 5% of the cases. This form results from heterozygous mutation of COL4A3 and COL4A4, encoding for α3(IV) and α4(IV). Patients with ADAS mostly present asymptomatic hematuria and slow progression of renal disease. [82, 83]

The overall incidence of AS is estimated at 1:50,000 live births. [84] In the USA, incidence ranges between 1:5,000 and 1:10,000 live births. According to USRD 2008, AS accounts for 3% of children and 0.2% of adults with ESRD. [85]

Pathogenesis

Basement membranes are sheet-like structures that support endothelial and epithelial cells and their major constituent is type IV collagen.

Each type IV collagen molecule is formed by 3 α-chains that are organized into a triple helical structure. There are 6 different types of α-chains [α1, α2, α3, α4, α5, α6 (IV)] forming type IV collagen. GBM is mainly formed by α3, α4, α5 chains, while Bowman's capsule expresses α5 and α6 chains. [86, 87] α3(IV), α4(IV), α5(IV) chains create an open network that interacts with laminin, midogen, heparan sulfate proteoglycans, to form and maintain the integrity of mature GBM.

In AS, mutations of the genes encoding for these chains results in incorrect folding or assembly of the triple helical structure, rendering them susceptible to proteolysis. Thus, there is loss of the normal function of the GBM and consecutive renal damage. To compensate for the loss α3, α4, and α5 chains, α1 and α2 chains accumulate in the GBM with resulting formation of thickened areas, alternating thinned areas.

In XLAS, expression of α3, α4 and α5 is completely absent, while in ARAS, α5 and α6 may be expressed in Bowman's capsule and distal tubules, although α3 and α4 are absent. In ADAS, there is complete or partial absence of expression of α3 and α4.

Renal Pathology

In early stages of the disease, light microscopy is unremarkable. As the disease advances, glomerular sclerosis, interstitial fibrosis and presence of interstitial foam cells can be observed. In severe cases, crescents and tubular atrophy may also be seen.

By standard immunofluorescence, IgM and C3 deposits may be observed in the mesangium and along the GBM. Indirect immunofluorescence of type IV collagen α chains in the kidney and in the skin shows absence of α3, α4, and α5 from GBM and Bowman's capsule, which is pathognomonic for Alport's syndrome.

Electron microscopy reveals alternating thinning and thickening of the GBM as well as splitting and lamellation of lamina densa, with irregular electron lucent areas containing electron dense granules of 20 to 90nm diameter. The thickened areas of the GBM may measure up to 1200nm (normal width 350nm) while thinned areas may measure 100nm.

There may also be effacement of the overlying foot processes of variable degrees.

Clinical manifestations

i. Renal Manifestations

Hematuria, microscopic or macroscopic, is the most common and earliest sign of GBM filter dysfunction in AS. All XLAS male patients present microscopic hematuria, which is usually persistent. More than 95% of females with the same form of AS also present microscopic hematuria, but it is typically intermittent. Macroscopic hematuria is not rare and can be intermittent or persistent in both males and females. In case of ARAS microscopic, hematuria is usually persistent in both males and females and it is present in 100% of the patients.

Hematuria is usually observed in the first years of life, especially after episodes of upper respiratory infection, where it presents as macroscopic hematuria. Albuminuria and non-selective proteinuria presents later than hematuria. Overt proteinuria is usually absent in childhood, but its onset may vary from early childhood to adolescence. All XLAS male patients and both ARAS male and female patients develop proteinuria.

Males usually present a transitional stage of microalbuminuria before overt proteinuria is established. Proteinuria increases progressively with age and in 30% of the cases, it is of nephrotic range. Nephrotic syndrome is more frequent in XLAS males, but it rarely occurs in females.

Hypertension is usually absent before the second decade of life and its incidence and severity increases with age and progression of the disease.

ESRD develops in all XLAS patients between adolescence and the third decade of life. 60% of XLAS males reach ESRD by age 30, and 90% by age of 40. [88] In the past, ESRD was considered quite rare in XLAS females, but a recent study demonstrated that 12% of females develop ESRD before 40 years of age, 30% by age of 60, and 40% by age 80. [89]

According the time of onset ESRD, two forms of XLAS are recognized; the "juvenile" type, and the "adult" type. [78] The juvenile type corresponds to the classical presentation of AS in childhood and progression to ESRD by age of 20, while in the adult type ESRD by age of 20, while in the adult type ESRD may develop after the third decade of life and in some cases after the 5th decade of life. Approximately 82% of XLAS patients present sensorineural hearing loss and 44% develop ocular abnormalities that accompany renal manifestations. [88] Juvenile onset of ESRD accompanied by 80% incidence of hearing loss and 40% incidence of ocular abnormalities is characterized as severe (S) type XLAS. XLAS patients that progress to ESRD by age of 26 and show lower incidence of extrarenal manifestations are classified into moderate-severe (MS) type XLAS, while patients with onset of ESRD after the age of 30, with 70% incidence of hearing loss and less than 30% incidence of ocular lesions, belong to moderate (M). [78]

ii. Hearing Defects

Sensorineural deafness is a characteristic but not universal feature of AS, presenting in approximately 80% of males, and 30% of females. Hearing impairment begins by late childhood or early adolescence on XLAS males, and both males and females with ARAS, before the onset of renal manifestations. [88, 89]

Hearing loss is never present at birth. In childhood, hearing defects can be detected only by audiometry. As disease advances, hearing loss progresses, and 50% of XLAS males show deafness by age of 25. By age of 40 years, more than 90% of XLAS patients are deaf.

iii. Ocular Manifestations

Anterior lenticonus is a pathognomonic feature of AS occurring in approximately 15-20% XLAS male patients. It is usually absent at birth, manifesting at the second or third decade of life. Anterior lenticonus shows a slow and progressive course, with deterioration of vision but without defects in color vision.

Another common ocular manifestation is the dot-and-fleck retinopathy that consists of multiple perimacular dots and flecks observed on indirect opthalmoscopy. This condition occurs in approximately 30% of AS patients. In XLAS male patients, dot and fleck retinopathy, shows an incidence of 85%. It rarely occurs in childhood and it usually presents in concomitance with the onset of renal failure.

Posterior polymorphous corneal dystrophy and temporal macular thinning are more rare, but may occur in XLAS patients.

iv. Leiomyomatosis

Diffuse leiomyomatosis of the esophagus and tracheobronchial tree has been reported in approximately 30 families with AS. [90] Patients are usually asymptomatic until late childhood. Symptoms include dysphagia, postprandial vomiting, epigastric pain, recurrent bronchitis, dyspnea, and cough.

v. Hematologic Disorders

In the past Epstein's syndrome and Flechner's syndrome, two hereditary conditions transmitted in autosomal dominant patterns, characterized by nephritis, macrothrombocytopenia, cytoplasmatic polymorphonuclear inclusions similar to Döhle bodies, and sensorineural deafness, were considered variants of AS.

The renal pathology of these syndromes is indistinguishable from AS, consisting of interstitial glomerulonephritis with mesangial expansion and glomerular sclerosis.

These syndromes are the result of mutations in the gene encoding for nonmuscle myosin heavy chain type IIA (MYHAII) localized to chromosome 22q12-13, a region where no collagen genes have been mapped. [88] Therefore, these syndromes are now considered as distinct forms of hereditary nephritis.

Diagnosis

Diagnosis of AS should result from the combination of clinical symptoms, pathologic findings and genetic testing. AS should be suspected when a patient presents hematuria and/or renal failure, and has a family history of hematuria in absence of other causes of hematuria. All patients with suspected AS should undergo audiometry and ophthalmologic examination, given the association of hearing and ophthalmologic defects to renal manifestations.

High frequency audiometry usually shows bilateral reduction in sensitivity to tones with frequencies between 200 to 800Hz in the early stages, and in other frequencies in more advanced stages.

Opthalmologic examination reveals the pathognomonic feature of AS, the anterior lenticonus, usually more marked into the anterior chamber of the eye.

Urinanalysis will reveal microscopic or macroscopic hematuria and microscope examination shows dysmorphic red blood cells and red blood cell casts. 24-hour urine collection is necessary for evaluating renal function and proteinuria.

Renal ultrasonography may be unremarkable but in most cases may show bilateral reduction of kidneys size, increased echogenicity, and cystis.

Confirmation of diagnosis of AS is obtained by renal biopsy, which shows the characteristic alternation of thickening and thinning zones of the GBM with splitting and lamellation of the lamina densa.

Skin biopsy with immunostaining for α5 chain of type IV collagen may be used as an alternative to renal biopsy especially in XLAS. Almost 80% of XLAS males and 60% of females present no α5(IV) in epidermal basement membranes. If skin biopsy does not confirm diagnosis of AS, renal biopsy is mandatory.

Genetic testing is useful when AS is suspected but cannot be confirmed with biopsy. It can also be useful in prenatal testing for pregnant women carriers of XLAS and in cases of increased risk for ARAS and ADAS.

Prenatal genetic testing can be performed by amniocentesis at 15-18 weeks of gestation or the 10th to 12th week of gestation by chorionic villus sampling. Preimplantation genetic testing is also an available option.

Differential diagnosis with thin basement membrane disease (TBMD) should be considered in cases of familial hematuria. Although renal biopsy shows diffuse thinning of GBM without zones of thickening, splitting of the lamina densa has also been described in TBMN. Of note, immunostaining of type IV collagen α chains in the kidney is unremarkable in cases of TBMN, despite familial TBMN results from COL4A3 and COL4A4 mutations. [91, 92]

Other conditions that should be considered in differential diagnosis of AS are hereditable glomerular diseases that manifest with hematuria such as IgA nephropathy, membranous nephropathy, membranoproliferative glomerulonephritis, and polycystic kidney disease.

Treatment

Given that no definitive treatment for AS exists, current clinical recommendations focus on delaying the progression of the disease to ESRD, with early introduction of RAS inhibitors. Angiotensin converting enzyme inhibitors (ACEIs) are chosen by nephrologists as first line therapy in AS patients with proteinuria and with or without hypertension.

According to the European Alport's registry, initiation of ACEIs before decline of GFR delays ESRD by years. [93, 94] If ACEIs treatment is administered after proteinuria is established, survival rates ameliorate to a lesser degree compared to early initiation. [95] It has been demonstrated that ACEIs reduce proteinuria in XLAS children. [96] Controlled and uncontrolled studies also showed that angiotensin-receptor blockers (ARBs) and aldosterone inhibitors reduce proteinuria in children with AS. [96-98].

A recent study showed that losartan was more efficient in reducing proteinuria compared to placebo or amlodipine. [98] Spironolactone combined with ACEIs was superior in reducing proteinuria over ACEIs combined to ARBs but adverse effects as hyperkaliemia may limit its use. [97] Aldosterone inhibition may be used as second line treatment or as an alternative to ARBs therapy.

Adverse effects associated with RAS blockade include orthostatic hypotension, hyperkaliemia, and reversible decline of GFR.

Cyclosporine A was recently studied in patients with AS, showing marked reduction or elimination of proteinuria and delay of progression of renal disease. [99, 100] Others suggest that cyclosporine A is effective in reducing proteinuria in patients with Alport syndrome, but this effect is temporary and they do not support its use in these patients. [101] On the other hand, use of cyclosporine A may accelerate interstitial fibrosis due to calcineurin-induced nephrotoxicity, accelerating progression of renal disease, therefore caution during its administration is recommended. [102]

Renal transplantation is indicated for AS patients with ESRD requiring renal replacement treatment. Survival rates and graft survival rates in XLAS patients were similar or better compared to other inherited renal diseases. [103]

Approximately 3 to 5% of transplanted males with Alport's syndrome develop anti-GBM nephritis. [104, 105] In most of the cases, this disorder develops within the first year from transplantation manifesting as rapidly progressive renal disease. However, incidence of anti-GBM disease is very low and given the excellent graft survival rates in AS patients, renal transplantation remains the optimal treatment option in AS.

References

[1] Aerts JM, Groener JE, Kuiper S, Donker-Koopman WE, Strijland A, Ottenhoff R, et al. Elevated globotriaosylsphingosine is a hallmark of Fabry disease. *Proc. Natl. Acad. Sci. U S A*. 2008 Feb 26;105(8):2812-7.

[2] Pastores GM, Lien YH. Biochemical and molecular genetic basis of Fabry disease. *J. Am. Soc. Nephrol.* 2002 Jun;13 Suppl 2:S130-3.

[3] Bernstein HS, Bishop DF, Astrin KH, Kornreich R, Eng CM, Sakuraba H, et al. Fabry disease: six gene rearrangements and an exonic point mutation in the alpha-galactosidase gene. *J. Clin. Invest.* 1989 Apr;83(4):1390-9.

[4] Wilcox WR, Oliveira JP, Hopkin RJ, Ortiz A, Banikazemi M, Feldt-Rasmussen U, et al; Fabry Registry. Females with Fabry disease frequently have major organ

involvement: lessons from the Fabry Registry. *Mol. Genet. Metab*. 2008 Feb;93(2): 112-28.

[5] Whybra C, Kampmann C, Willers I, Davies J, Winchester B, Kriegsmann J, et al. Anderson-Fabry disease: clinical manifestations of disease in female heterozygotes. *J. Inherit. Metab. Dis*. 2001 Dec;24(7):715-24.

[6] MacDermot KD, Holmes A, Miners AH. Anderson-Fabry disease: clinical manifestations and impact of disease in a cohort of 60 obligate carrier females. *J. Med. Genet.* 2001 Nov;38(11):769-75.

[7] Deegan PB, Baehner AF, Barba Romero MA, Hughes DA, Kampmann C, Beck M; European FOS Investigators. Natural history of Fabry disease in females in the Fabry Outcome Survey. *J. Med. Genet.* 2006 Apr;43(4):347-52.

[8] Hopkin RJ, Bissler J, Banikazemi M, Clarke L, Eng CM, Germain DP, et al. Characterization of Fabry disease in 352 pediatric patients in the Fabry Registry. *Pediatr. Res.* 2008 Nov;64(5):550-5.

[9] Schiffmann R. Fabry disease. *Pharmacol Ther*. 2009 Apr;122(1):65-77.

[10] Eng CM, Fletcher J, Wilcox WR, Waldek S, Scott CR, Sillence DO, et al. Fabry disease: baseline medical characteristics of a cohort of 1765 males and females in the Fabry Registry. *J. Inherit. Metab. Dis*. 2007 Apr;30(2):184-92.

[11] Desnick RJ, Brady R, Barranger J, Collins AJ, Germain DP, Goldman M, et al. Fabry disease, an under-recognized multisystemic disorder: expert recommendations for diagnosis, management, and enzyme replacement therapy. *Ann. Intern. Med.*. 2003 Feb 18;138(4):338-46.

[12] MacDermot KD, Holmes A, Miners AH. Anderson-Fabry disease: clinical manifestations and impact of disease in a cohort of 98 hemizygous males. *J. Med. Genet*. 2001 Nov;38(11):750-60.

[13] Germain DP. Fabry disease. Orphanet. *J. Rare Dis*. 2010 Nov 22;5:30.

[14] Mehta A, Ricci R, Widmer U, Dehout F, Garcia de Lorenzo A, Kampmann C, et al. Fabry disease defined: baseline clinical manifestations of 366 patients in the Fabry Outcome Survey. *Eur. J. Clin. Invest*. 2004 Mar;34(3):236-42.

[15] Branton MH, Schiffmann R, Sabnis SG, Murray GJ, Quirk JM, Altarescu G, et al. Natural history of Fabry renal disease: influence of alpha-galactosidase A activity and genetic mutations on clinical course. *Medicine (*Baltimore). 2002 Mar;81(2):122-38.

[16] Nakao S, Kodama C, Takenaka T, Tanaka A, Yasumoto Y, Yoshida A, et al. Fabry disease: detection of undiagnosed hemodialysis patients and identification of a "renal variant" phenotype. *Kidney Int.* 2003 Sep;64(3):801-7.

[17] Cabrera-Salazar MA, O'Rourke E, Charria-Ortiz G, Barranger JA. Radiological evidence of early cerebral microvascular disease in young children with Fabry disease. *J. Pediatr*. 2005 Jul;147(1):102-5.

[18] Ramaswami U, Whybra C, Parini R, Pintos-Morell G, Mehta A, Sunder-Plassmann G, et al; FOS European Investigators. Clinical manifestations of Fabry disease in children: data from the Fabry Outcome Survey. *Acta. Paediatr.* 2006 Jan;95(1):86-92.

[19] Orteu CH, Jansen T, Lidove O, Jaussaud R, Hughes DA, Pintos-Morell G, et al; FOS Investigators. Fabry disease and the skin: data from FOS, the Fabry outcome survey. *Br J. Dermatol.* 2007 Aug;157(2):331-7.

[20] Shelley ED, Shelley WB, Kurczynski TW. Painful fingers, heat intolerance, and telangiectases of the ear: easily ignored childhood signs of Fabry disease. *Pediatr. Dermatol.* 1995 Sep;12(3):215-9.

[21] Sodi A, Ioannidis AS, Mehta A, Davey C, Beck M, Pitz S. Ocular manifestations of Fabry's disease: data from the Fabry Outcome Survey. *Br. J. Ophthalmol.* 2007 Feb;91(2):210-4. Epub 2006 Sep 14.

[22] Keilmann A, Hajioff D, Ramaswami U; FOS Investigators. Ear symptoms in children with Fabry disease: data from the Fabry Outcome Survey. *J. Inherit. Metab. Dis.* 2009 Dec;32(6):739-44.

[23] Meikle PJ, Hopwood JJ, Clague AE, Carey WF. Prevalence of lysosomal storage disorders. *JAMA*. 1999 Jan 20;281(3):249-54.

[24] Spada M, Pagliardini S, Yasuda M, Tukel T, Thiagarajan G, Sakuraba H, et al. High incidence of later-onset Fabry disease revealed by newborn screening. *Am. J. Hum. Genet.* 2006 Jul;79(1):31-40.

[25] Lin HY, Chong KW, Hsu JH, Yu HC, Shih CC, Huang CH, et al. High incidence of the cardiac variant of Fabry disease revealed by newborn screening in the Taiwan Chinese population. *Circ. Cardiovasc. Genet.* 2009 Oct;2(5):450-6.

[26] Branton M, Schiffmann R, Kopp JB. Natural history and treatment of renal involvement in Fabry disease. *J. Am. Soc. Nephrol.* 2002 Jun;13 Suppl 2:S139-43.

[27] Elleder M, Poupětová H, Kozich V. [Fetal pathology in Fabry's disease and mucopolysaccharidosis type I]. Cesk Patol. 1998 Jan;34(1):7-12. [Article in Czech]

[28] Sessa A, Toson A, Nebuloni M, Pallotti F, Giordano F, Battini G, et al. Renal ultrastructural findings in Anderson-Fabry disease. *J. Nephrol.* 2002 Mar-Apr;15(2):109-12.

[29] Alroy J, Sabnis S, Kopp JB. Renal pathology in Fabry disease. *J. Am. Soc. Nephrol.* 2002 Jun;13 Suppl 2:S134-8.

[30] Kojima Y, Fukumoto S, Furukawa K, Okajima T, Wiels J, Yokoyama K, et al. Molecular cloning of globotriaosylceramide/CD77 synthase, a glycosyltransferase that initiates the synthesis of globo series glycosphingolipids. *J. Biol. Chem.* 2000 May 19;275(20):15152-6.

[31] Ergonul Z, Clayton F, Fogo AB, Kohan DE. Shigatoxin-1 binding and receptor expression in human kidneys do not change with age. *Pediatr. Nephrol.* 2003 Mar;18(3):246-53.

[32] Thomaidis T, Relle M, Golbas M, Brochhausen C, Galle PR, Beck M, et al. Downregulation of alpha-galactosidase A upregulates CD77: functional impact for Fabry nephropathy. *Kidney Int.* 2009 Feb;75(4):399-407.

[33] Fischer EG, Moore MJ, Lager DJ. Fabry disease: a morphologic study of 11 cases. *Mod Pathol.* 2006 Oct;19(10):1295-301.

[34] Klionsky DJ, Abdalla FC, Abeliovich H, Abraham RT, Acevedo-Arozena A, Adeli K, et al. Guidelines for the use and interpretation of assays for monitoring autophagy. *Autophagy.* 2012 Apr;8(4):445-544.

[35] Liebau MC, Braun F, Höpker K, Weitbrecht C, Bartels V, Müller RU, et al. Dysregulated autophagy contributes to podocyte damage in Fabry's disease. *PLoS. One.* 2013 May 17;8(5):e63506.

[36] Kiselyov K, Jennigs JJ Jr, Rbaibi Y, Chu CT. Autophagy, mitochondria and cell death in lysosomal storage diseases. *Autophagy.* 2007 May-Jun;3(3):259-62.

[37] Vitner EB, Platt FM, Futerman AH. Common and uncommon pathogenic cascades in lysosomal storage diseases. *J. Biol. Chem*. 2010 Jul 2;285(27):20423-7.

[38] Ravikumar B, Sarkar S, Davies JE, Futter M, Garcia-Arencibia M, Green-Thompson ZW, et al. Regulation of mammalian autophagy in physiology and pathophysiology. *Physiol Rev*. 2010 Oct;90(4):1383-435.

[39] Cinà DP, Onay T, Paltoo A, Li C, Maezawa Y, De Arteaga J, et al. Inhibition of MTOR disrupts autophagic flux in podocytes. *J. Am. Soc. Nephrol*. 2012 Mar;23(3):412-20.

[40] Sanchez-Niño MD, Sanz AB, Carrasco S, Saleem MA, Mathieson PW, Valdivielso JM, et al. Globotriaosylsphingosine actions on human glomerular podocytes: implications for Fabry nephropathy. *Nephrol Dial Transplant*. 2011 Jun;26(6):1797-802.

[41] Shen JS, Meng XL, Moore DF, Quirk JM, Shayman JA, Schiffmann R, et al. Globotriaosylceramide induces oxidative stress and up-regulates cell adhesion molecule expression in Fabry disease endothelial cells. *Mol Genet Metab*. 2008 Nov;95(3):163-8.

[42] Sessa A, Meroni M, Battini G, Maglio A, Brambilla PL, Bertella M, et al. Renal pathological changes in Fabry disease. *J. Inherit. Metab. Dis*. 2001;24 Suppl 2:66-70; discussion 65.

[43] Valbuena C, Carvalho E, Bustorff M, Ganhão M, Relvas S, Nogueira R, et al. Kidney biopsy findings in heterozygous Fabry disease females with early nephropathy. *Virchows Arch.* 2008 Oct;453(4):329-38.

[44] Thurberg BL, Rennke H, Colvin RB, Dikman S, Gordon RE, Collins AB, et al. Globotriaosylceramide accumulation in the Fabry kidney is cleared from multiple cell types after enzyme replacement therapy. *Kidney Int*. 2002 Dec;62(6):1933-46.

[45] Fogo AB, Bostad L, Svarstad E, Cook WJ, Moll S, Barbey F, et al; all members of the International Study Group of Fabry Nephropathy (ISGFN). Scoring system for renal pathology in Fabry disease: report of the International Study Group of Fabry Nephropathy (ISGFN). *Nephrol. Dial. Transplant*. 2010 Jul;25(7):2168-77.

[46] Wornell P, Dyack S, Crocker J, Yu W, Acott P. Fabry disease and nephrogenic diabetes insipidus. *Pediatr Nephrol*. 2006 Aug;21(8):1185-8.

[47] Sessa A, Meroni M, Battini G, Righetti M, Maglio A, Tosoni A, et al. Renal involvement in Anderson-Fabry disease. *J. Nephrol*. 2003 Mar-Apr;16(2):310-3.

[48] Ries M, Gupta S, Moore DF, Sachdev V, Quirk JM, Murray GJ, et al. Pediatric Fabry disease. *Pediatrics*. 2005 Mar;115(3):e344-55.

[49] Wanner C, Oliveira JP, Ortiz A, Mauer M, Germain DP, Linthorst GE, et al. Prognostic indicators of renal disease progression in adults with Fabry disease: natural history data from the Fabry Registry. *Clin. J. Am. Soc. Nephrol*. 2010 Dec;5(12):2220-8.

[50] Ortiz A, Oliveira JP, Waldek S, Warnock DG, Cianciaruso B, Wanner C; Fabry Registry. Nephropathy in males and females with Fabry disease: cross-sectional description of patients before treatment with enzyme replacement therapy. *Nephrol. Dial Transplant.* 2008 May;23(5):1600-7.

[51] Kleinert J, Dehout F, Schwarting A, de Lorenzo AG, Ricci R, Kampmann C, et al. Prevalence of uncontrolled hypertension in patients with Fabry disease. *Am. J. Hypertens*. 2006 Aug;19(8):782-7.

[52] Jain G, Warnock DG. Blood pressure, proteinuria, and nephropathy in Fabry disease. *Nephron. Clin*. Pract. 2011;118(1):c43-8.

[53] Andrade J, Waters PJ, Singh RS, Levin A, Toh BC, Vallance HD, et al. Screening for Fabry disease in patients with chronic kidney disease: limitations of plasma alpha-

galactosidase assay as a screening test. *Clin. J. Am. Soc. Nephrol.* 2008 Jan;3(1): 139-45.

[54] Schiffmann R, Kopp JB, Austin HA 3rd, Sabnis S, Moore DF, Weibel T, et al. Enzyme replacement therapy in Fabry disease: a randomized controlled trial. *JAMA.* 2001 Jun 6;285(21):2743-9.

[55] Eng CM, Guffon N, Wilcox WR, Germain DP, Lee P, Waldek S, et al; International Collaborative Fabry Disease Study Group. Safety and efficacy of recombinant human alpha-galactosidase A--replacement therapy in Fabry's disease. *N. Engl. J.* Med. 2001 Jul 5;345(1):9-16.

[56] Mehta A, Clarke JT, Giugliani R, Elliott P, Linhart A, Beck M, et al; FOS Investigators. Natural course of Fabry disease: changing pattern of causes of death in FOS - Fabry Outcome Survey. *J. Med. Genet.* 2009 Aug;46(8):548-52.

[57] West M, Nicholls K, Mehta A, Clarke JT, Steiner R, Beck M, et al. Agalsidase alfa and kidney dysfunction in Fabry disease. *J. Am. Soc. Nephrol.* 2009 May;20(5):1132-9.

[58] Ries M, Clarke JT, Whybra C, Timmons M, Robinson C, Schlaggar BL, et al. Enzyme-replacement therapy with agalsidase alfa in children with Fabry disease. *Pediatrics.* 2006 Sep;118(3):924-32.

[59] Banikazemi M, Bultas J, Waldek S, Wilcox WR, Whitley CB, McDonald M, et al; Fabry Disease Clinical Trial Study Group. Agalsidase-beta therapy for advanced Fabry disease: a randomized trial. *Ann. Intern. Med.* 2007 Jan 16;146(2):77-86.

[60] Schwarting A, Dehout F, Feriozzi S, Beck M, Mehta A, Sunder-Plassmann G; European FOS Investigators. Enzyme replacement therapy and renal function in 201 patients with Fabry disease. *Clin. Nephrol.* 2006 Aug;66(2):77-84.

[61] Vedder AC, Linthorst GE, Houge G, Groener JE, Ormel EE, Bouma BJ, et al. Treatment of Fabry disease: outcome of a comparative trial with agalsidase alfa or beta at a dose of 0.2 mg/kg. *PLoS One.* 2007 Jul 11;2(7):e598.

[62] García de Lorenzo A; en nombre del grupo de enfermedad de FABRY-GETER. [Consensus for the study and treatment of Fabry disease. GETER Foundation*]. Med Clin* (Barc). 2011 Jul 9;137(4):178-83. [Article in Spanish]

[63] Eng CM, Germain DP, Banikazemi M, Warnock DG, Wanner C, Hopkin RJ, et al. Fabry disease: guidelines for the evaluation and management of multi-organ system involvement. *Genet. Med.* 2006 Sep;8(9):539-48.

[64] Kosch M, Koch HG, Oliveira JP, Soares C, Bianco F, Breuning F, et al. Enzyme replacement therapy administered during hemodialysis in patients with Fabry disease. *Kidney Int.* 2004 Sep;66(3):1279-82.

[65] Mignani R, Panichi V, Giudicissi A, Taccola D, Boscaro F, Feletti C, et al. Enzyme replacement therapy with agalsidase beta in kidney transplant patients with Fabry disease: a pilot study. *Kidney Int.* 2004 Apr;65(4):1381-5.

[66] Sessa A, Meroni M, Battini G, Righetti M, Mignani R. Chronic renal failure, dialysis, and renal transplantation in Anderson-Fabry disease. *Semin. Nephrol.* 2004 Sep;24(5):532-6.

[67] Germain DP, Waldek S, Banikazemi M, Bushinsky DA, Charrow J, Desnick RJ, et al. Sustained, long-term renal stabilization after 54 months of agalsidase beta therapy in patients with Fabry disease. *J. Am. Soc. Nephrol.* 2007 May;18(5):1547-57.

[68] Schiffmann R, Ries M, Timmons M, Flaherty JT, Brady RO. Long-term therapy with agalsidase alfa for Fabry disease: safety and effects on renal function in a home infusion setting. *Nephrol Dial Transplant*. 2006 Feb;21(2):345-54.

[69] Fuller M, Lovejoy M, Brooks DA, Harkin ML, Hopwood JJ, Meikle PJ. Immunoquantification of alpha-galactosidase: evaluation for the diagnosis of Fabry disease. *Clin. Chem*. 2004 Nov;50(11):1979-85.

[70] Bodensteiner D, Scott CR, Sims KB, Shepherd GM, Cintron RD, Germain DP. Successful reinstitution of agalsidase beta therapy in Fabry disease patients with previous IgE-antibody or skin test reactivity to the recombinant enzyme. *Genet Med*. 2008 May;10(5):353-8.

[71] Linthorst GE, Hollak CE, Donker-Koopman WE, Strijland A, Aerts JM. Enzyme therapy for Fabry disease: neutralizing antibodies toward agalsidase alpha and beta. *Kidney Int*. 2004 Oct;66(4):1589-95.

[72] Vedder AC, Breunig F, Donker-Koopman WE, Mills K, Young E, Winchester B, et al. Treatment of Fabry disease with different dosing regimens of agalsidase: effects on antibody formation and GL-3. *Mol Genet. Metab*. 2008 Jul;94(3):319-25.

[73] Ishii S, Chang HH, Yoshioka H, Shimada T, Mannen K, Higuchi Y, et al. Preclinical efficacy and safety of 1-deoxygalactonojirimycin in mice for Fabry disease. *J. Pharmacol. Exp. Ther*. 2009 Mar;328(3):723-31.

[74] Porto C, Pisani A, Rosa M, Acampora E, Avolio V, Tuzzi MR, et al. Synergy between the pharmacological chaperone 1-deoxygalactonojirimycin and the human recombinant alpha-galactosidase A in cultured fibroblasts from patients with Fabry disease. *J. Inherit. Metab. Dis*. 2012 May;35(3):513-20.

[75] Germain DP, Fan JQ. Pharmacological chaperone therapy by active-site-specific chaperones in Fabry disease: in vitro and preclinical studies. *Int. J. Clin. Pharmacol. Ther*. 2009;47 Suppl 1:S111-7.

[76] Giugliani R, Waldek S, Germain DP, Nicholls K, Bichet DG, Simosky JK, et al. A Phase 2 study of migalastat hydrochloride in females with Fabry disease: selection of population, safety, and pharmacodynamic effects. *Mol. Genet. Metab*. 2013 May;109(1):86-92.

[77] Alport AC. Hereditary Familial Congenital Haemorrhagic Nephritis. *Br. Med. J*. 1927 Mar 19;1(3454):504-6.

[78] Gross O, Netzer KO, Lambrecht R, Seibold S, Weber M. Meta-analysis of genotype-phenotype correlation in X-linked Alport syndrome: impact on clinical counselling. *Nephrol. Dial. Transplant*. 2002 Jul;17(7):1218-27.

[79] Bekheirnia MR, Reed B, Gregory MC, McFann K, Shamshirsaz AA, Masoumi A, et al. Genotype-phenotype correlation in X-linked Alport syndrome. *J. Am. Soc. Nephrol*. 2010 May;21(5):876-83.

[80] Boye E, Mollet G, Forestier L, Cohen-Solal L, Heidet L, Cochat P, et al. Determination of the genomic structure of the COL4A4 gene and of novel mutations causing autosomal recessive Alport syndrome. *Am. J. Hum. Genet*. 1998 Nov;63(5):1329-40.

[81] Heidet L, Arrondel C, Forestier L, Cohen-Solal L, Mollet G, Gutierrez B, et al. Structure of the human type IV collagen gene COL4A3 and mutations in autosomal Alport syndrome. *J. Am. Soc. Nephrol*. 2001 Jan;12(1):97-106.

[82] van der Loop FT, Heidet L, Timmer ED, van den Bosch BJ, Leinonen A, Antignac C, et al. Autosomal dominant Alport syndrome caused by a COL4A3 splice site mutation. *Kidney Int.* 2000 Nov;58(5):1870-5.

[83] Ciccarese M, Casu D, Ki Wong F, Faedda R, Arvidsson S, Tonolo G, et al. Identification of a new mutation in the alpha4(IV) collagen gene in a family with autosomal dominant Alport syndrome and hypercholesterolaemia. *Nephrol. Dial Transplant.* 2001 Oct;16(10):2008-12.

[84] Levy M, Feingold J. Estimating prevalence in single-gene kidney diseases progressing to renal failure. *Kidney Int.* 2000 Sep;58(3):925-43.

[85] Collins AJ, Foley RN, Herzog C, Chavers B, Gilbertson D, Ishani A, et al. United States Renal Data System 2008 Annual Data *Report. Am. J. Kidney Dis.* 2009 Jan;53(1 Suppl):S1-374.

[86] Kashtan CE, Michael AF. Alport syndrome. *Kidney Int.* 1996 Nov;50(5):1445-63.

[87] Kashtan CE, Kleppel MM, Gubler MC. Immunohistologic findings in Alport syndrome. *Contrib. Nephrol.* 1996;117:142-53.

[88] Jais JP, Knebelmann B, Giatras I, De Marchi M, Rizzoni G, Renieri A, et al. X-linked Alport syndrome: natural history in 195 families and genotype- phenotype correlations in males. *J. Am. Soc. Nephrol.* 2000 Apr;11(4):649-57.

[89] Jais JP, Knebelmann B, Giatras I, De Marchi M, Rizzoni G, Renieri A, et al. X-linked Alport syndrome: natural history and genotype-phenotype correlations in girls and women belonging to 195 families: a "European Community Alport Syndrome Concerted Action" study. *J. Am. Soc. Nephrol.* 2003 Oct;14(10):2603-10.

[90] Antignac C, Heidet L. Mutations in Alport syndrome associated with diffuse esophageal leiomyomatosis. *Contrib. Nephrol.* 1996;117:172-82.

[91] Lemmink HH, Nillesen WN, Mochizuki T, Schröder CH, Brunner HG, van Oost BA, et al. Benign familial hematuria due to mutation of the type IV collagen alpha4 gene. *J. Clin. Invest.* 1996 Sep 1;98(5):1114-8.

[92] Savige J, Rana K, Tonna S, Buzza M, Dagher H, Wang YY. Thin basement membrane nephropathy. *Kidney Int.* 2003 Oct;64(4):1169-78.

[93] Gross O, Licht C, Anders HJ, Hoppe B, Beck B, Tönshoff B, et al. Early angiotensin-converting enzyme inhibition in Alport syndrome delays renal failure and improves life expectancy. *Kidney Int.* 2012 Mar;81(5):494-501.

[94] Temme J, Peters F, Lange K, Pirson Y, Heidet L, Torra R, et al. Incidence of renal failure and nephroprotection by RAAS inhibition in heterozygous carriers of X-chromosomal and autosomal recessive Alport mutations. *Kidney Int.* 2012 Apr;81(8):779-83.

[95] Gross O, Beirowski B, Koepke ML, Kuck J, Reiner M, Addicks K, et al. Preemptive ramipril therapy delays renal failure and reduces renal fibrosis in COL4A3-knockout mice with Alport syndrome. *Kidney Int.* 2003 Feb;63(2):438-46.

[96] Proesmans W, Van Dyck M. Enalapril in children with Alport syndrome. *Pediatr Nephrol.* 2004 Mar;19(3):271-5.

[97] Kaito H, Nozu K, Iijima K, Nakanishi K, Yoshiya K, Kanda K, et al. The effect of aldosterone blockade in patients with Alport syndrome. *Pediatr. Nephrol.* 2006 Dec;21(12):1824-9.

[98] Webb NJ, Lam C, Shahinfar S, Strehlau J, Wells TG, Gleim GW, et al. Efficacy and safety of losartan in children with Alport syndrome--results from a subgroup analysis of

a prospective, randomized, placebo- or amlodipine-controlled trial. *Nephrol. Dial Transplant.* 2011 Aug;26(8):2521-6.

[99] Callís L, Vila A, Nieto J, Fortuny G. Effect of cyclosporin A on proteinuria in patients with Alport's syndrome. *Pediatr. Nephrol.* 1992 Mar;6(2):140-4.

[100] Callís L, Vila A, Carrera M, Nieto J. Long-term effects of cyclosporine A in Alport's syndrome. *Kidney Int.* 1999 Mar;55(3):1051-6.

[101] Massella L, Muda AO, Legato A, Di Zazzo G, Giannakakis K, Emma F. Cyclosporine A treatment in patients with Alport syndrome: a single-center experience. *Pediatr. Nephrol.* 2010 Jul;25(7):1269-75.

[102] Charbit M, Gubler MC, Dechaux M, Gagnadoux MF, Grünfeld JP, Niaudet P. Cyclosporin therapy in patients with Alport syndrome. Pediatr. *Nephrol. 2007 Jan;22(1):57-63.*

[103] Temme J, Kramer A, Jager KJ, Lange K, Peters F, Müller GA, et al. Outcomes of male patients with Alport syndrome undergoing renal replacement therapy. *Clin. J. Am. Soc. Nephrol.* 2012 Dec;7(12):1969-76.

[104] Kashtan CE. Renal transplantation in patients with Alport syndrome. *Pediatr. Transplant.* 2006 Sep;10(6):651-7.

[105] Fleming SJ, Savage CO, McWilliam LJ, Pickering SJ, Ralston AJ, Johnson RW, et al. Anti-glomerular basement membrane antibody-mediated nephritis complicating transplantation in a patient with Alport's syndrome. *Transplantation.* 1988 Dec;46(6):857-9.

Images of Glomerulonephritis

Nakopoulou Lydia
University of Athens, Medical School, Department of Pathology

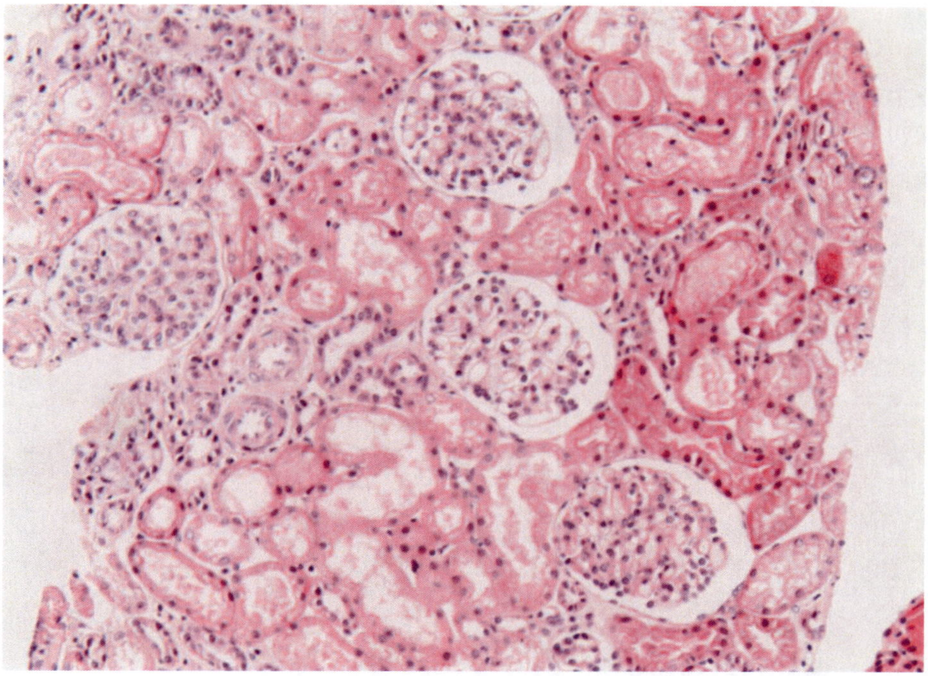

Figure 1. Minimal change disease (MCD). Four glomeruli with normal size and no glomerular changes (H/E, x250).

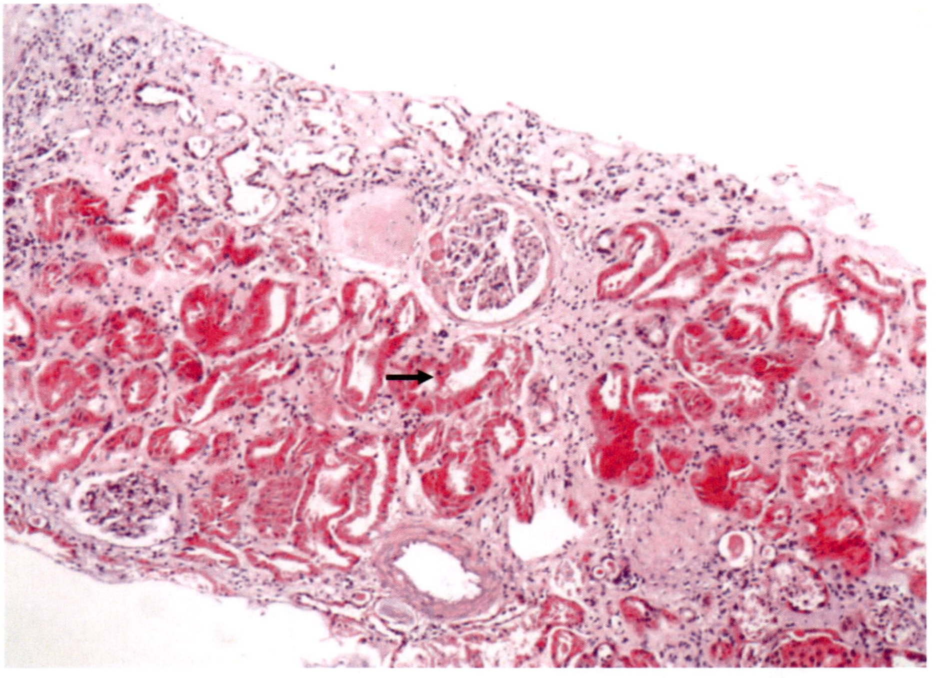

Figure 2. Focal segmental glomerulosclerosis. There is a glomerulus with a segmental acellular area with hyalinosis lesions (arrow) (H/E, x250).

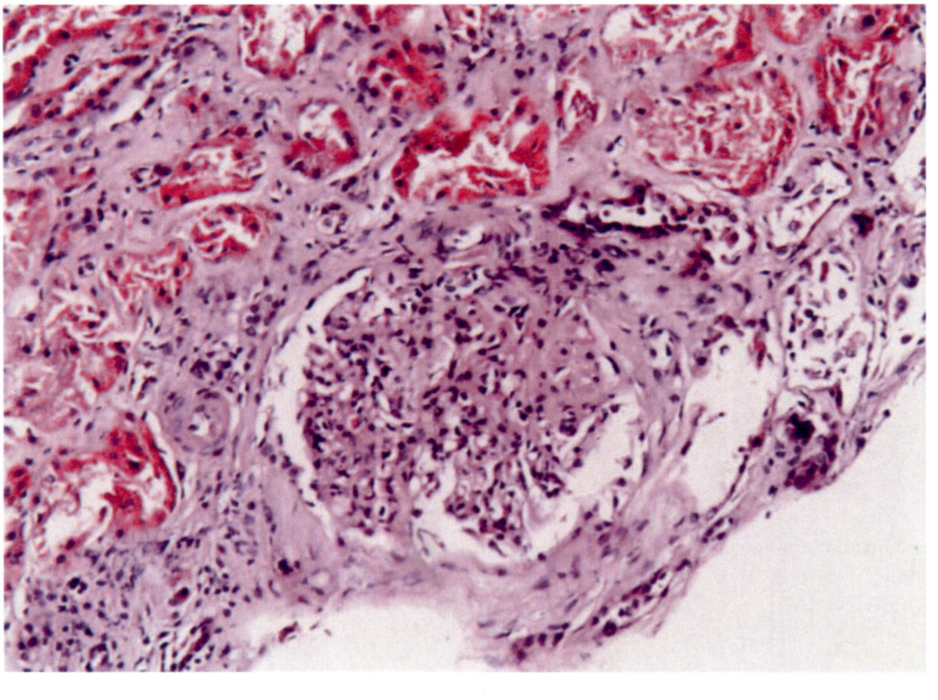

Figure 3. Focal segmental glomerulosclerosis. There is segmental acellular eosinophilic matrix (H/E, x400).

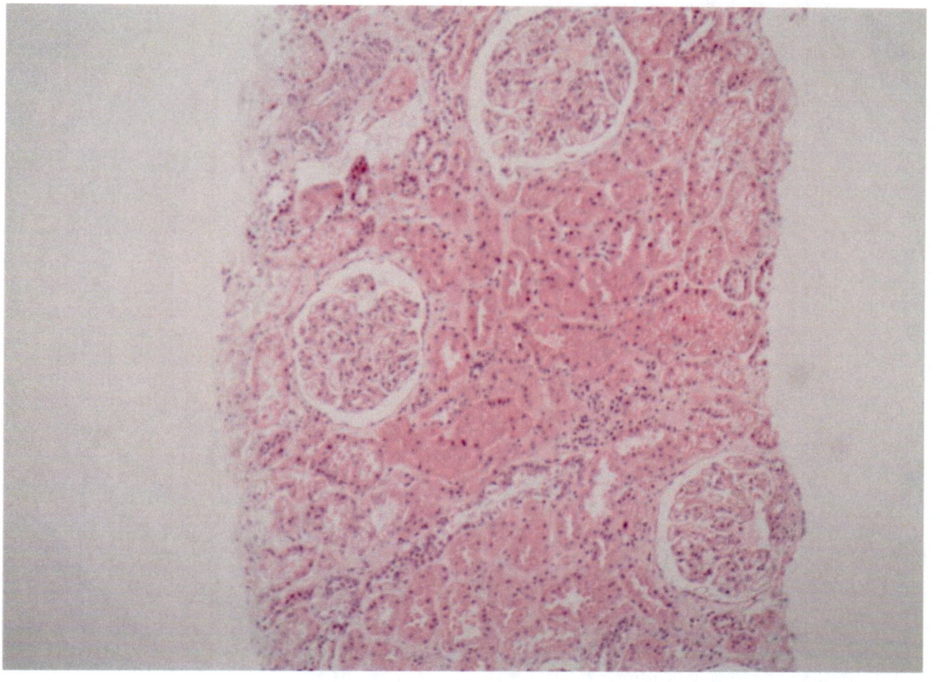

Figure 4. Membranous glomerulonephritis stage II. Three glomeruli with mild diffuse thickening of glomerular capillaries (H/E, x250).

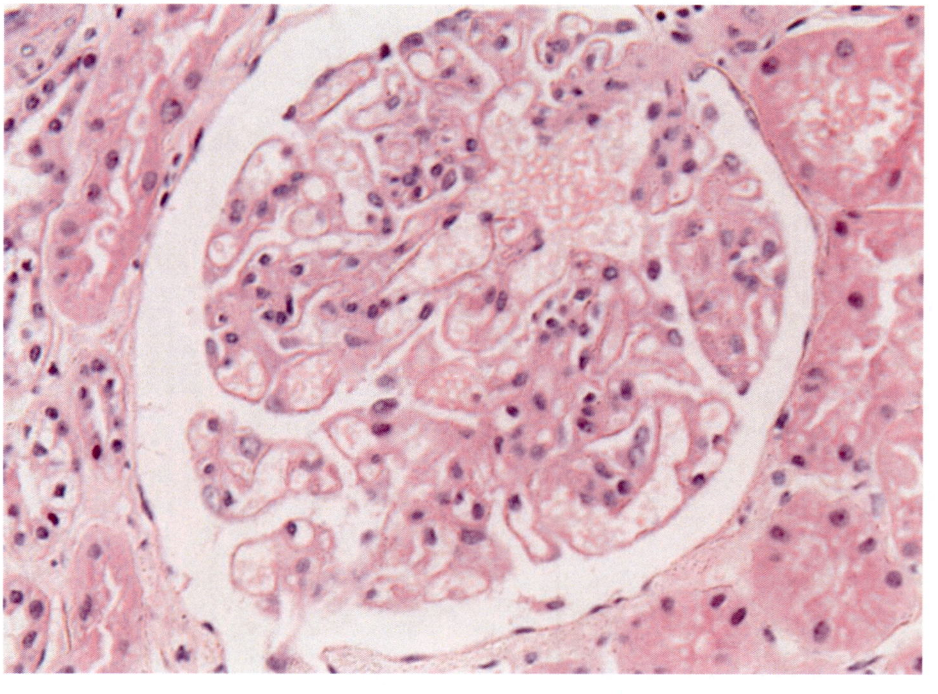

Figure 5. Membranous glomerulonephritis stage II. One glomerulus with mild diffuse thickening of glomerular capillaries (H/E, x400).

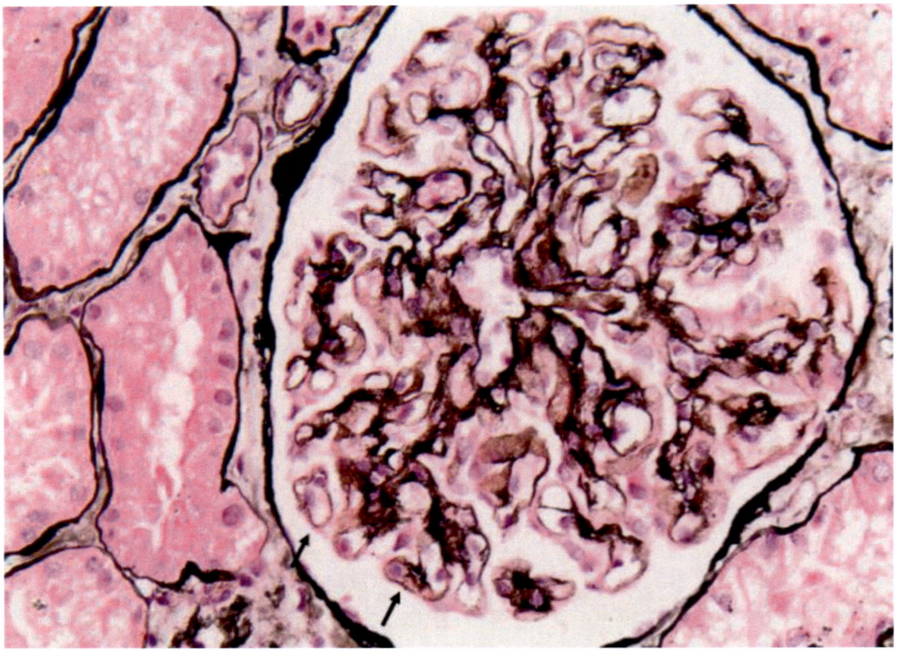

Figure 6. Membranous glomerulonephritis stage II. Focal subepithelial spikes formation (arrows) (Jone's methenamine silver stain, x400).

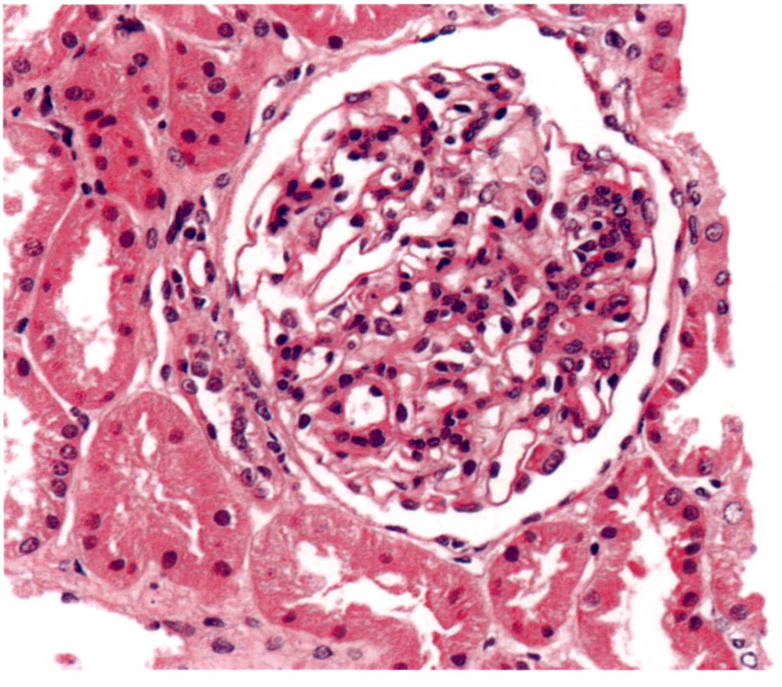

Figure 7. IgA nephropathy. Moderate to severe hyperplasia of mesangial cells, with increase of mesangial matrix (H/E, x400).

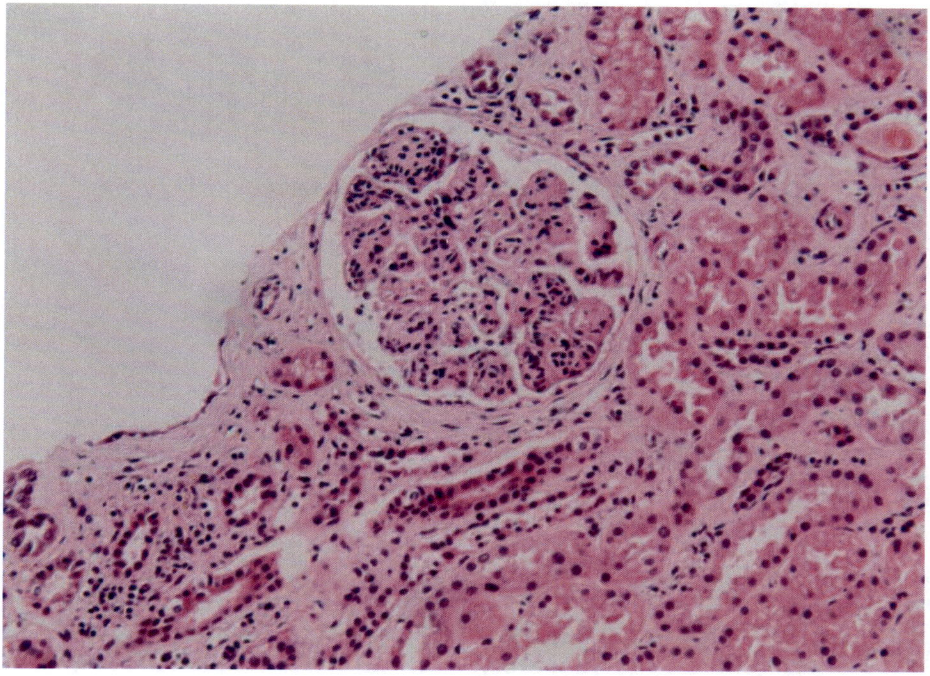

Figure 8. Membranoproliferative glomerulonephritis (MPGN) type I. A glomerulus with increased lobulation, hypercellularity, with obliteration of capillary lumen caused by proliferation of endothelial cells, as well as infiltration by leucocytes (H/E, x250).

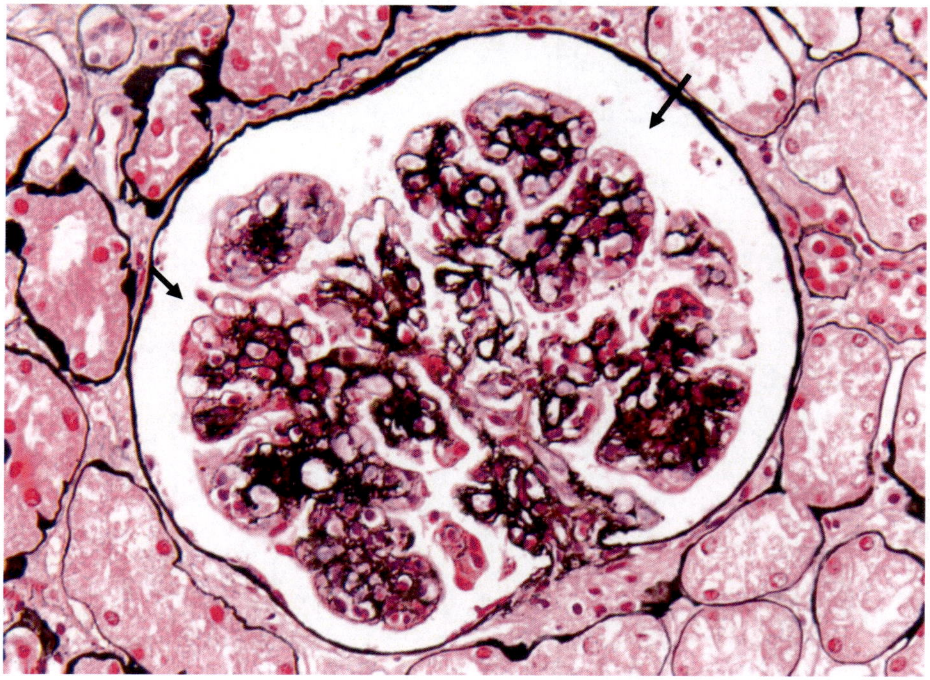

Figure 9. MPGN type I. GBM with segmental duplication (arrows) and cellular interposition (Jone's methenamine silver stain, x400).

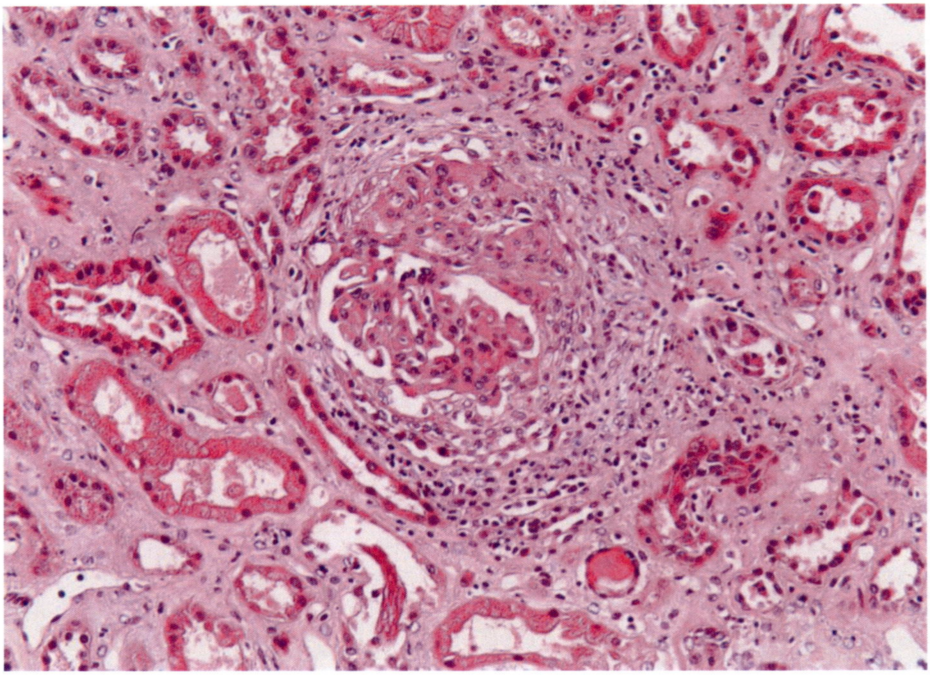

Figure 10. Pauci-immune (ANCA) crescentic glomerulonephritis. There is a glomerulus compressed by a large circumferential cellular crescent. There is inflammation in the adjacent tissue (H/E, x250).

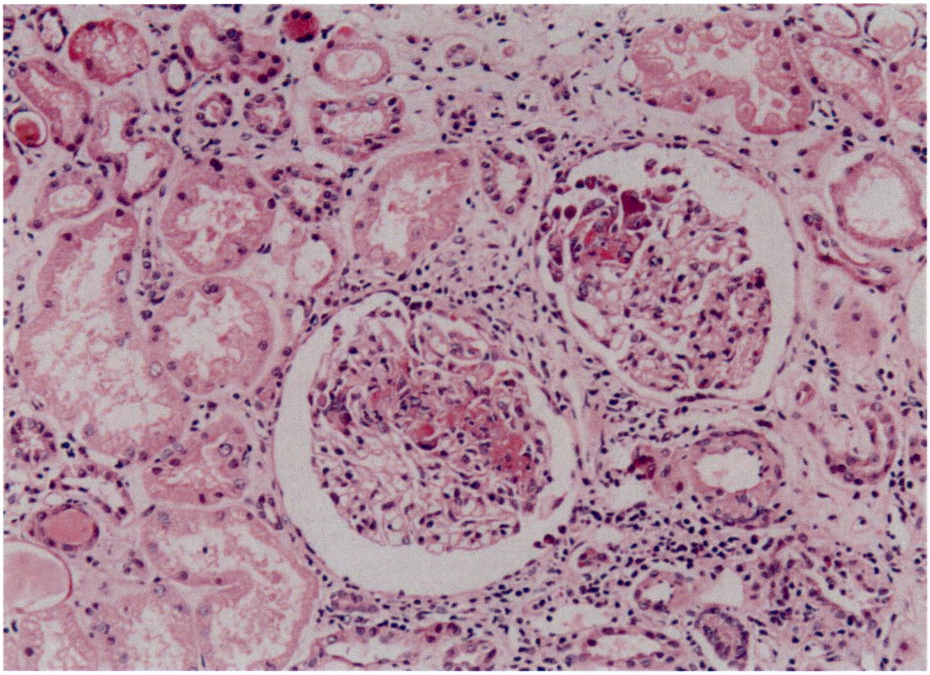

Figure 11. Pauci-immune (ANCA) crescentic glomerulonephritis. Two glomeruli with segmental fibrinoid necrosis (H/E, x250).

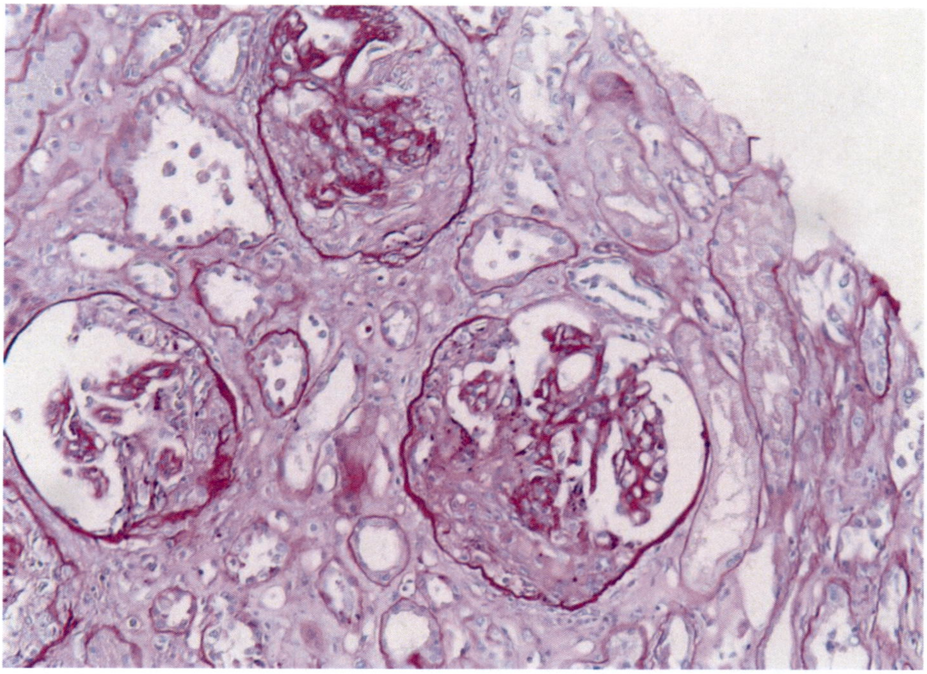

Figure 12. Pauci-immune (ANCA) crescentic glomerulonephritis. Three glomeruli with circumferential cellular crescents of different size (PAS stain, x250).

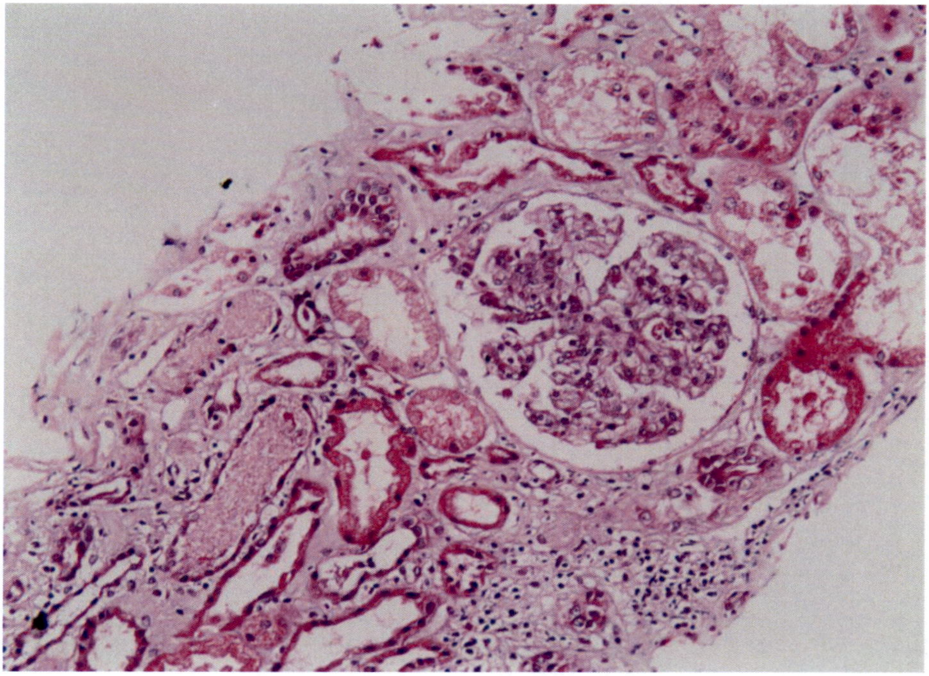

Figure 13. Mesangioproliferative glomerulonephritis. A glomerulus with moderate mesangial prominence, with increase of mesangial matrix and mesangial cells (PAS stain, x250).

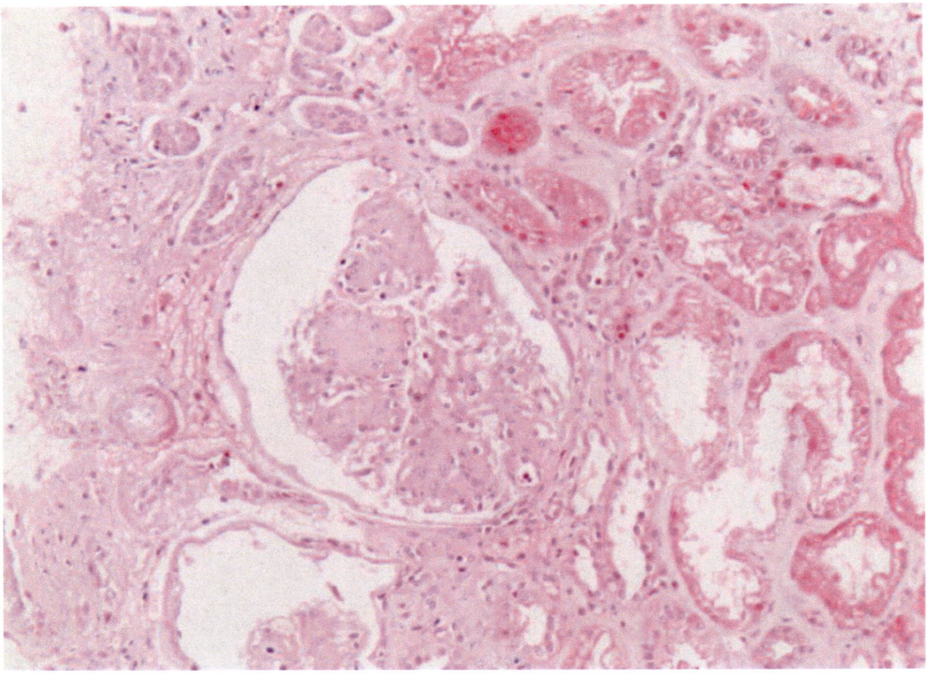

Figure 14. Nodular diabetic nephrosclerosis. Mesangial nodules (classic Kimmelstiel-Wilson nodules) (H/E, x250).

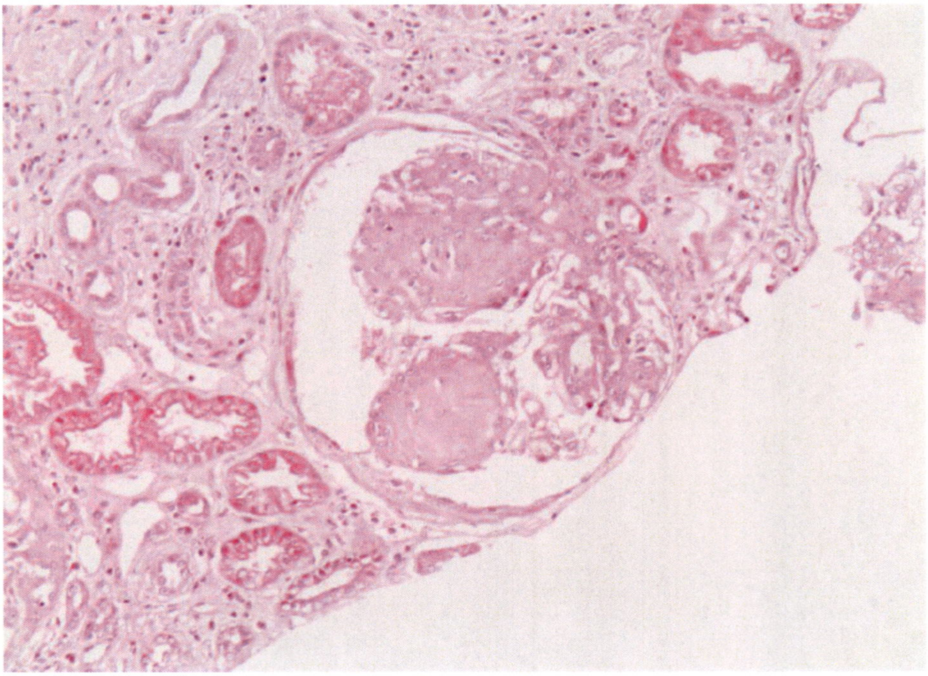

Figure 15. Nodular diabetic nephrosclerosis. Two large mesangial nodules (H/E, x400).

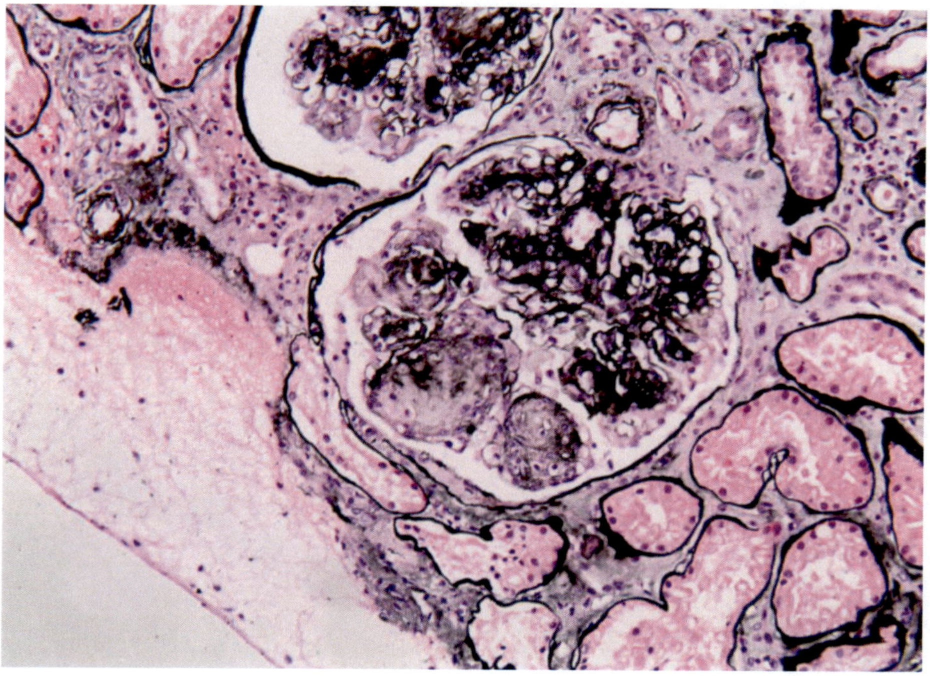

Figure 16. Nodular diabetic nephrosclerosis. Mesangial nodules of different size (Jone's methenamine silver stain, x400).

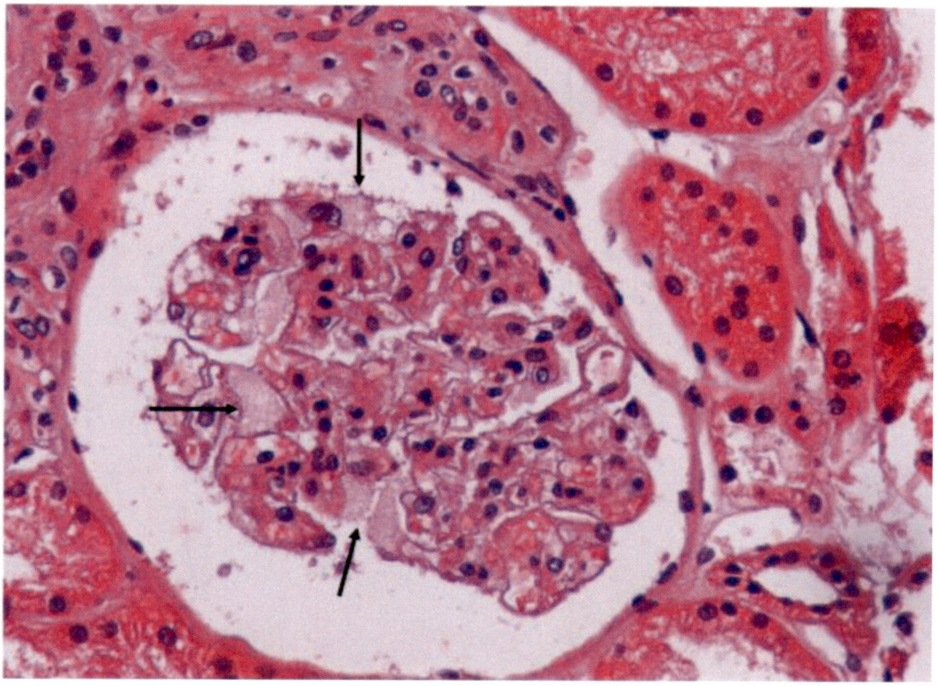

Figure 17. Fabry's disease. Podocytes with foaming protoplasm (arrows) (H-E x400).

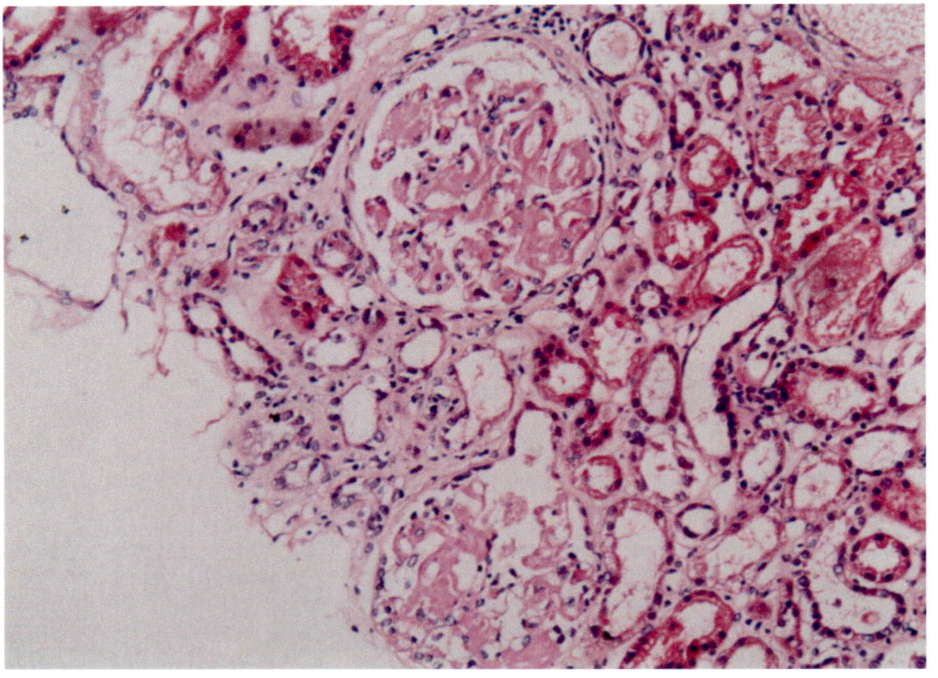

Figure 18. AL Amyloidosis. Two glomeruli with amorphous eosinophilic material present in mesangial areas and focally in peripheral capillary walls (H/E, x250).

Author's Contact Information

Dr. Foteini Lamprianou, MD
Nephrology Department,
General Hospital of Rhodes,
Agioi Apostoloi,
Rhodes P.C 85100, Greece
Tel: 00302241080048
Email: f_lamprianou@yahoo.com

Index

B

C

D

E

F

G

H

I

J

K

L

M

N

O

P

Q

R

S

T

U

V

W

X

Y

Z